D1761316

...al Liverpool University Hospital – Staff Library

Breast Core Biopsy

Commissioning Editor: William Schmitt
Development Editor: Sheila Black
Editorial Assistant: Liz MacSween
Project Manager: Cheryl Brant
Design Manager: Sarah Russell
Illustration Manager: Gillian Richards
Illustrator: Ian Ramsdon
Marketing Managers: Matt Latuchie (US), John Canelon (UK)

Breast Core Biopsy

A Pathologic–Radiologic Correlative Approach

Ira J. Bleiweiss MD
Professor of Pathology
Mount Sinai School of Medicine;
Attending Pathologist, Chief of Surgical Pathology
and Director, Division of Breast Pathology
Mount Sinai Medical Center
New York, USA

Shabnam Jaffer MD
Assistant Professor of Pathology
Mount Sinai School of Medicine;
Assistant Attending Pathologist
Mount Sinai Medical Center
New York, USA

Susan R. Drossman MD
Assistant Professor of Radiology
Mount Sinai School of Medicine;
Schaffer, Schonholz and Drossman
New York, USA

SAUNDERS
ELSEVIER

SAUNDERS
ELSEVIER

Saunders is an imprint of Elsevier Inc.

© 2008, Elsevier Inc. All rights reserved.

First published 2008

No part of this publication may be reproduced, stored in a retrieval system, or transmitted in any form or by any means, electronic, mechanical, photocopying, recording or otherwise, without the prior permission of the Publishers. Permissions may be sought directly from Elsevier's Health Sciences Rights Department, 1600 John F. Kennedy Boulevard, Suite 1800, Philadelphia, PA 19103-2899, USA: phone: (+1) 215 239 3804; fax: (+1) 215 239 3805; or, e-mail: healthpermissions@elsevier.com. You may also complete your request on-line via the Elsevier homepage (http://www.elsevier.com), by selecting 'Support and contact' and then 'Copyright and Permission'.

ISBN: 978-1-4160-0026-6

British Library Cataloguing in Publication Data
A catalogue record for this book is available from the British Library

Library of Congress Cataloging in Publication Data
A catalog record for this book is available from the Library of Congress

Notice
Medical knowledge is constantly changing. Standard safety precautions must be followed, but as new research and clinical experience broaden our knowledge, changes in treatment and drug therapy may become necessary or appropriate. Readers are advised to check the most current product information provided by the manufacturer of each drug to be administered to verify the recommended dose, the method and duration of administration, and contraindications. It is the responsibility of the practitioner, relying on experience and knowledge of the patient, to determine dosages and the best treatment for each individual patient. Neither the Publisher nor the author assume any liability for any injury and/or damage to persons or property arising from this publication.

The Publisher

ELSEVIER your source for books, journals and multimedia in the health sciences
www.elsevierhealth.com

Working together to grow libraries in developing countries
www.elsevier.com | www.bookaid.org | www.sabre.org
ELSEVIER BOOK AID International Sabre Foundation

The publisher's policy is to use **paper manufactured from sustainable forests**

Printed in China
Last digit is the print number: 9 8 7 6 5 4 3 2 1

Contents

Foreword

Drs Bleiweiss, Jaffer, and Drossman have written a comprehensive and highly instructive review of core biopsy technique and interpretation. The authors emphasize the importance of collaboration and communication between the radiologist and pathologist, and they show how this is fundamental to diagnostic accuracy of benign and malignant breast disease. While the book is primarily intended for those two practitioners of core biopsy, it is equally relevant to surgeons, others in clinical practice, and even to informed patients, and this reflects the significance which core biopsy has attained in the past ten to fifteen years. Although the radiologist and pathologist may seem to be in the wings or even anonymous to the patient being evaluated for possible breast disease, these specialists have come to play the principal role in diagnosis. Furthermore, their upfront work with core biopsy guides the subsequent treatment, particularly with regard to surgical planning. The benefit to the patient is clear. Surgery can be avoided when there is radiologic and pathologic concordance of benignity. And, when surgery is indicated, the approach is directed and fine-tuned by findings on core biopsy, minimizing the need for re-excision or treatment changes in mid stream. In this volume, the authors delve into several such clinical scenarios, including the importance of searching for multifocality and radiographically occult disease when core biopsy shows invasive lobular or related histology; planning appropriate margin resection or considering mastectomy if extensive or multifocal DCIS is detected on core biopsy (or biopsies); and planning for extent of axillary lymph node sampling based on core biopsy findings such as tumor grade, lymphatic invasion, or micropapillary disease. Thankfully the days of intraoperative frozen section diagnosis and surgical decision making with the patient under anesthesia are long over. In sharp contrast, the information provided by core biopsy brings the patient into the communication between surgeon, radiologist and pathologist, and enables informed treatment planning long before going to the operating room.

As the paradigm for surgical treatment of breast cancer has shifted away from the standard knee-jerk reaction of mastectomy for all histologic types toward individualized operative planning, this richly illustrated book represents an important guide. Furthermore, the finely tuned treatment strategy which core biopsy allows is an early step toward what will hopefully be the future of multimodality breast cancer treatment, namely customized chemotherapeutic, hormonal, and other treatment based on molecular and genetic fingerprinting of the individual's tumor biology. Already, in fact, core biopsy plays a role in this context, providing hormone and Her-2 information which impacts treatment for patients undergoing neoadjuvant therapy. And, as the authors point out, the future possibilities are limitless.

Having had the privilege of working closely with the authors of this volume for the past several years, I have been guided by and benefited from their coordinated expertise in core biopsy. I am indebted to them on behalf of myself and our mutual patients.

Christina Weltz, MD
Assistant Professor of Surgery
Mount Sinai School of Medicine, New York, NY
Summer 2007

Preface

It was in the latter part of 1994 that the core biopsy began to play an increasingly important role in my daily practice as a surgical pathologist specializing in breast disease. At that time sonographic evaluation of the breast had undergone great technical improvements, as had mammography in the immediately prior years. Similarly the means to accurately target and sample ever smaller lesions of the breast stereotactically and via ultrasound also became a reality. Its ease of use, relative noninvasiveness as compared to surgical alternatives, cost effectiveness, and its advantages both real and potential all contributed to the popularity of the procedure. In short, it took off exponentially, as did our volume, to the point where we currently evaluate 15 to 25 core biopsy specimens daily. The idea of getting more and more information out of less and less tissue had moved from the realm of the cytologist to that of the surgical pathologist.

I realized early on, however, that if the dual goals of proper surgical planning for malignancies and avoidance of unnecessary surgery for benign lesions were to be met, a level of diagnostic precision was necessary such that simple histologic interpretation would not suffice; i.e., it would not be enough to just read the slides without a concomitant awareness of the target's imaging findings. Obviously this requires close collaboration and communication with the person performing the biopsy. In this regard I was extremely fortunate to already have had close working relationships with a number of radiologists, relationships forged over the years in dealing with wire localized surgical biopsies. This cooperation is not only intellectually satisfying, but, more than anything else, it is responsible for the great accuracy which can be achieved with this technique. That is what this book is really about. It will depict our methods of correlation of radiologic and pathologic findings gleaned from over 10 years of experience and over 15,000 cases, but in the end it is really about communication between the pathologist and the radiologist (or surgeon[1]) and what specific information needs to be shared. In order to best achieve this goal, the book will be structured so as to reflect the way lesions present clinically, rather than chapters devoted to specific pathologic entities. Thus the titles of the chapters will be the imaging characteristics, while the respective pathologic entities will be discussed therein, mirroring the journey from recognition of imaging abnormality to core biopsy to pathologic diagnosis. Finally, although we have substantial experience with MRI-directed core biopsies, we have consciously omitted a discussion of this topic, since, to our knowledge, there are no specific histologic correlates of increased vascular flow-the basic abnormality identified with MRI.

Ira J Bleiweiss, MD

[1] While surgeons are increasingly performing core biopsies themselves, especially those utilizing sonography, radiologists are still responsible for the vast majority of the procedures. Thus, the term "radiologist" will be used but those surgeons reading this book should feel free to substitute "surgeon". The need for communication and correlation is the same regardless of the specialty of the physician performing the biopsy. No offense to the surgeons is meant.

Acknowledgements

Our sincerest thanks go to the following radiologists for their additional imaging contributions: Ulana Suprun, Helene Tapper, and Miriam Levy of Medical Imaging of Manhattan; George Hermann and JoLinda Mester of Mount Sinai Medical Center; Barry Berson of Maklansky Imaging; and Stacy Tashman, Stephanie Zalasin, Stacey Vitiello, Orna Hadar, Barbara Baskin, and Julie Mitnick of Murray Hill Radiology and Mammography.

Dedication

To our respective families:
Stephanie and Jason
Gulzar Meghyi and Sadique Jaffer
Adam, Eliana, Julia, and Gabriel
For their love, support, and endless patience

and

In memory of Caren Bleiweiss-Slomin
whose valiant struggle with breast cancer ended all too soon

CHAPTER 1

Introduction and general considerations

The perfection of the technology of image-directed core biopsy of the breast has radically altered patterns of care in the diagnosis and treatment of breast lesions. No longer does a surgical specimen typically yield the initial diagnosis; rather, the core biopsy has rapidly become the diagnostic standard in many institutions.[1] The popularity and cost effectiveness of this technique has thereby increased the frequency of the core biopsy as a routine specimen in surgical pathology. The modern day pathologist is called upon to make increasingly specific diagnoses on rapidly shrinking amounts of tissue. Breast core biopsies are a perfect example of this phenomenon, and it behooves both the practicing surgical pathologist and the physician performing the biopsy to be aware of both their diagnostic utility and limitations. Accuracy in core biopsy interpretation results in proper surgical planning,[2,3] as well avoidance of surgery for benign lesions.[4–6] In order to maximize their diagnostic yield and accuracy, it is necessary for pathologic findings to be correlated with radiologic features.[7] This is best accomplished by ongoing communication between the pathologist and radiologist.

The radiologist should provide the pathologist with abbreviated imaging characteristics for each lesion biopsied. The pathologist needs a basic working knowledge of breast imaging, however, in order to put this information to its best use diagnostically. Likewise a greater familiarity with pathologic aspects increases the imaging acumen of the radiologist. Thus the remainder of this chapter will consist of sections specifically geared to the opposite specialty.

BASIC RADIOLOGIC CONSIDERATIONS – A PRIMER FOR THE PATHOLOGIST

An increase in the use of screening mammography and the more frequent use of whole breast ultrasound have had a major impact on the size and stage of image-detected breast cancers. A number of new technologies, including minimally invasive breast procedures have revolutionized breast cancer diagnosis over the last ten years.[8,9] The clinically oriented interventional breast radiologist can take the primary responsibility of directing the workup of breast problems from detection of the lesion on screening studies to obtaining a specific tissue diagnosis. The entire diagnostic process including biopsy can be accomplished in one or two office visits.

A number of advantages have been demonstrated for core biopsy over other techniques. The specific and accurate histologic diagnosis yielded by image-guided large core biopsy procedures[10–14] allows for definitive planning of one-step surgical procedures, surgery can be avoided for lesions proven to be benign, and excision of the core biopsy site is typically more accurate than after surgical incisional biopsy since there is less tissue reaction and hematoma formation. In addition, core biopsy has been shown to be more cost-effective than surgical biopsy in the evaluation of indeterminate nonpalpable breast lesions.[15] It is in the management of BIRADS 4 lesions (those with suspicious features-see below) that the use of core biopsy yields the greatest cost savings.[16] The use of stereotactic core biopsy rather than surgical biopsy for highly suspicious calcifications decreases the number of operations and thus the overall cost.[17]

The selection of an image guidance modality for minimally invasive breast biopsy is generally dictated by the lesion type and sometimes by the lesion location. Most masses can be biopsied using ultrasound guidance, and most microcalcifications and areas of asymmetry should be sampled stereotactically.

Breast ultrasound

Ultrasound guided core biopsy provides a quicker, easier, and less expensive modality than stereotactic core biopsy and is used in almost all patients who have a mass seen sonographically. The patient is scanned in a supine position, ipsilateral arm above the patient's head and often obliqued to facilitate needle placement. Ultrasound guided biopsy requires a sampling instrument; we use a Bard Biopty gun, an automated tru cut, 14 gauge needle, obtaining multiple (at least four) passes through the lesion.[18,19] The skin is cleansed with betadine, and 1% lidocaine is used for anesthesia. A small nick is made in the skin with an 11-blade scalpel, a 13-gauge introducer is positioned at the leading edge of the lesion and several

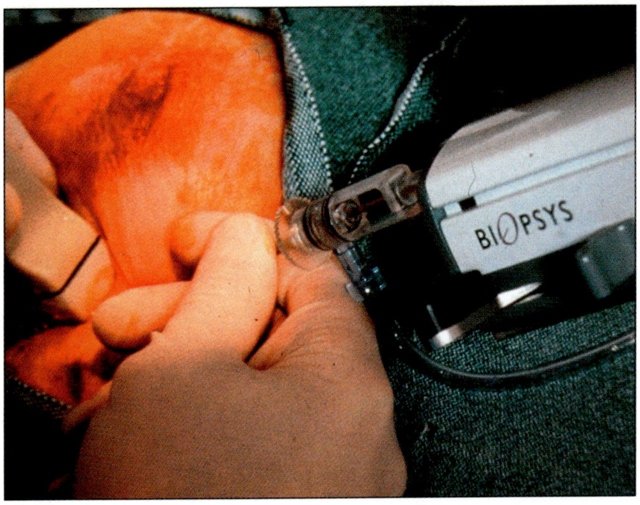

FIGURE 1.1 Ultrasound-guided core biopsy is performed free hand. The biopsy instrument may be an automated gun or a vacuum assisted biopsy instrument. (Courtesy of Ethicon Endo-Surgery, Inc. of Johnson and Johnson).

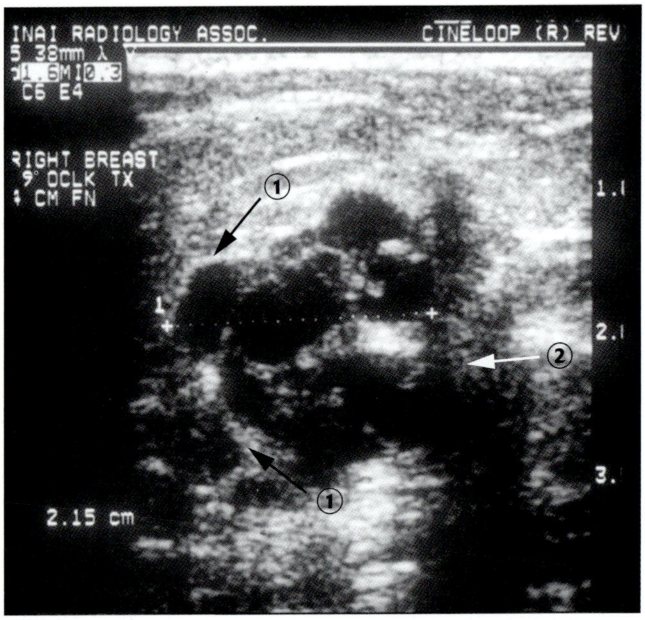

FIGURE 1.2 Sonography demonstrates a complex cystic and solid multilobulated mass. There are cystic, anechoic areas that demonstrate posterior through transmission (arrows 1), and other solid areas that demonstrate posterior shadowing (arrow 2).

passes are then made (Fig. 1.1). Compression is applied for hemostasis, steristrips are placed over the skin nick, and the patient is informed of the results approximately 24 hours later.

Breast ultrasound relies on the transmission of specialized sound waves using a high frequency transducer to penetrate through and image the underlying tissue. Varying rates of reflection and refraction between the sound waves and tissue structures and interfaces results in the formation of an image.

All the descriptive terms that follow are relative to the echotexture of mammary fat that is gray. Sonographically distinguishable tissue types within the breast include skin, fat, stromal fibrous elements and Cooper's ligaments, fibroglandular tissue, and mammary ducts. Lesions that are darker than fat are hypoechoic, specifically tumors. Lesions that are anechoic are often cystic, and lesions that are hyperechoic include skin, suspensory ligaments, and dense fibroglandular tissue and are almost always benign. Isoechoic nodules have the same echodensity as fat. When the internal nature of a lesion is homogeneous, sound waves can pass easily through it giving the sonographic appearance of posterior through-transmission which appears as an area of white or bright echoes behind the lesion (Fig 1.2). When the internal nature of the lesion is heterogeneous or densely packed with non-uniform cells, the sound waves cannot easily pass through and are reflected at a different rate, producing a dark area behind the lesion known as posterior shadowing (Figs 1.2, 1.3).

Ultrasound is primarily a method for differentiating cystic lesions from solid masses; however, there are specific sonographic characteristics that can distinguish some benign solid masses from malignant ones. There are

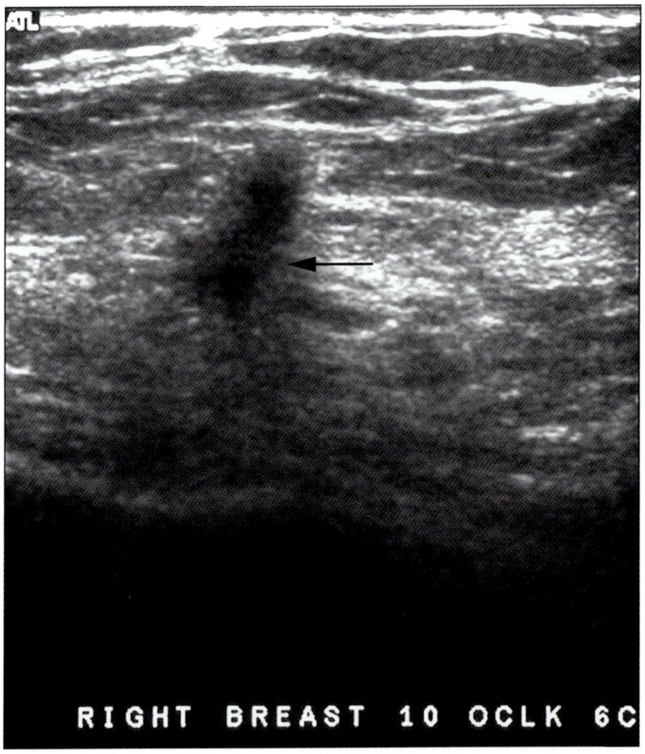

FIGURE 1.3 In the breast, fat is isoechoic or gray. Glandular breast tissue and Coopers' ligaments are echogenic, and solid masses are often hypoechoic to fat. Sonography demonstrates a hypoechoic, taller than wide, microlobulated mass (arrow). There is some posterior shadowing.

several sonographic features that are suggestive of malignancy (Box 1.1). These include lesions that are taller than wide, a finding which implies that the lesion is growing across tissue planes. Normal tissue planes in a supine patient run in a horizontal direction. The majority of breast cancers are markedly hypoechoic with respect to the surrounding breast fat. Shadowing, spiculation, and microlobulation are all suspicious sonographic findings (Fig. 1.4). Ductal extension, angulation, a branching pattern, and microlobulation may suggest an intraductal location, and these are all worrisome for malignancy. Calcifications seen on sonography are more likely to be malignant than benign. Since most breast cancers are iso-hypoechoic they contrast with the punctate hyperechoic nature of the calcifications. Some cancers have thick echogenic irregular rims which represent a fibroelastotic host reaction to the tumor. The imaging findings in breast ultrasound often reflect the gross morphology and to a lesser extent the dominant histological features of the lesion being evaluated. Most circumscribed malignant nodules represent either special type tumors such as intracystic papillary, mucinous, medullary carcinomas, or high-grade invasive duct carcinomas. The latter two lesions tend to be highly cellular and fast growing and do not allow enough time for a host desmoplastic reaction. They typically show a host inflammatory response composed of lymphocytes and plasma cells. Most circumscribed lesions show evidence of enhanced posterior through transmission, a result of the lack of desmoplastic reaction and the uniformity of the host inflammatory response. Spiculated lesions are more often low to intermediate grade invasive duct carcinomas, invasive lobular carcinoma, or tubular carcinoma (Fig. 1.5). They grow more slowly, creating a desmoplastic reaction which does not allow sound to penetrate through the lesion, resulting in the marked posterior acoustic shadowing seen sonographically.

The classical fibroadenoma is well circumscribed and perfectly smoothly ellipsoid in shape with a horizontal diameter that is greater than its anteroposterior diameter. The lesion parallels tissue planes, and a thin echogenic capsule suggests a pushing, noninvasive leading edge, a

BOX 1.1 Sonographic findings suspicious for malignancy (see also Fig 1.5)

- Shadowing
- Solid nodule
- Spiculation
- Angular margins
- Thick echogenic halo
- Microlobulation
- Taller than wide
- Hypoechogenic
- Calcification
- Duct extension and branching pattern

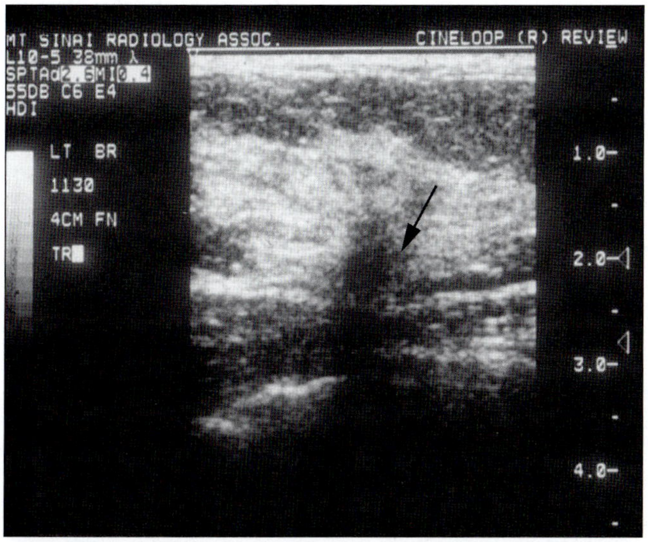

FIGURE 1.4 Sonography of a typical invasive breast cancer. The lesion is microlobulated (arrow), hypoechoic to fat, and demonstrates angulated margins and posterior shadowing.

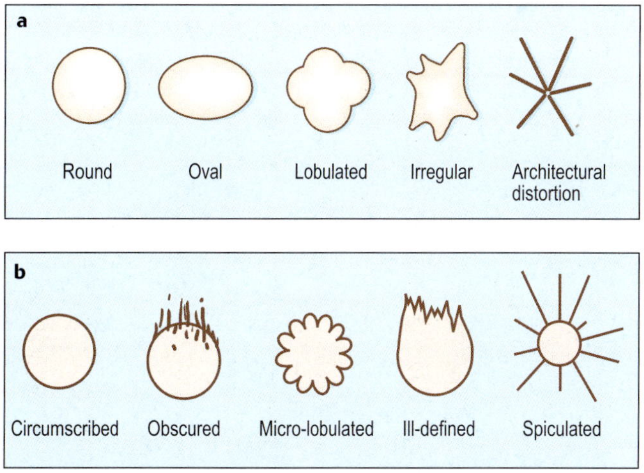

FIGURE 1.5 (a) Mass shape, as defined by the American College of Radiology Breast Imaging Reporting and Data System, can be divided into five shapes-round, oval, lobulated, irregular (though not strictly a mass) architectural distortion. **(b)** A mass can have one of five margins. The American College of Radiology Breast Imaging Reporting and Data System defines these, as represented by this schematic-circumscribed, obscured, microlobulated, ill defined, and speculated. (Originally published in Kopans DB, Breast Imaging, 2nd Ed., 1998, Lippincott-Raven, Philadelphia, pp. 275 and 277, redrawn with permission.)

benign finding (Fig. 1.6). Such nodules have a less than 1% chance of malignancy; similarly, a small percentage of benign breast lesions are spiculated. Regardless of the imaging characteristics, the ideal core biopsy sample skewers the lesion through and through so that lesional tissue is central in the core with uninvolved breast tissue seen on either end (Fig. 1.7).

Stereotactic core biopsy

Stereotactic breast biopsies are performed with radiologic imaging; thus, any type of breast lesion that can be imaged mammographically can be biopsied with this technique. Radiologic findings which are suspicious for malignancy are similar to those seen sonographically regarding shapes of lesions (Box 1.2). Lesion localization is done by triangulation. Principles of stereotaxis rely on the apparent movement of a lesion in two stereo views (parallax shift principles) to calculate the coordinates of a lesion in three planes: horizontal, vertical, and depth.

We use a Fischer Mammotest Stereotactic Breast Biopsy system. In most systems the patient is placed prone on the table with her breast protruding through an aperture in the table (Fig. 1.8). The breast is placed in compres-

BOX 1.2	Mammographic findings suspicious for malignancy (see also Figs 1.5 and 1.13)
	Mass
	Nodule
	Spiculation
	Irregular margins
	Indistinct margins
	Microlobulation
	Architectural distortion
	Asymmetric density
	Calcification
	Developing density

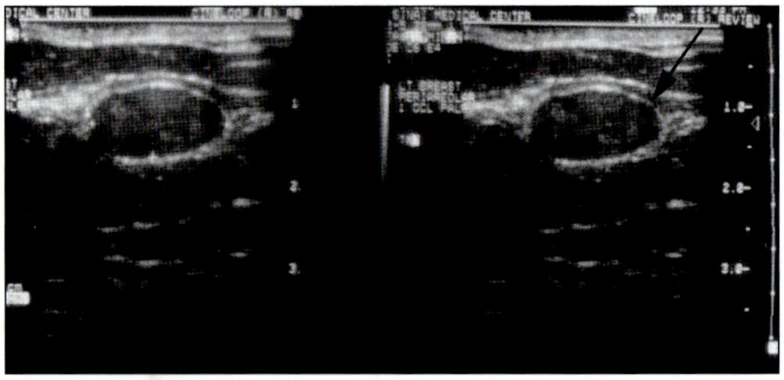

FIGURE 1.6 Sonography shows a solid, oval, hypoechoic mass with a thin echogenic capsule (arrow). The lesion parallels the tissue planes and is characteristic of a fibroadenoma.

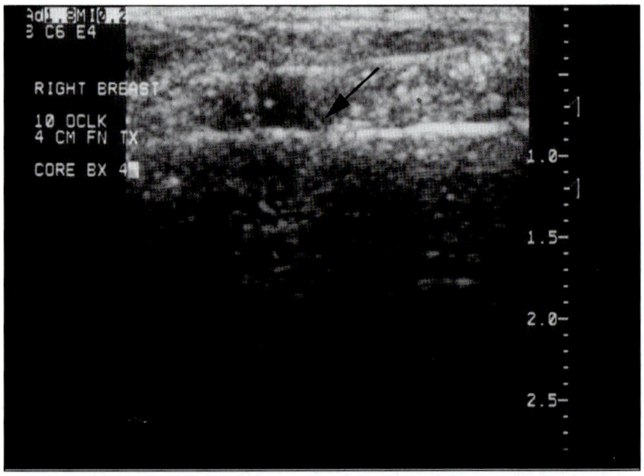

FIGURE 1.7 The ideal ultrasound guided core biopsy (arrow) spears the lesion and takes a cross section so that the pathologist sees normal breast tissue, lesion, and normal breast tissue.

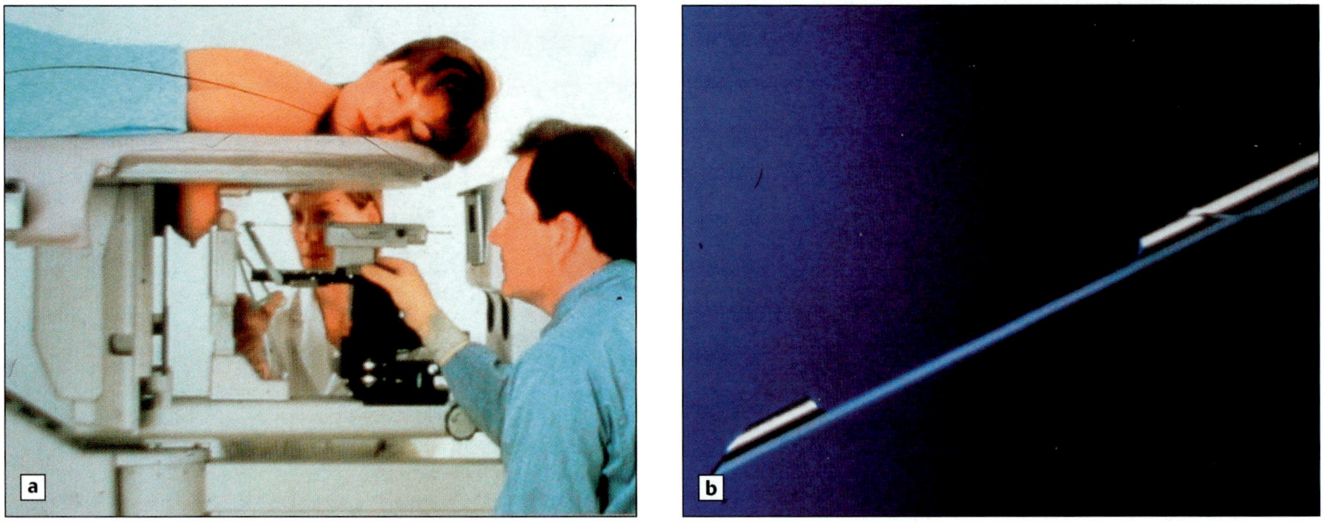

FIGURE 1.8 Stereotactic core biopsy. The patient is placed prone on a table with a hole in the center for the breast to hang dependent. The breast is in compression, and the physician works beneath the table. (From an original supplied courtesy of Ethicon Endo-Surgery, Inc. of Johnson and Johnson.)

sion, and the table rises approximately four feet off the floor. The physician and assistant are seated on stools, and the operator workspace is under the patient's chest and head. A scout view (zero degrees) is obtained, followed by two stereo views (15 degree obliques +15, −15); these are used to calculate the lesion's position. Once the coordinates are obtained, the skin is cleansed with betadine, and local anesthesia is administered with 1% lidocaine. Deep anesthesia is achieved with a combination of lidocaine plus epinephrine. A small (4 mm) skin nick is made with an 11-blade scalpel. Tissue is suctioned into a collecting chamber where it is cut by a shearing device and then resuctioned into a retrieval chamber (Fig. 1.9). The biopsy instrument is positioned, and samples are obtained by rotating the vacuum assisted directional sampling instrument in a clockwise fashion. A total of at least 15 contiguous samples with the 11-gauge probe are made to acquire a total of 1500 mg of tissue. While fewer cores are obtained with the 8-gauge vacuum assisted biopsy device, a greater overall volume of tissue is sampled. Following this, an air cavity is made by suctioning the biopsy site, and a post-stereo pair of mammograms is obtained to visualize the air filled cavity and to judge the adequacy of the procedure. Specimen radiography is essential for all calcification cases in order to ensure adequate sampling. Cores containing calcifications are isolated from those without calcifications and placed in separate formalin bottles. Once the lesion is thoroughly sampled (or in some cases completely removed) a small stainless steel clip (or other marking device[20]) is placed to document lesion position (Fig. 1.10). This allows easy

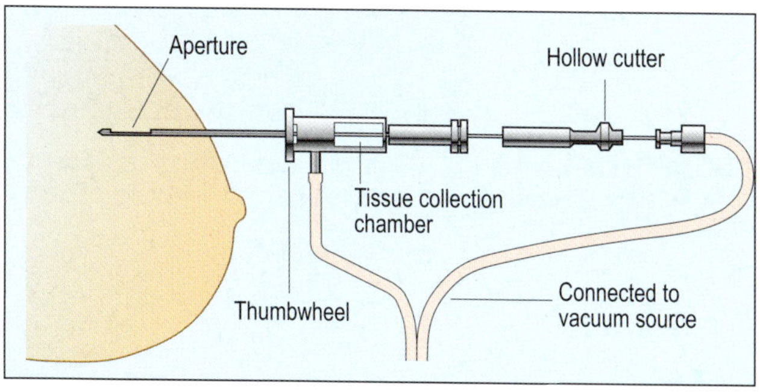

FIGURE 1.9 Stereotactic core biopsy. The procedure is performed with a vacuum assisted directional biopsy system. Specimen retrieval is quick and easy. (Redrawn from an original supplied courtesy of Ethicon Endo-Surgery, Inc. of Johnson and Johnson.)

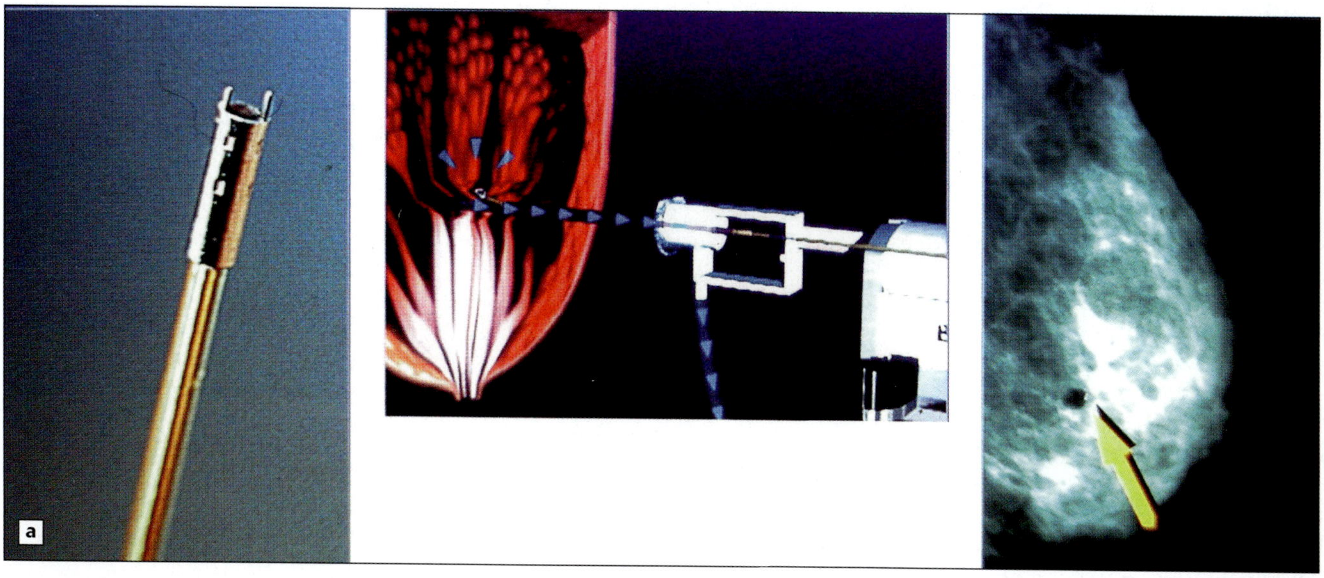

FIGURE 1.10 A clip or marker is placed at the biopsy site to mark the location of the procedure. This can be localized if preoperative wire localization is necessary. Many different types of markers are available, **(a)** including stainless steel clips.

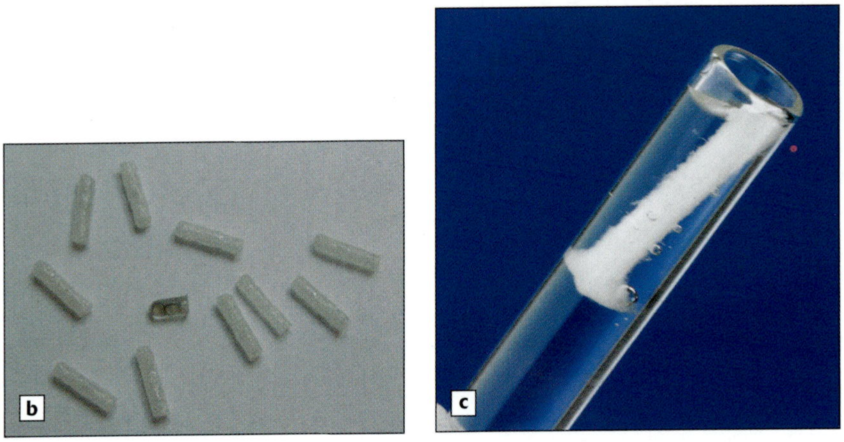

FIGURE 1.10—cont'd **(b)** air impregnated vicryl pellets, **(c)** or single collagen pellets. (**a,** from an original supplied courtesy of Ethicon Endo-Surgery, Inc. of Johnson and Johnson; **b,** courtesy of SenoRx Corp. **c,** courtesy of Ethicon Endo-Surgery, Inc. of Johnson and Johnson.)

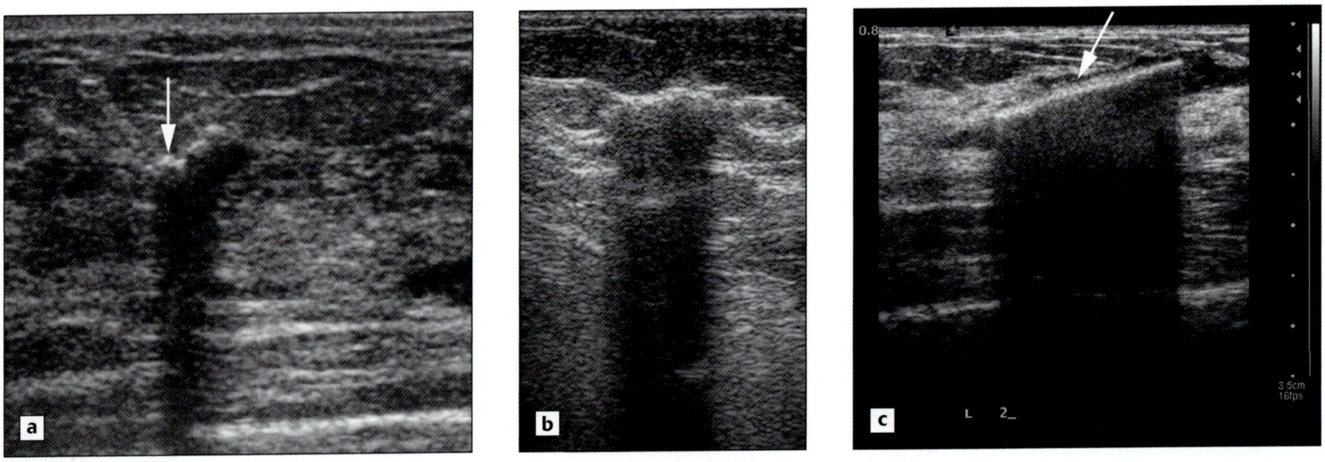

FIGURE 1.11 Many markers are visualized under ultrasound as an echogenic linear component with dense posterior shadowing (arrows). Sonographic localization for surgery represents a major advantage over mammographic techniques in that it is simpler for the radiologist and less uncomfortable for the patient. (**a,b** Courtesy of SenoRx Corp., **c** courtesy of Ethicon Endo-Surgery, Inc. of Johnson and Johnson.)

sonography-guided relocalization of the area (Fig. 1.11) if therapeutic lumpectomy becomes necessary, particularly if the mammographic abnormality has been removed by the cores. Post clip stereo views are obtained followed by a post biopsy unilateral mammogram to show that the clip resides where the lesion was formerly located and to serve as the patient's new baseline mammogram. Hemostasis is achieved with manual compression, and the small skin nick is covered with steri-stripes.

The procedure is highly efficient because it can obtain multiple specimens in a contiguous fashion with a single insertion. The specimens are large (11-gauge) (Fig. 1.12), and tissue can be acquired from outside the line of fire, thus decreasing the underestimation of problem lesions such as atypical duct hyperplasia (ADH) and duct carcinoma in situ (DCIS).

Types of calcification requiring percutaneous biopsy include granular, dense pleomorphic with ductal distri-

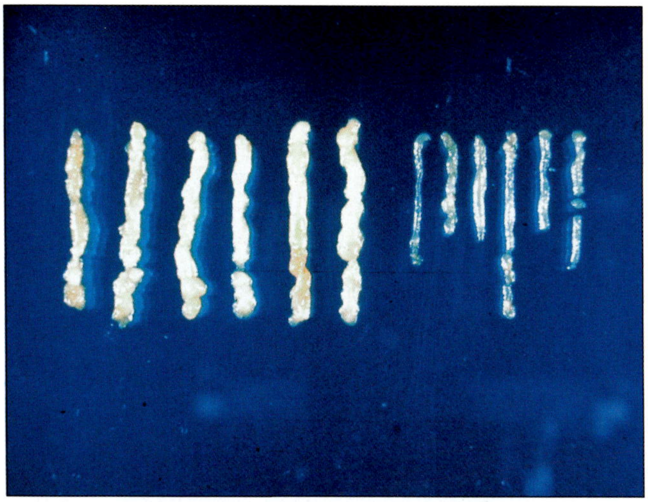

FIGURE 1.12 Specimens vary in size depending on the gauge of the biopsy instrument. On the left are specimens from an 11–gauge vacuum assisted biopsy instrument, while those on the right derive from a 14–gauge automated biopsy gun.

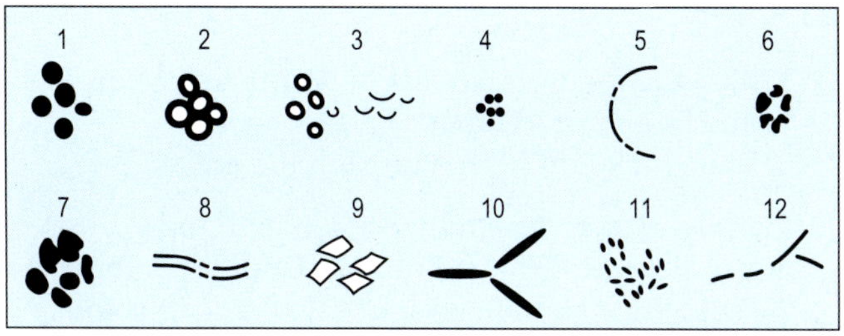

FIGURE 1.13 This schematic represents many of the types of calcifications that can be seen by mammography. (1) Calcified debris in ducts; (2) dense, lucent-centered calcifications in fat necrosis; (3) precipitated calcifications in small cysts (milk of calcium); (4) concretions in small, cystically dilated lobules; (5) rim calcifications in the wall of a cyst; (6) early deposits in an involuting fibroadenoma; (7) large deposits in an involuting fibroadenoma; (8) vascular calcifications; (9) skin calcifications; (10) calcified rods in secretory disease; (11) pleomorphic deposits in intraductal cancer; (12) fine linear calcifications found in comedocarcinoma. (Originally published in Kopans DB, Breast Imaging, 2nd Ed., 1998, Lippincott-Raven, Philadelphia, p. 317, reprinted with permission.)

bution, and dense pleomorphic with lobular distribution (Fig. 1.13).

The American College of Radiology has established a reporting system or lexicon to aid in the clear, concise transmission of results and interpretations of mammograms.[21] This terminology provides standardized language and decision-oriented recommendations in the assessment of the mammographic findings. This system, known as BIRADS (Breast Imaging Reporting and Data System), has become the basis for the reporting of both screening (the evaluation of asymptomatic women in the search for unsuspected breast cancers) and diagnostic (symptomatic patients or women requiring additional evaluation because of abnormal screening studies) breast imaging. The mammographic features are described using the breast imaging lexicon, and a final assessment and classification is assigned. There are six possible decision categories including:

- 0 – needs additional imaging evaluation;
- 1 – negative;
- 2 – benign finding;
- 3 – probably benign-short interval follow-up with mammography every 6 months for a total of 2 years;
- 4 – suspicious abnormality-biopsy should be considered; and
- 5 – highly suggestive of malignancy-appropriate action should be taken.

The ability of image-guided core biopsy to replace surgical biopsy for initial diagnosis clearly depends on the accuracy of histological results. In most cases, 14–gauge biopsy specimens are adequate; this is almost always the case for noncalcified masses which are homogeneous on ultrasound, in which sampling of one part of the lesion is representative of the whole. However, in lesions which are heterogeneous, sampling of multiple areas, specifically the solid components, is necessary for a definitive diagnosis.

For lesions that present as calcifications, the size of the specimens and amount of tissue retrieved greatly influence the accuracy of the diagnosis. This is due to the fact that atypical duct hyperplasia, ductal carcinoma in situ, and invasive duct carcinoma (IDC) are part of a continuum of changes often seen adjacent to each other. Essentially they may coexist in the same lesion, all of which manifests itself radiographically as pleomorphic calcifications. Thus, the larger the core size and the more cores obtained, the higher the likelihood of identifying the most aggressive components of the lesion, decreasing the chances of underestimation of ADH from DCIS, and DCIS from IDC.

PATHOLOGY FOR RADIOLOGISTS – SPECIMEN HANDLING, EVALUATION, AND REPORTING

Breast core biopsies are processed in a manner identical with other types of tissue biopsies. In general, while fatty breast tissue may require a longer period of formalin fixation, the cores need a minimum of several hours in formalin prior to additional processing. While some institutions embed each core cylinder into an individual paraffin block, we believe this practice is unnecessary and wasteful of resources. Regardless of whether they derive from a stereotactic or sonographic procedure the contents

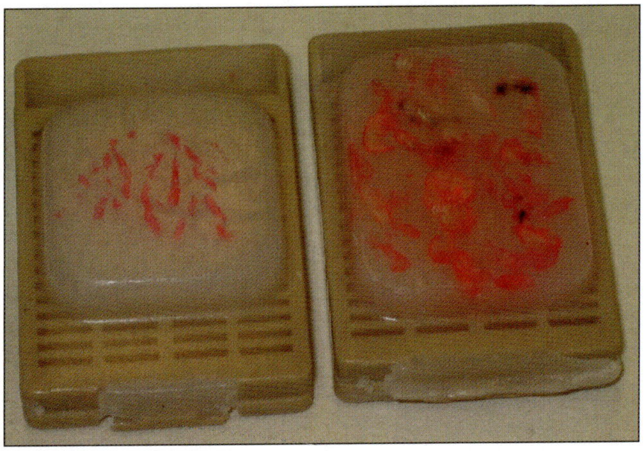

FIGURE 1.14 Paraffin blocks containing sonograpically obtained core biopsies on the left and stereotactically obtained larger cores on the right. All of the individual core cylinders have been embedded at the same level in the blocks, allowing for adequate sectioning of each in each resultant slide.

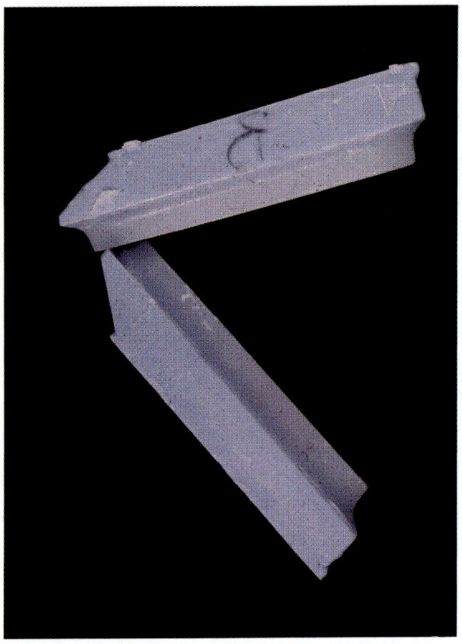

FIGURE 1.15 Paraffin block viewed on edge, demonstrating that numerous sections can be prepared from the thickness of the paraffin and the tissue embedded within it.

of an individual formalin bottle are entirely embedded into a single paraffin block, although larger volume mammotome-derived specimens may occasionally require a second block (Fig. 1.14). If one's histology technologists are adept at embedding multiple cores at the same level within the paraffin block, as is the case in our laboratory with regard to prostatic chips or needle biopsies, this skill can be similarly applied to breast core biopsies. Cores taken in order to investigate calcifications are treated identically; however, we find it helpful for the radiologist, after performing the specimen radiograph, to place those cores containing the target calcifications in one bottle and the remaining cores in a separate container. This assists us greatly in later finding the targeted calcifications. We routinely examine an initial hematoxylin and eosin stained slide and 3 deeper levels (cut at 20–25 micron intervals, depending on the thickness of the tissue) from each paraffin block; however, occasionally blocks require far more levels to be cut for complete diagnostic accuracy, and radiologists should realize that numerous sections can be taken of an individual paraffin block (Fig 1.15).

Before reaching a conclusive diagnosis, it is essential that the pathologist be made aware of the imaging characteristics of the lesion.[22] The following basic information should be provided by the radiologist, ideally from the outset:

1. Is the lesion well circumscribed or does it have irregular borders?
2. Is the lesion solid, cystic, or partially solid and partially cystic?
3. What is the size of the lesion?
4. Has the lesion been stable over time, grown, or have its imaging characteristics changed?
5. Did the lesion disappear or shrink in size during the biopsy procedure?
6. Has the lesion been entirely removed?

In the case of stereotactically performed biopsies, it is not sufficient for the radiologist to simply inform the pathologist that evaluation of calcifications is the reason for the procedure. The radiologist should circle with a wax pencil the cores containing the target calcifications on the specimen radiograph, and the pathologist should receive and view the specimen radiograph him(or her)self so as to directly compare the number and pattern of calcifications removed with those found histologically.[21] To evaluate these biopsies without the benefit of the specimen radiograph is akin to looking for a needle in a haystack without knowing the appearance of a needle, and, as examples to follow will demonstrate, can lead to diagnostic inaccuracy, unnecessary surgical biopsies, and may be potentially dangerous, both clinically and medico-legally. Although not essential, it is useful for the radiologist to provide the following information in cases of calcifications:

1. Are the calcifications new or old but increasing in number?
2. Are any calcifications linear or linear and branching?
3. Have the targeted calcifications been entirely removed?

Diagnostically speaking, accuracy of sonographically directed cores is maximized when both peripheral edges

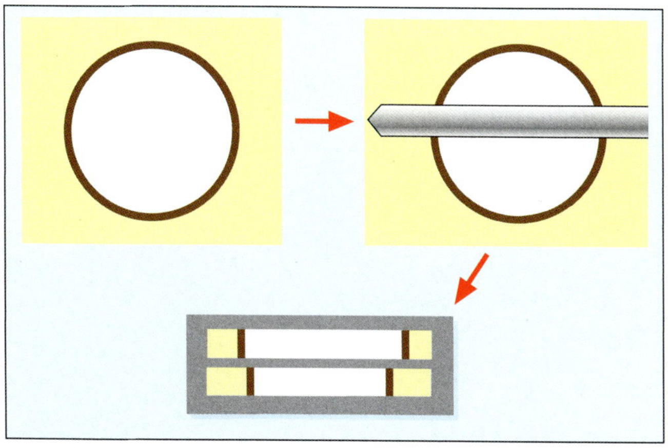

FIGURE 1.16 Diagrammatic representation of an adequate core biopsy sample. The lesion (white) has been transected by the biopsies, leaving uninvolved tissue (yellow) on either end of the core cylinders. This not only allows the pathologist to examine the periphery of the lesion, a diagnostically important area, but also enables him to be certain that lesional tissue has been sampled.

of the lesion can be clearly demarcated on the individual cores, i.e., the core has gone completely through the lesion (Fig. 1.16). In cases targeting calcifications, we first evaluate the specimen radiograph for number of calcifications removed, size and clustering of the calcifications, presence of linear and/or branching forms, and associated radiodense tissue. If the histology of the initial four slides does not correlate with the radiograph, we perform radiographs of the paraffin blocks and cut deeper levels if the calcifications are still evident on these radiographs. This is the situation in approximately 10–15% of our cases, perhaps not a surprising result given the small size of some calcifications and the huge number of sections derivable from even a core biopsy of narrow gauge. We report the specific location of the calcifications as to whether the underlying process they represent is intraductal carcinoma, fibroadenoma, fibrocystic changes, duct hyperplasia, atypical duct hyperplasia, etc. To simply report "calcifications are present" renders insufficient information for diagnostic, treatment, follow-up, and, potentially, even medico-legal purposes.

The above approach allows the pathologist in the vast majority of cases to render diagnoses much more specific than "benign breast tissue", "fibrosis", or "fibrocystic changes" (which, however, may be both adequate and accurate under certain circumstances). It also allows the pathologist to identify those cases in which the lesion has not been adequately sampled or in which the target has been missed completely. Finally an intellectually satisfying rapport develops between the pathologist and radiologist, leading to better communication and, we are certain, better patient care.[23]

REFERENCES

Note that many of the following articles discuss aspects of core biopsies additional to those of the sections in which they are referred to. These articles are marked with an asterisk (*).

1. Verkooijen HM. Diagnostic accuracy of stereotactic large-core needle biopsy for nonpalpable breast disease: Results of a multicenter prospective study with 95% surgical confirmation. Int J Cancer 99,853–859,2002.
2. Verkooijen HM, Rinkes HM, Peeters PHM, et al. Impact of stereotactic large-core needle biopsy on diagnosis and surgical treatment of non-palpable breast cancer. EJSO 27:244–249,2001.
3. Carmon M, Rivkin L, Abu-Dalo R, et al. Increased mammographic screening and use of percutaneous image-guided core biopsy in non-palpable breast cancer: impact on surgical treatment. Isr Med Assoc J 6:326–328,2004.
4. Acheson MB, Patton RG, Howisey RL, et al. Histologic correlation of image-guided core biopsy with excisional biopsy of nonpalpable breast lesions. Arch Surg 132:815–821,1997.
5. Stolier AJ. Stereotactic breast biopsy: A surgical series. J Am Coll Surg 185:224–228,1997.
*6. Acheson MB, Patton RG, Howisey RL, et al. Three- to six- year followup for 379 benign image-guided large-core needle biopsies of nonpalpable breast abnormalities. J Am Coll Surg 195:462–466,2002.
7. Crystal P, Koretz M, Shcharynsky S, et al. Accuracy of sonographically guided 14-gauge core-needle biopsy: results of 715 consecutive breast biopsies with at least two-year follow-up of benign lesions. J Clin Ultrasound 33:47–52,2005.
8. Liberman L. Percutaneous image-guided core breast biopsy. Radiol Clin N Am 40:483–500,2002.
9. Philpotts LE. Controversies in core-needle breast biopsy. Sem Roentgenol 36:270–283,2001.
10. Brenner RJ, Bassett LW, Fajardo LL, et al. Stereotactic core-needle breast biopsy: A multi-institutional prospective trial. Radiology 218:866–872,2001.
11. Cipolla C, Fricano S, Vieni S, et al. Validity of needle core biopsy in the characterization of mammary lesions. Breast 15:76–80,2006.
12. Bolovar AV, Alonso-Bartolome P, Garcia EO, Ayensa FG. Ultrasound-guided core needle biopsy of non-palpable breast lesions: a prospective analysis in 204 cases. Acta Radiol 46:690–695,2005.
13. Dillon MF, Hill AD, Quinn CM, et al. The accuracy of ultrasound, stereotactic, and clinical core biopsies in the diagnosis of cancer, with an analysis of false-negative cases. Ann Surg 242:701–707,2005.
14. Crowe JP, Patrick RJ, Rybicki LA, et al. Does ultrasound core breast biopsy predict histologic finding on excisional biopsy? Am J Surg 186:397–399,2003.
15. Golub RM, Bennett CL, Stinson T, et al. Cost minimization study of image-guided core biopsy versus surgical excisional biopsy for women with abnormal mammograms. 22:2430–2437,2004.
16. Fahy BN, BoldRJ, Schneider PD, et al. Cost-benefit analysis of biopsy methods for suspicious mammographic lesions. Arch Surg 136:990–994,2001.
17. Liberman L, Gougoutas CA, Zakowski MF, et al. Calcifications highly suggestive of malignancy: comparison of breast biopsy methods. Am J Roentgenol 177:165–172,2001.
18. Morris EA, Liberman L, Trevisan SG, et al. Histologic heterogeneity of masses at percutaneous breast biopsy. The Breast Journal 8:187–191,2002.
19. Fishman JE, Milikowski C, Ramsinghani R, et al. US-guided core-needle biopsy of the breast: how man y specimens are necessary? Radiology 226:779–782,2003.
20. Rosen EL, Baker JA, Soo MS. Accuracy of a collagen-plug biopsy site marking device deployed after stereotactic core needle breast biopsy. 181:1295–1299,2003.
21. Bassett L, Winchester DP, Caplan RB, et al. Stereotactic core-needle biopsy of the breast: A report of the joint task force of the American College of Radiology, American College of Surgeons, and College of American Pathologists. CA 47:171–190,1997.
22. Berg WA, Hruban RH, Kumar D, et al. Lessons from mammographic-histopathologic correlation of large-core needle breast biopsy. RadioGraphics 16:1111–1130,1996.
23. Bleiweiss IJ, Drossman S, Hermann G. Accuracy in mammographically directed breast biopsies. Communication is Key. Arch Pathol Lab Med 121:11–18,1997.

CHAPTER 2

Well-circumscribed solid lesions

One of the great advances of core biopsy technology is that it allows benign lesions to be followed rather than excised. Nowhere is this more apparent than in the workup of a well-circumscribed solid lesion of low radiographic suspicion. The most common such entity in the female breast, fibroadenoma, is also the most frequent diagnosis to be made on core biopsy.

Mammographically, these lesions are typically well circumscribed, oval, or lobulated. Margins may be well defined or partially obscured by surrounding tissue (Fig. 2.1), and they are frequently multiple and bilateral. They most often develop in young women and rarely arise or grow after menopause. In postmenopausal women, fibroadenomas undergo atrophy and will frequently calcify, aiding in their mammographic diagnosis. The calcifications are typically coarse, popcorn-like, and sharply marginated (see Chaps 10 and 12). On ultrasound, the lesion is solid and hypoechoic to the surrounding breast parenchyma; it does not traverse tissue planes, and it is parallel to the pectoralis muscle (Fig. 2.2). There is often a well-defined hypoechoic capsule. Internal echoes are homogenous; thus, there is often good posterior through transmission and, less frequently, shadowing posterior to the lesion. The more lobulated and angulated the borders of the lesion, the more suspicious the lesion is for malignancy. When sampling these lesions, the radiologist should target the more angulated and inhomogeneous portions (Fig. 2.3). The biopsy instrument is placed at the leading edge of the mass when utilizing an automated spring loaded gun and beneath the lesion when using a vacuum assisted device. Multiple passes are often taken to ensure adequate lesion sampling.

While the imaging characteristics of fibroadenomata are relatively consistent, their microscopic appearance can be quite variable, in part depending on the age of the patient when diagnosed. As the name implies the lesions contain a combined proliferation of benign glands and stroma in which the stroma typically dominates by pushing glandular elements into compressed curvilinear patterns (Fig. 2.4a,b). The glandular component retains the normal two cell layer epithelial/myoepithelial structure of benign breast tissue. Myxoid fibroadenomata tend to occur in younger patients, retaining this growth pattern but exhibiting a loose, paucicellular stroma with abundant myxoid material (Fig. 2.4c). These lesions have been associated with myxomas in other sites, most notably cardiac myxomas, in an inherited disorder known as Carney's Syndrome;[1] therefore, correctly classifying fibroadenomata in this way is important because it can alert the clinician to the latter, a potentially life-threatening albeit rare condition. Partially myxoid fibroadenomata are not uncommon. With increasing age fibroadenomata tend to hyalinize, calcify, and even ossify and sometimes may only be recognizable as such because their basic stromal growth pattern is maintained, despite the occasional near complete loss of their glandular element (Fig. 2.4d).

Fibroadenomata may also contain any of the histologic elements of fibrocystic changes, either singly or in combination. The term complex fibroadenoma has been applied to lesions which combine the usual growth patterns with sclerosing adenosis (Fig. 2.4e), cysts, papillary apocrine metaplasia (Fig. 2.4f), and/or epithelial calcifications. This designation is not a trivial one, as some studies have demonstrated an increased risk for the development of invasive breast carcinoma in individuals with complex fibroadenoma.[2] Somewhat paradoxically, usual, florid (Fig. 2.4g) or even atypical duct hyperplasia contained within a fibroadenoma does not seem to increase risk any more than that associated with identical hyperplasia seen in non-fibroadenomatous breast tissue. Occasional cases of fibroadenomata containing in situ lobular carcinoma (LCIS), atypical lobular hyperplasia (ALH) (fig 2.4h), atypical duct hyperplasia (ADH), or intraductal carcinoma (DCIS) are, in our opinion, probably "guilt by association", meaning that they are secondarily involved by a process that primarily is occurring (and probably arising) in the tissue adjacent to the fibroadenoma. Therefore we feel that in the rare instances in which these diagnoses are made on core biopsy, the recommendations for excision should be identical with those for the same diagnoses on non-fibroadenomatous core biopsies (see Chap. 10). Thus we believe that fibroadenomata harboring DCIS or ADH warrant excision to evaluate the surrounding tissue for DCIS and/or invasive carcinoma, whereas those containing ALH or LCIS can safely be followed with the caveat that the patient is at increased risk for the development of invasive carcinoma.

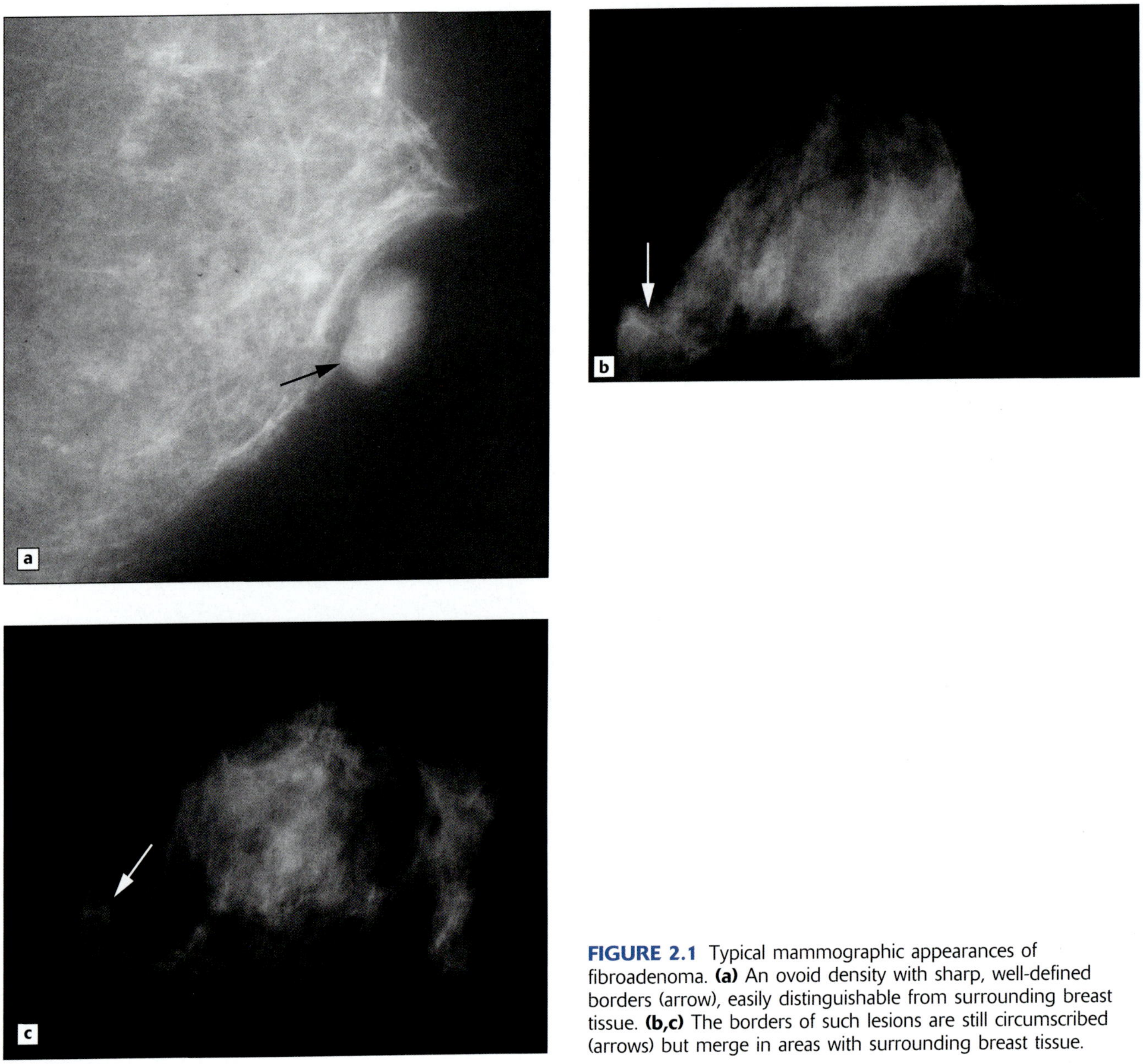

FIGURE 2.1 Typical mammographic appearances of fibroadenoma. **(a)** An ovoid density with sharp, well-defined borders (arrow), easily distinguishable from surrounding breast tissue. **(b,c)** The borders of such lesions are still circumscribed (arrows) but merge in areas with surrounding breast tissue.

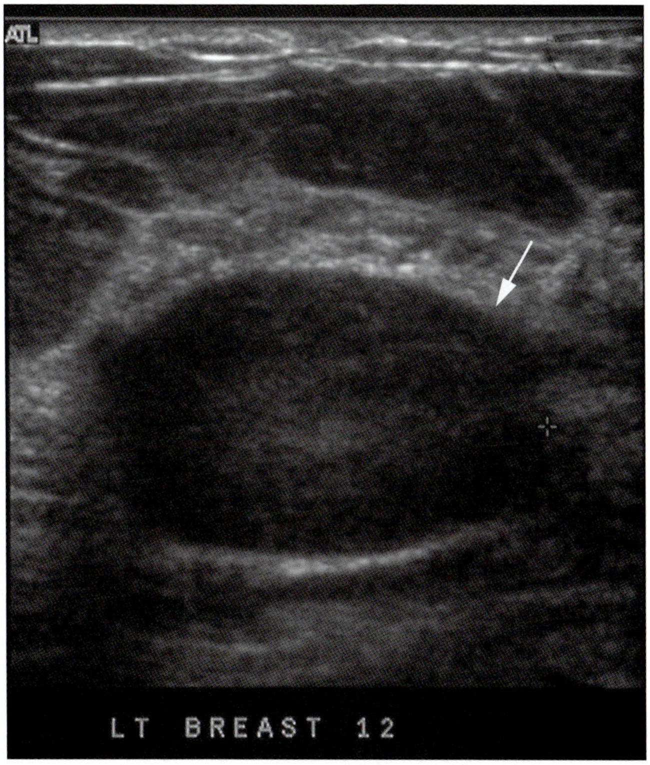

FIGURE 2.2 Ultrasound appearance of fibroadenoma. Sonography demonstrates an oval, solid, hypoechoic mass. The lesion's long axis parallels the tissue planes, and it has homogeneous internal echoes, a thin echogenic capsule (arrow), and some posterior through transmission.

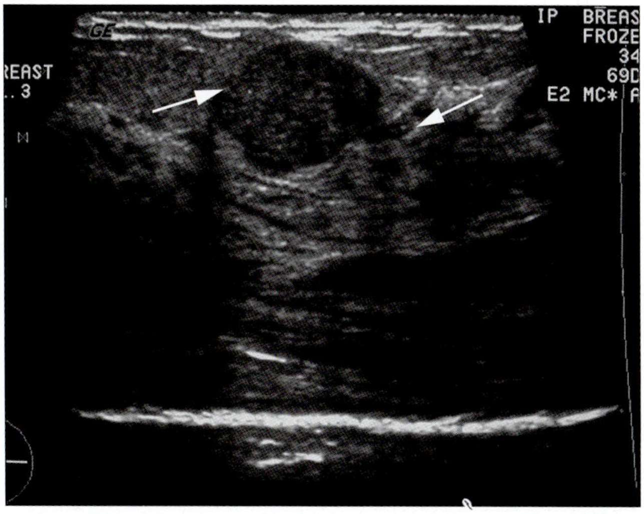

FIGURE 2.3 Targeting. Proper ultrasound-guided core biopsy should selectively target the less homogeneous area of a circumscribed but slightly lobulated solid mass. Arrows point out the areas that should be targeted.

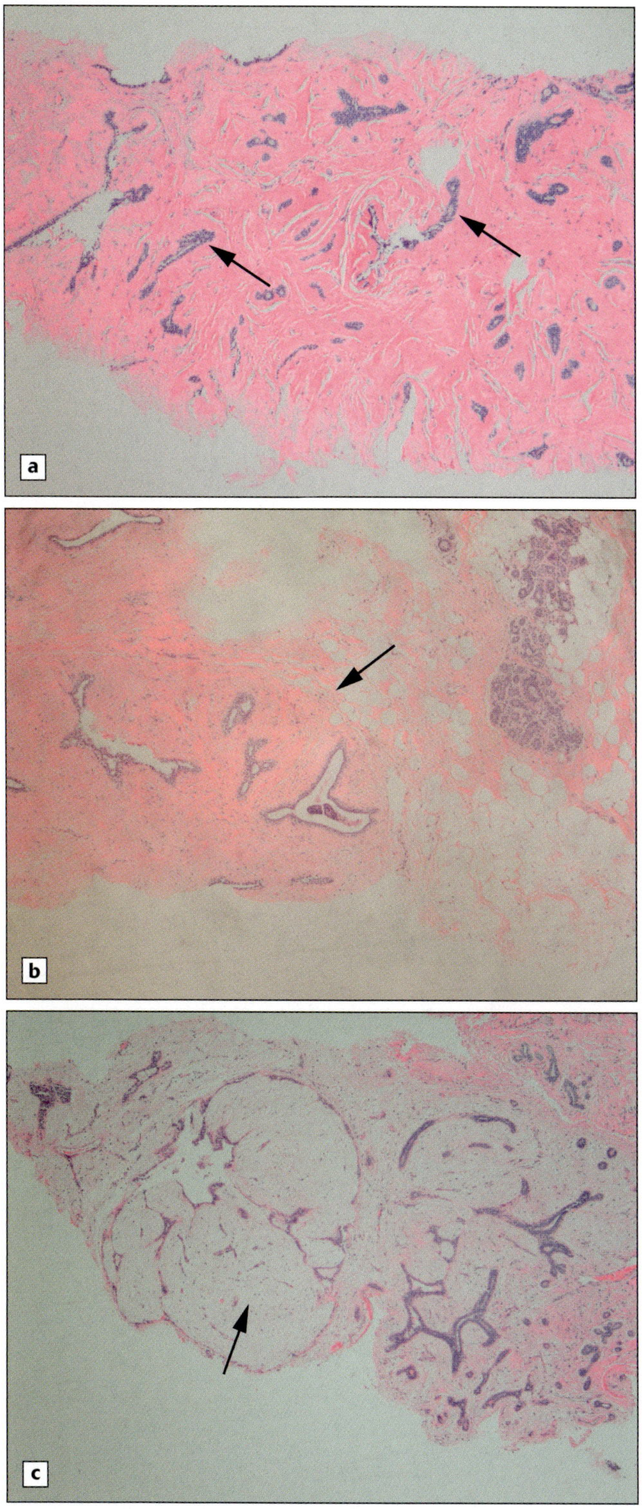

FIGURE 2.4 Variable but typical histology of core biopsies of fibroadenoma. Mixtures of these patterns are not infrequent. **(a)** Nodular aggregates of fibrous tissue are separated by benign glands, composed of epithelial and myoepithelial cells. The glands are typically elongated and compressed (arrows). **(b)** Note the sharply demarcated edge (arrow) of the fibroadenoma relative to surrounding breast tissue. **(c)** Myxoid fibroadenoma: the pattern of glandular proliferation is identical; however, the stroma is loosely cellular and composed of minimally staining matrix (arrow).

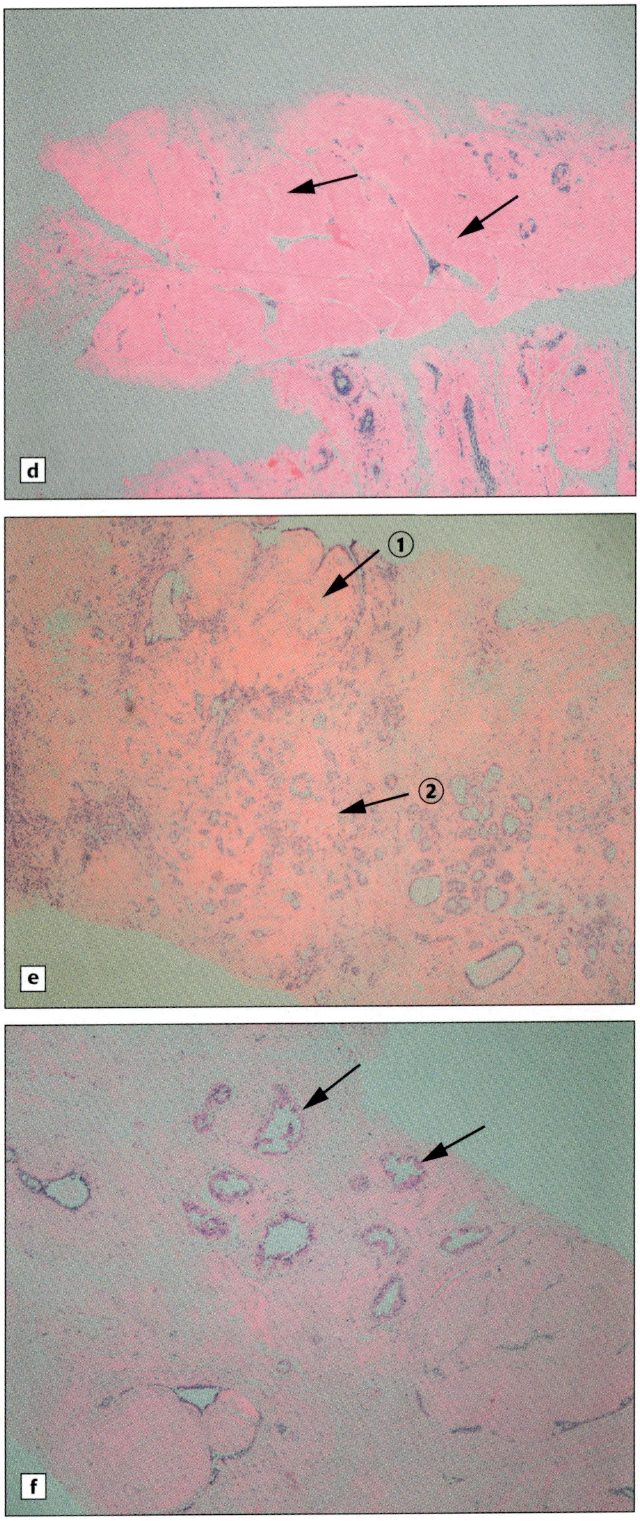

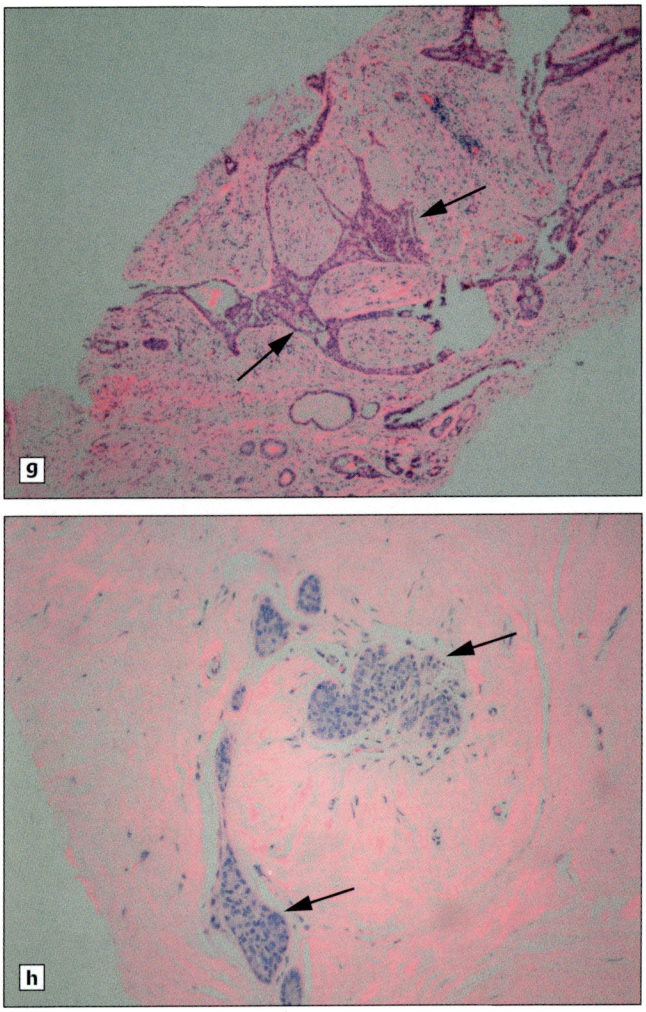

FIGURE 2.4—cont'd (d) Hyalinized fibroadenoma: again the overall pattern is maintained, but in this variation the stroma is completely acellular and composed of dense fibrous tissue (arrows). **(e)** Complex fibroadenoma: the compressed glandular pattern typical of fibroadenoma (arrow 1) is combined with a pattern of sclerosing adenosis (small tightly clustered glands, separated by fibrous stroma-arrow 2). **(f)** Complex fibroadenoma: in this example the compressed glands with hyalinized stroma (bottom) are joined by apocrine metaplasia composed of cells with granular, brightly eosinophilic cytoplasm (arrows) creating tiny papillary formations. **(g)** Fibroadenoma: the compressed glands contain an epithelial proliferation in a pattern typical of florid duct hyperplasia (arrows). **(h)** Fibroadenoma containing lobular neoplasia: the compressed and partially dilated glands contain a uniform small cell proliferation typical of in situ lobular carcinoma (arrows).

While the above histologic patterns in fibroadenomata do not correlate to specific imaging characteristics, occasional cases will on sonography show focal internal cystic areas. Some of these lesions are more lobulated, demonstrate slight irregularity to their borders, or do not have the typical through transmissions seen in classic fibroadenomas (Fig. 2.5a–d). Such cases usually correspond histologically to apocrine metaplasia-lined cyst walls admixed with more conventional fibroadenomatous patterns (Fig. 2.5e). The imaging management for these and

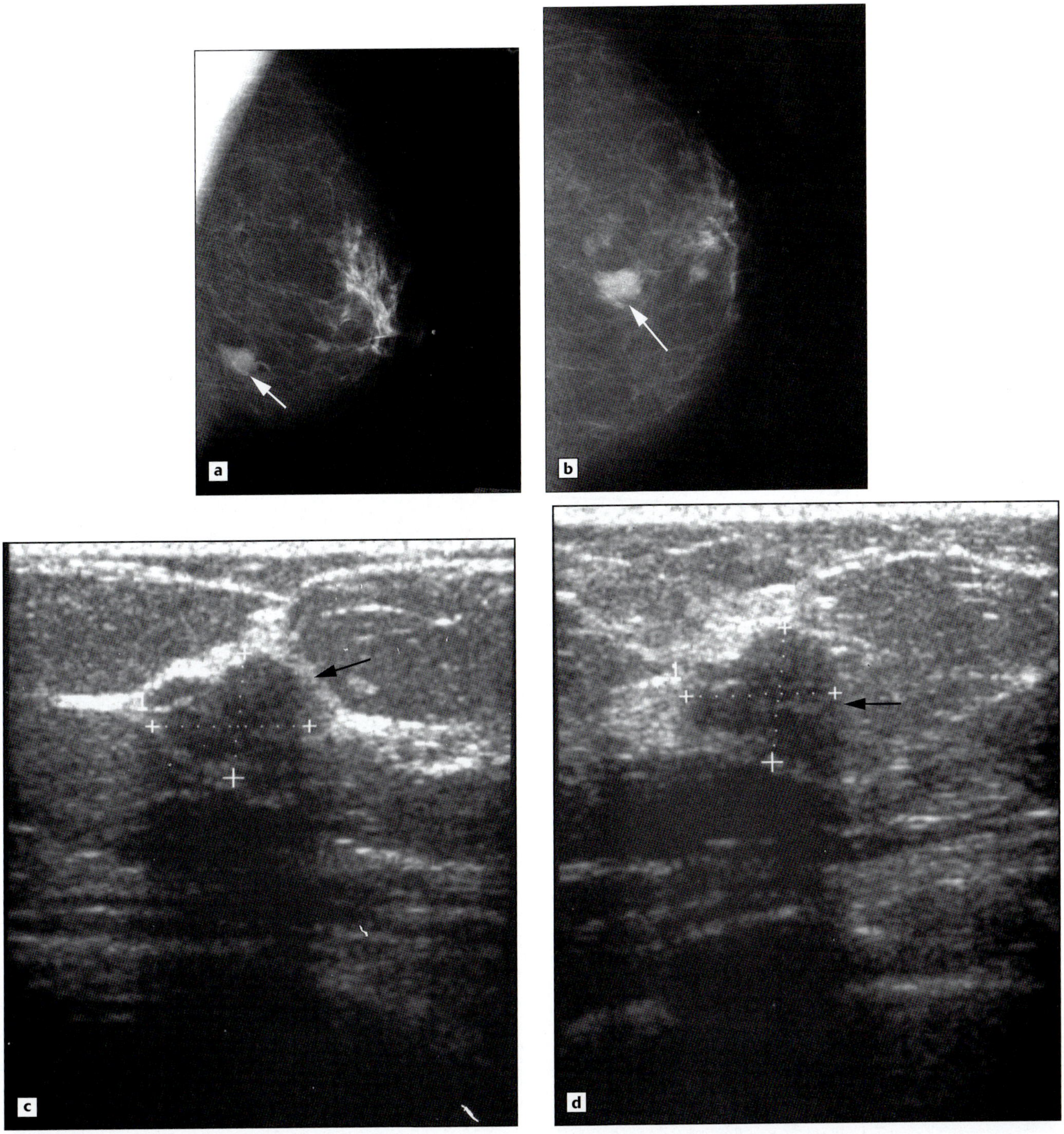

FIGURE 2.5 Fibroadenoma containing cystic apocrine metaplasia. **(a,b)** Mammogram-Baseline MLO and CC view demonstrates an oval, intermediate density, gently lobulated mass (arrows). **(c,d)** Sonography demonstrates a solid macrolobulated mass, homogeneous internal echoes (arrows) and some posterior shadowing.

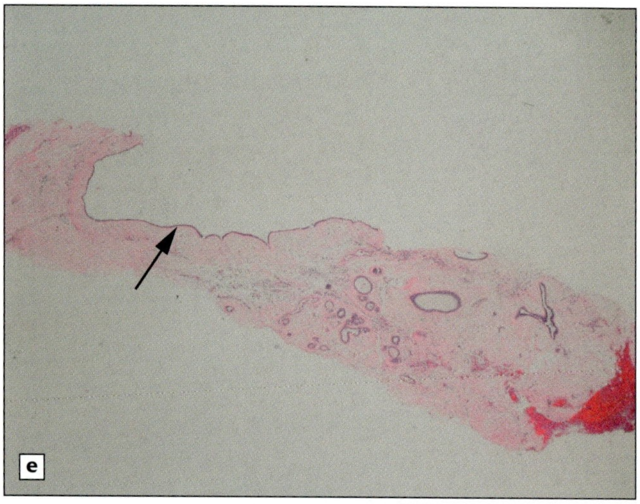

FIGURE 2.5—cont'd (e) This core shows a solid fibrous component with compressed fibroadenomatous glands and an adjacent cyst wall lined by apocrine metaplasia (arrow). The cyst wall lines the edge of the core cylinder.

other complex fibroadenomata, once the diagnosis is established, is similar to that for conventional fibroadenoma.

A fibroepithelial lesion related to fibroadenoma is the phyllodes tumor. These lesions are also hypoechoic with respect to surrounding breast tissue and may demonstrate more peripheral lobulations than the typical fibroadenoma, suggesting that different components of the mass are growing at different rates (histologically evident by the heterogeneity of stromal cellularity and mitotic rate typical of phyllodes). Phyllodes tumors can also have areas of slit-like anechoic spaces, hence the name cystosarcoma phyllodes. There is a large degree of overlap sonographically between a fibroadenoma and a phyllodes tumor;[3] however, phyllodes tumors usually demonstrate rapid growth,[4] maintaining their circumscription (Fig. 2.6). This overlap extends to histology as, for all practical purposes, it is impossible to histologically distinguish phyllodes tumor from fibroadenomata with cellular stroma (cellular fibroadenoma;

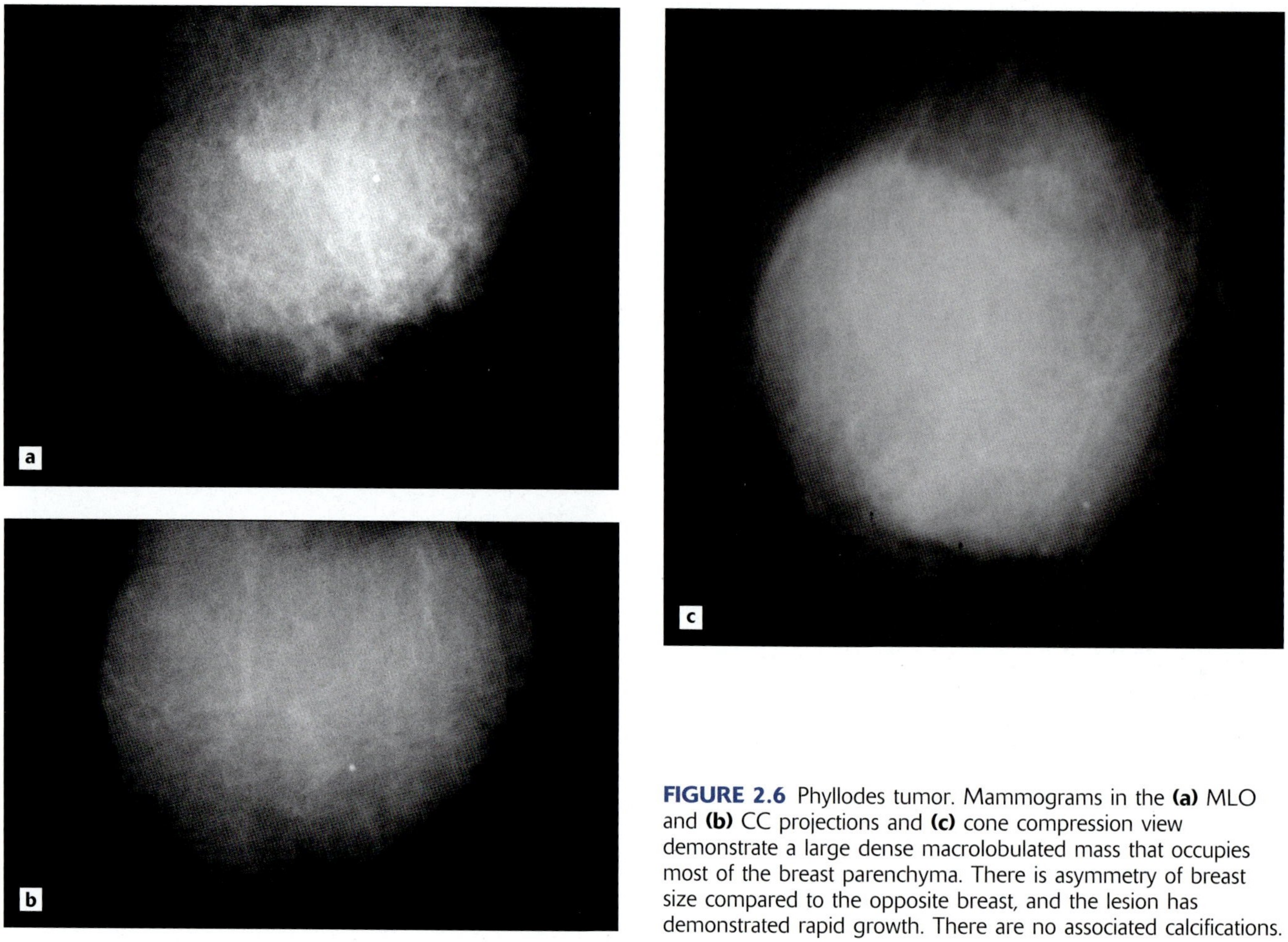

FIGURE 2.6 Phyllodes tumor. Mammograms in the **(a)** MLO and **(b)** CC projections and **(c)** cone compression view demonstrate a large dense macrolobulated mass that occupies most of the breast parenchyma. There is asymmetry of breast size compared to the opposite breast, and the lesion has demonstrated rapid growth. There are no associated calcifications.

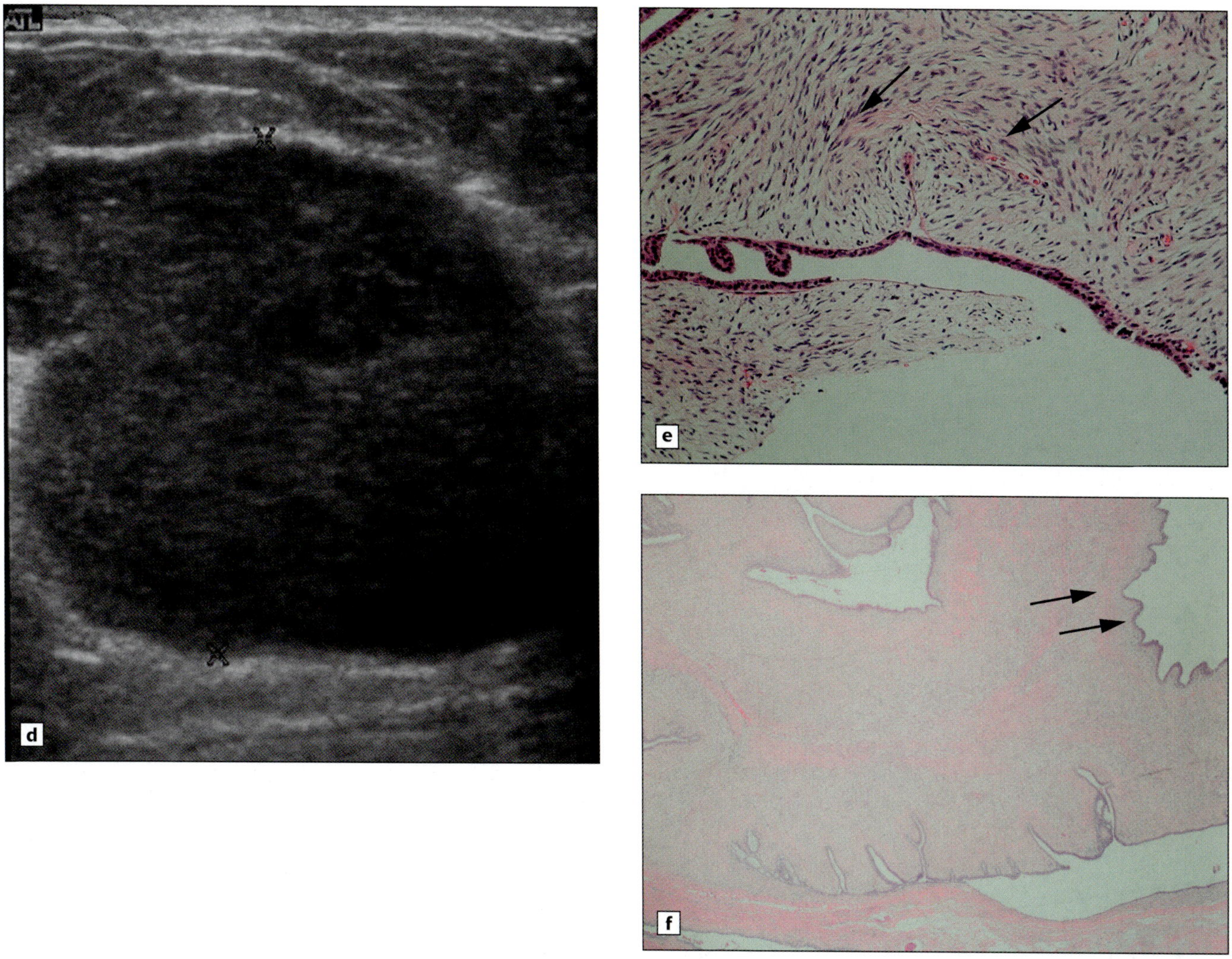

FIGURE 2.6—cont'd **(d)** Sonography demonstrates a large heterogeneous solid mass with some anechoic areas and some through transmission. There is a thick echogenic capsule. **(e)** Core biopsy reveals benign epithelium covering a cellular stroma composed of uniform spindle cells (arrows). Phyllodes tumor cannot be distinguished from cellular fibroadenoma based on this histology alone (see Fig. 2.7d). **(f)** Surgical excision reveals broad based, leaf-like structures with histologically benign but cellular stroma, diagnostic for phyllodes tumor. Note that the variability of stromal cellularity is most evident on excision, illustrating part of the problem of limited sampling afforded by core biopsy. Subepithelial stromal condensation (Cambian layer) is focally apparent (arrows).

Fig. 2.7) on core biopsy alone, although some authors have stated that any mitoses identified on core are highly predictive of phyllodes.[5] Cellular fibroadenoma is a far more common lesion than phyllodes tumor and microscopically is comprised of a typical fibroadenomatous pattern of benign elongated glandular structures compressed by a stromal proliferation which shows a somewhat increased but extremely variable cellularity. Although not pathognomonic, condensation of this stromal cellularity in areas directly underlying the epithelium, a so-called Cambian layer, is more frequently seen in phyllodes tumors. No stromal atypia or mitotic activity is evident in cellular fibroadenomas. The distinction between the two lesions may be difficult even on excision specimens.

There are no specific size cutoffs to distinguish between phyllodes tumor and fibroadenoma; however, phyllodes tumors generally exhibit rapid growth and therefore, have typically been diagnosed at relatively large size (average 4–5 cm) when already palpable.[6] This, however, is based largely on data from the pre-mammographic era, and we fully expect that mammographic screening will decrease the average size of phyllodes tumors at time of diagnosis in the same way that it has affected that of invasive carcinoma.

The distinction of cellular fibroadenoma from phyllodes tumor exemplifies a somewhat problematic situation specifically brought about by the era of mammographic screening and is, in our view, one which can only be resolved with communication between the pathologist

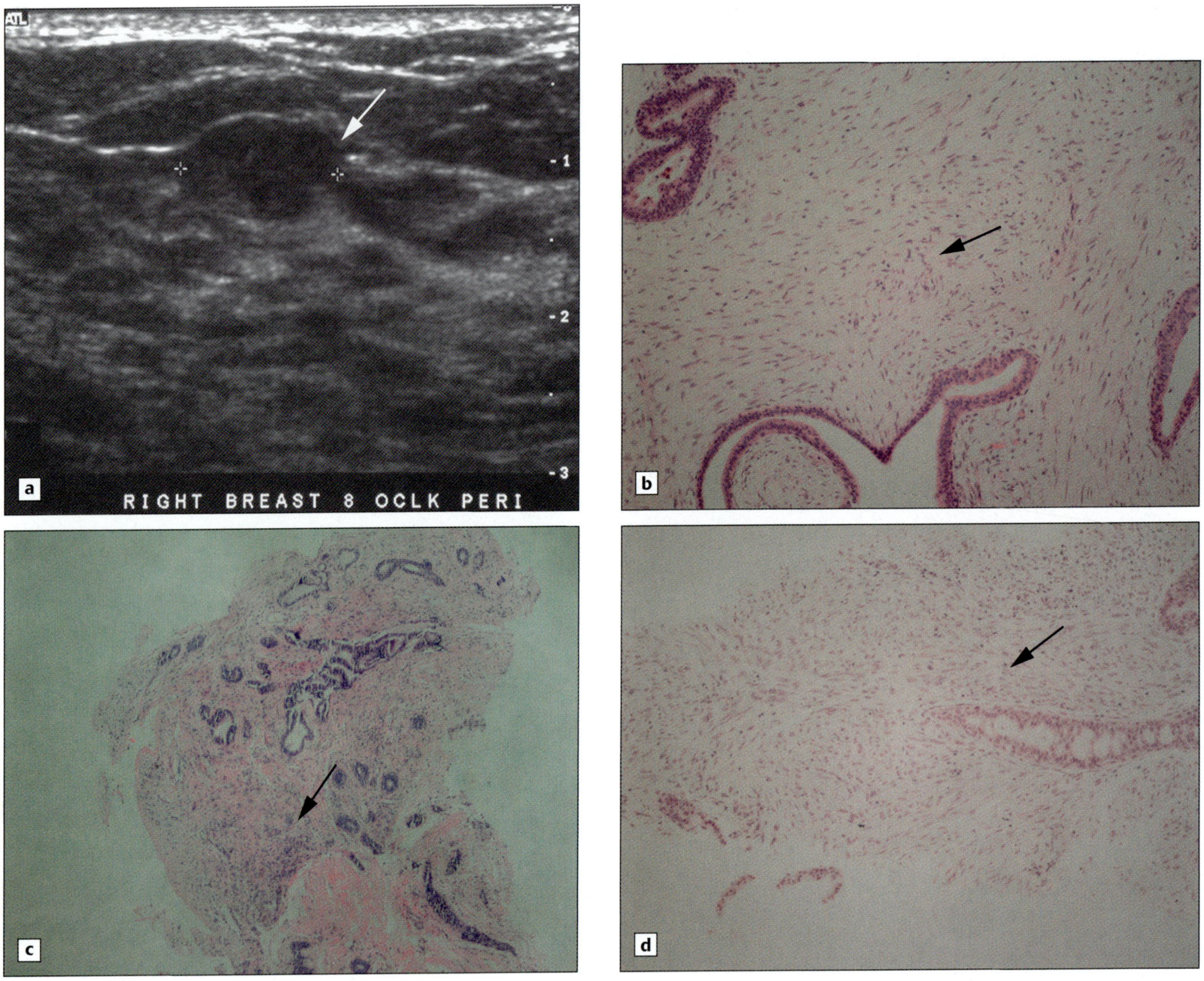

FIGURE 2.7 Cellular fibroadenoma. **(a)** Sonography demonstrates a homogeneous solid mass with a thin echogenic capsule (arrow) and a somewhat rounder than oval appearance. **(b,c)** Core biopsies reveals benign glands and increasingly cellular stroma (arrows), which in areas **(d)** are indistinguishable (arrow) from that possible in phyllodes tumor (see Fig. 2.6e).

and radiologist. Essentially we are faced with a differential diagnosis which can be difficult on surgical excision and, in the typical case, is virtually impossible on core biopsy. Since the main distinguishing feature between them is the latter's rapid growth, we feel that it is not necessary to surgically remove all such core-biopsied lesions provided that there is careful radiologic and clinical follow-up in a time interval commensurate with the level of suspicion (Figs 2.8 and 2.9). Cellular fibroadenomata are certainly far more common lesions than phyllodes tumors. There is no evidence that they are premalignant or prone to local recurrence, and surgical removal is unnecessary unless performed for cosmetic purposes. Careful radiologic follow-up would prevent such surgery. Furthermore, size alone does not appear to be a prognostic factor in phyllodes tumor; thus, the change in size ascribed to the follow-up interval would have no bearing on the patient's outcome. Since a nonpalpable phyllodes tumor is by nature small, the growth allowed by short interval follow-up should not be sufficiently large that a more disfiguring lumpectomy (or mastectomy) would be needed to achieve negative margins. Thus we believe it is safe and justifiable to reserve surgical excision for those lesions which enlarge either radiologically, clinically, or both.

Phyllodes tumor of the breast is, as alluded to, nearly an impossible diagnosis to make on core biopsy alone unless one sees heterologous malignant stromal elements

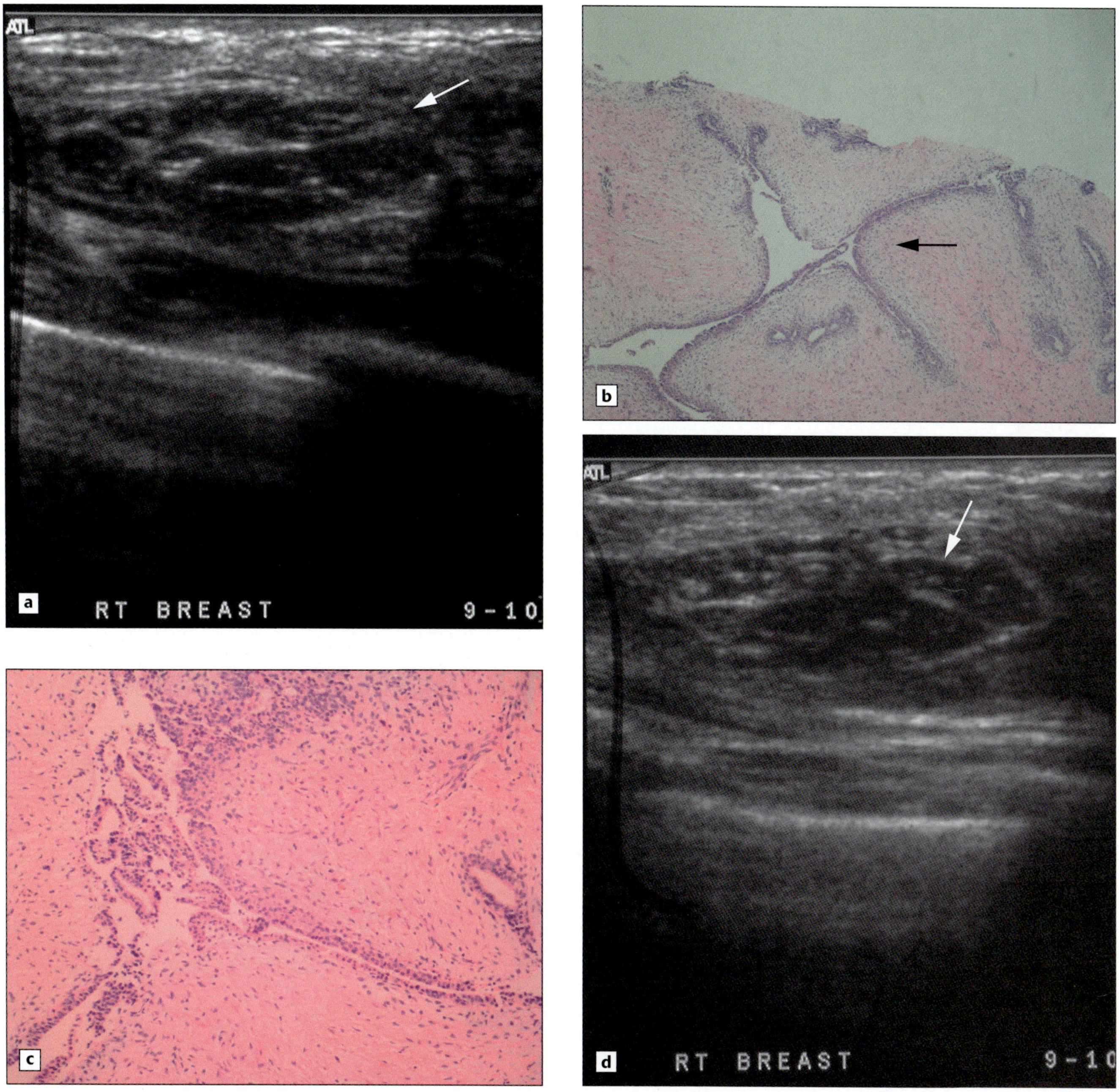

FIGURE 2.8 Follow-up imaging of cellular fibroepithelial lesion-stability. **(a)** Sonography revealing a well-circumscribed solid hypoechoic mass (arrow). **(b)** Core biopsy shows a fibroepithelial lesion with very cellular stroma and an accentuated papillary pattern reminiscent of phyllodes (arrow). **(c)** Higher power reveals a lack of subepithelial stromal condensation and absence of mitosis. **(d)** Follow up sonography six months later reveals stability in terms of size of the lesion (arrow), consistent with cellular fibroadenoma.

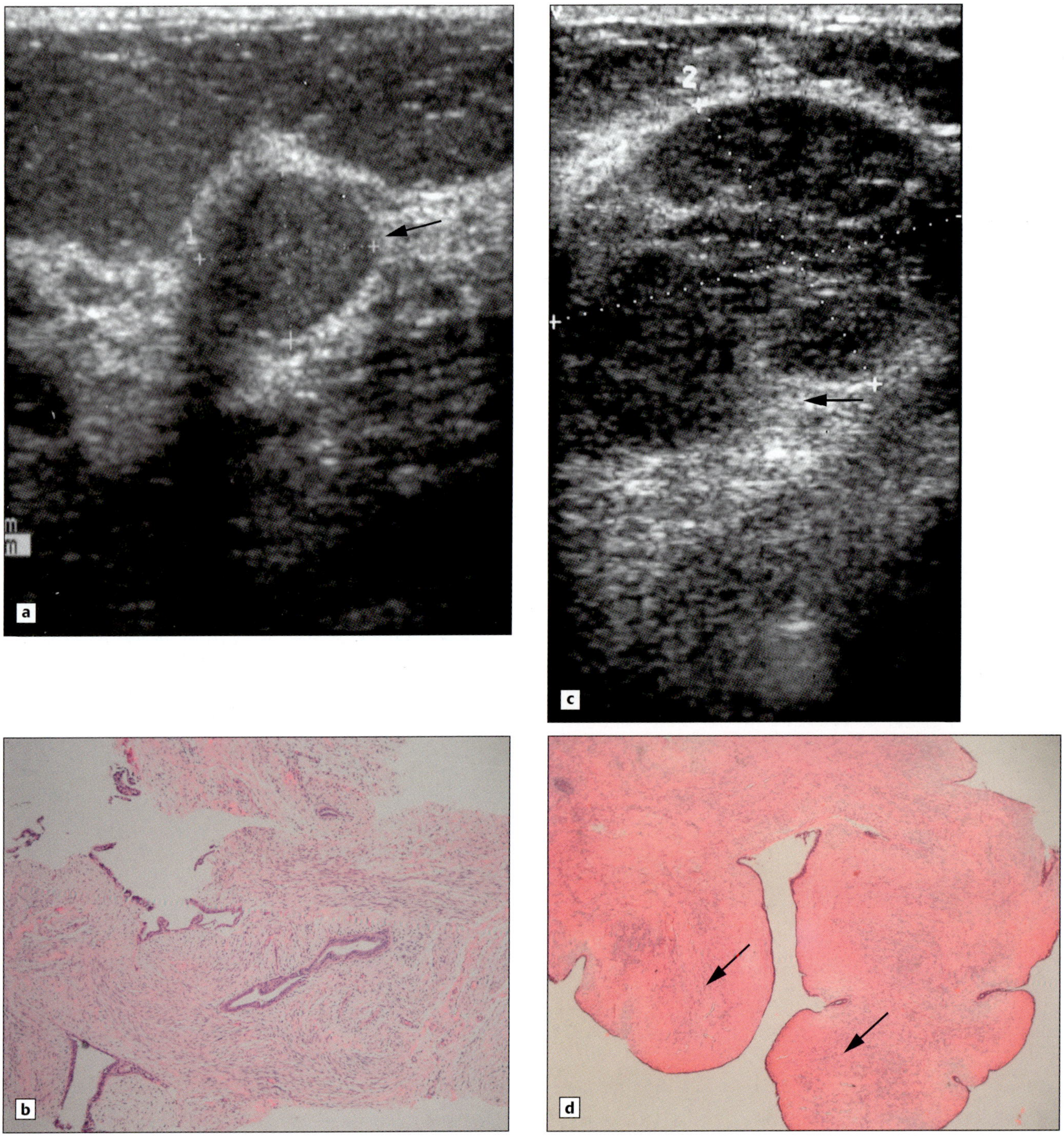

FIGURE 2.9 Follow-up imaging of cellular fibroepithelial lesion-growth. **(a)** Sonography showing a solid round-oval mass (arrow) with a thin capsule and predominantly homogeneous echoes. **(b)** Ultrasound-guided cored biopsy demonstrates findings of a cellular fibroadenoma. **(c)** Sonographic follow-up in six months demonstrated interval increase in size. The lesion has macrolobulated margins and central slit-like anechoic spaces (arrow). **(d)** Surgical excision demonstrates a phyllodes tumor with typical broad papillary structures containing the cellular stroma (arrows).

such as liposarcoma (Fig. 2.10). Such cases are extremely uncommon; however, certainly one may suspect the diagnosis based on extreme stromal cellularity accompanying a typical fibroadenomatoid/phyllodes histology combined with a clinical history of rapid growth. Phyllodes tumors have been classified as histologically benign, borderline, and malignant based on numerous histologic factors (mitotic activity, necrosis, size, etc.); however, histologic and nonhistologic factors that would be accurately predictive of benign or malignant clinical behavior are still lacking (even on complete surgical excision). The most consistently predictive factors are the presence or absence of "stromal overgrowth"[7] and the status of surgical resection margins. Clearly none of the above factors are evaluable on core biopsy alone.

The core biopsy differential diagnosis of fibroadenoma is not limited to phyllodes tumor. Fibrocystic changes, usually composed of sclerosing adenosis, can occasionally form a radiographic and/or clinical mass, corresponding to the synonymous terms nodular fibrocystic change, nodular sclerosing adenosis,[8] or, in older terminology, adenosis tumor. The imaging findings of such lesions are similar to those of fibroadenoma with the exception that they show slightly irregular borders and often do not

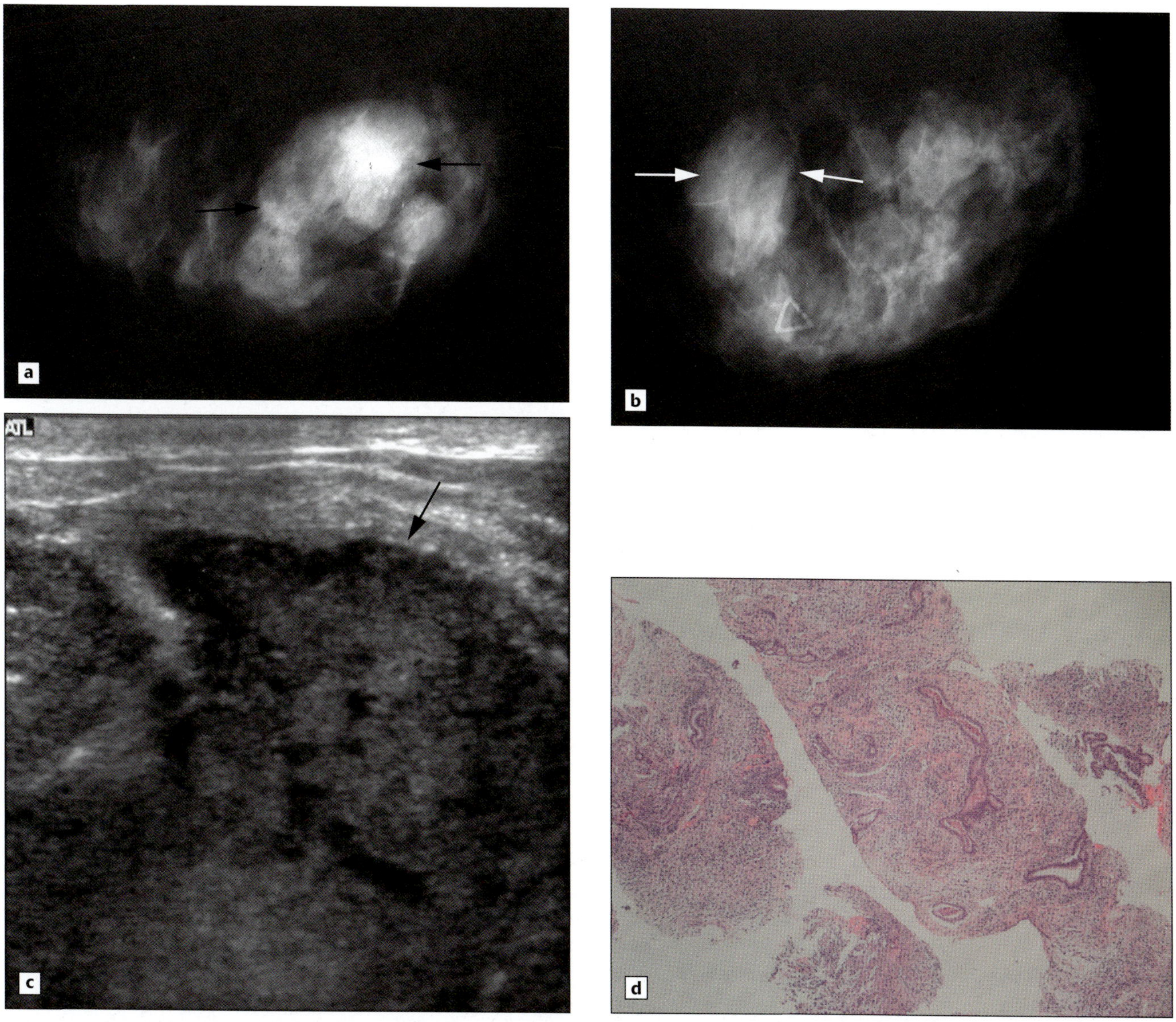

FIGURE 2.10 Malignant phyllodes tumor. **(a,b)** Mammogram demonstrates a dense lobulated mass (arrows) which demonstrated rapid growth. The lesion has some indistinct margins but no associated calcifications. **(c)** Sonography demonstrates a solid macrolobulated mass with inhomogenous internal echoes (arrow). There are areas of shadowing and other areas of through transmission. **(d)** Core biopsies demonstrate benign epithelium lined by extremely cellular and

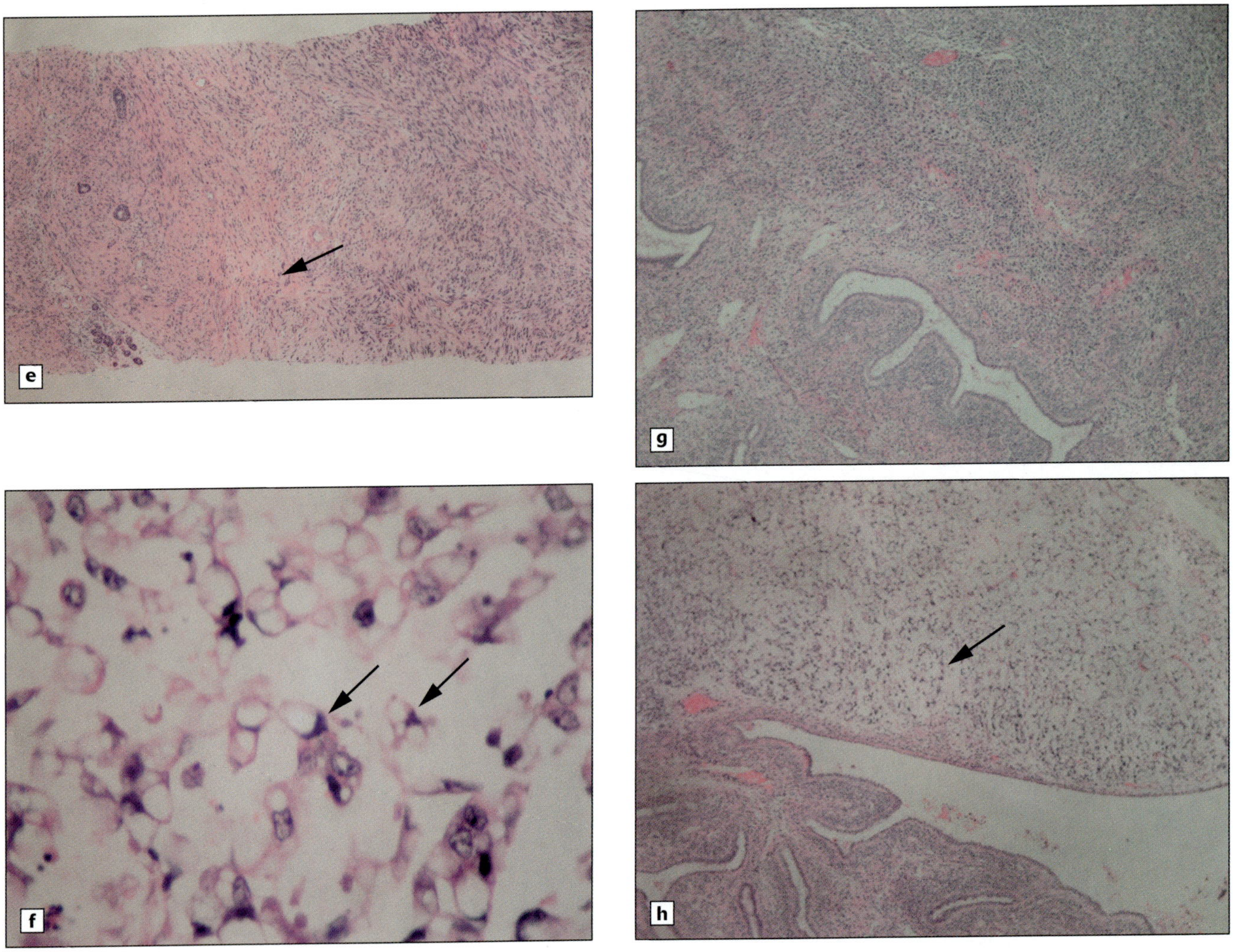

FIGURE 2.10—cont'd **(e)** cytologically malignant spindle cell stroma with numerous mitoses (arrow) and **(f)** focal liposarcomatous differentiation (arrows). Surgical excision confirms the diagnosis with **(g)** nonspecific stromal malignancy and **(h)** liposarcoma (arrow).

demonstrate the thin peripheral echogenic capsule which is so characteristic of fibroadenoma (Fig. 2.11). In evaluating resultant core biopsies, it is important to be aware of the entity because one might otherwise be concerned that the lesion had been missed and generate a rather nonspecific report of "benign breast tissue" or "fibrocystic changes". The diagnosis of "nodular fibrocystic change" can be confidently made when fatty breast tissue is identified on both edges of areas of sclerosing adenosis on individual cores, i.e., the core has gone completely through the lesion. This assures the radiologist that the lesion has been "hit", and an unnecessary surgical procedure is averted. In our experience, core biopsies of nodular fibrocystic change may be occasionally be difficult to distinguish from sclerosing intraductal papillomata because the central portion of the former typically may have a radial fibrotic pattern. We have found additional histologic levels to be of great value in this regard (Fig. 2.11d,e). The imaging characteristics may be helpful in such instances as sclerosing papillomata are often seen sonographically as regions of distortion, vague shadowing or even spiculation.. Sometimes, however, the imaging characteristics overlap as well and, in such cases, it is probably prudent to recommend excision, as with intraductal papillomata (see Chap. 5).

Fibroadenomata sometimes will contain small amounts of adipose tissue, probably an involutional change which occurs most frequently in elderly patients. The adipose tissue is most prevalent at the periphery of such lesions and accounts for the slightly irregular contours which may be seen sonographically (Fig. 2.12) or as a change in a lesion being followed over the long term. Such lesions can be differentiated from hamartoma (see Chap. 3) by the presence of compressed, usually hyalinized, typical fibroadenomatous stromal growth patterns amidst the fat. On sonographic imaging

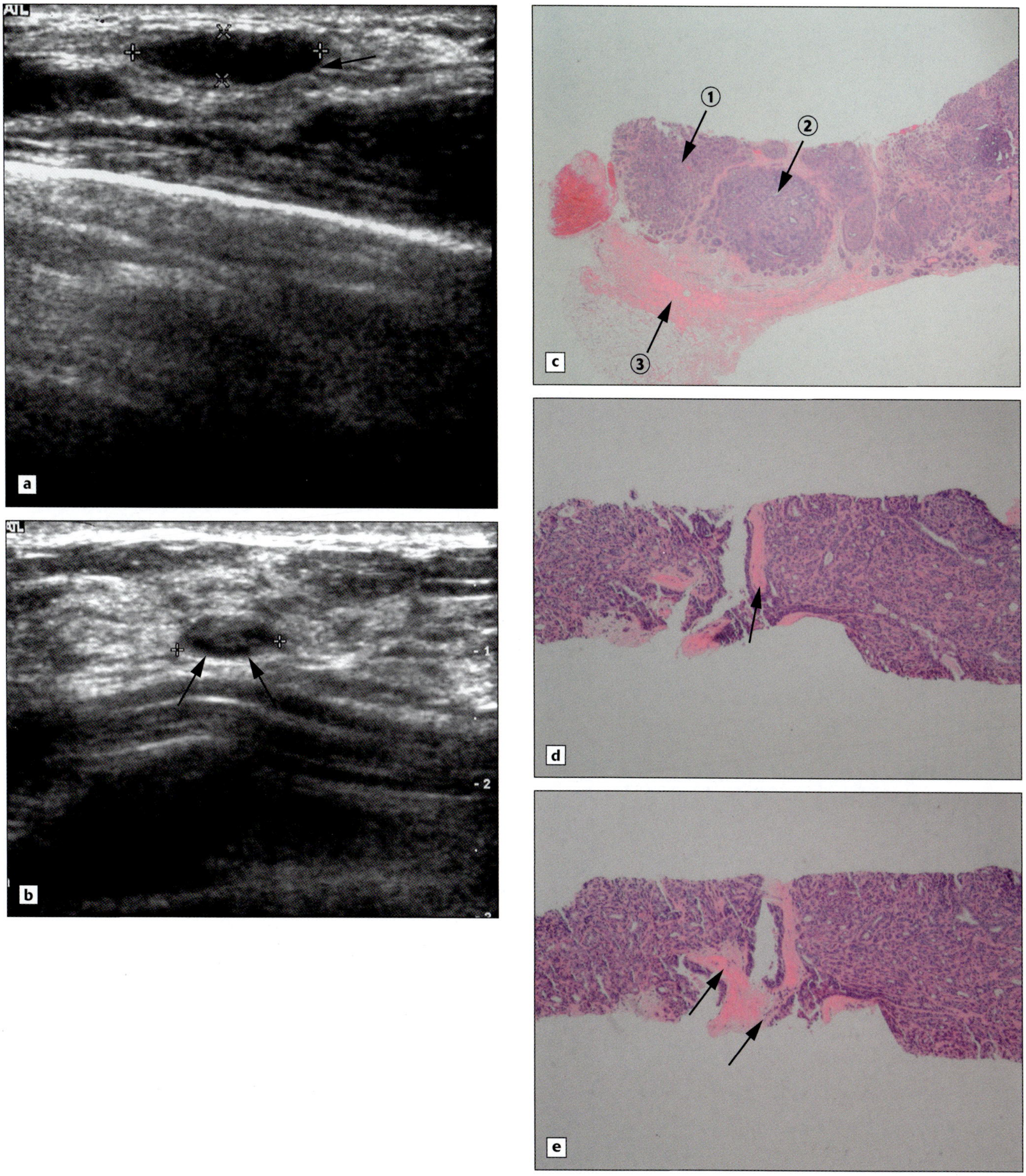

FIGURE 2.11 Nodular sclerosing adenosis, two examples. **(a)** Sonography of the left breast/axillary tail shows a focal hypoechoic oval mass with smooth margins (arrow) and minimal border irregularities. The lesion is oriented parallel with tissue planes. **(b)** Right sonography: there is an oval hypoechoic mass in the right breast at the 7 o'clock axis 1 cm from the nipple. This has internal areas which appear anechoic (arrows). **(c)** Core biopsy reveals multiple nests of sclerosing adenosis (arrows 1 and 2). Note the sharp border between the lesion (arrow 3) and adjacent adipose tissue and the lack of a fibrous capsule. The central portion of such lesions tends to be somewhat more fibrotic with a retracting appearance. **(d)** Occasional cases can be difficult to distinguish from papillomas because of the central fibrosis (arrow). Deeper sections of the paraffin block **(e)** often are helpful in this distinction, here showing that the fibrous areas connect (arrows) in a pattern typical of the center of nodular sclerosing adenosis, rather than showing the epithelial growth surrounding papillary structures of a sclerosing papilloma.

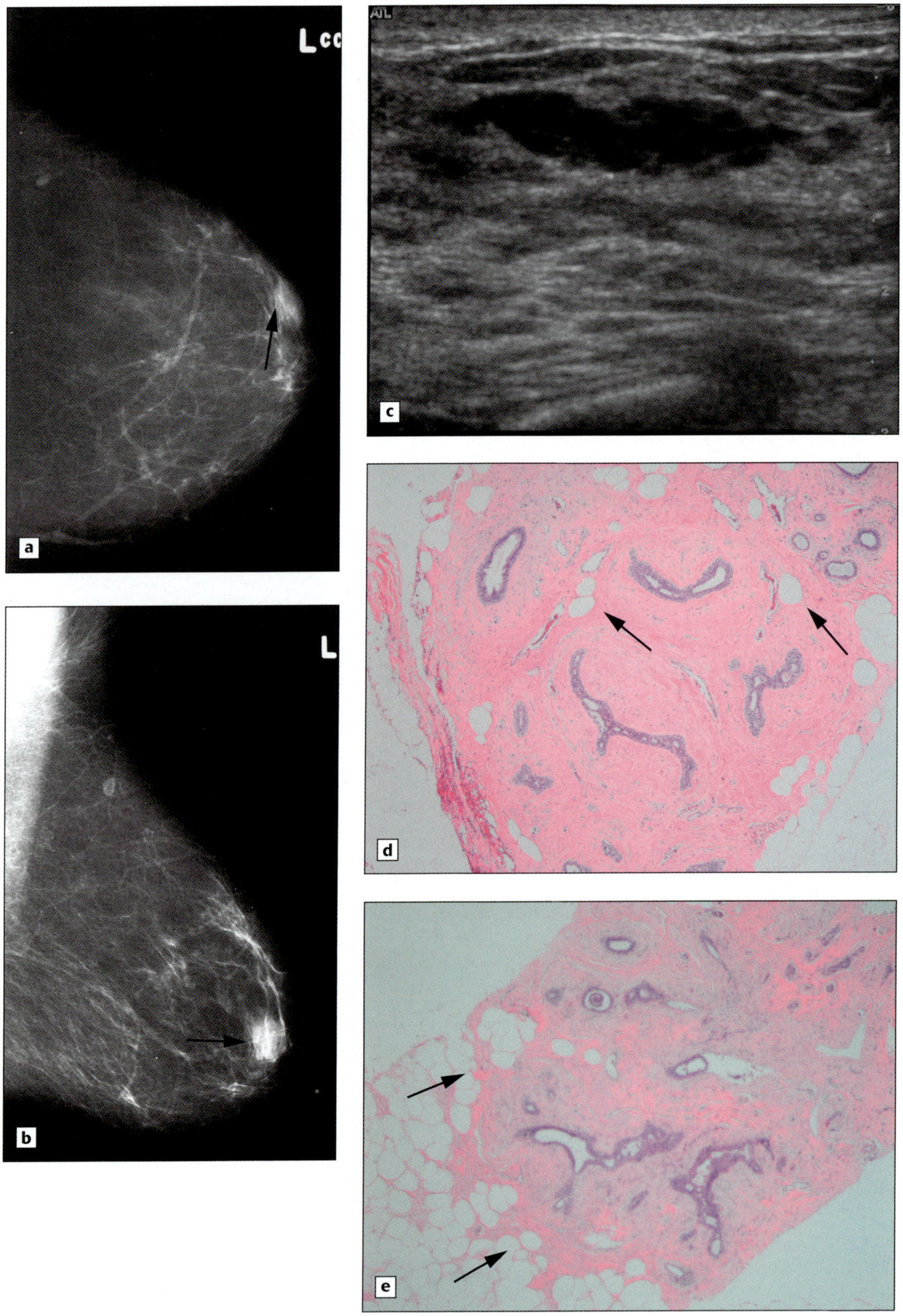

FIGURE 2.12 Fibroadenoma with fatty infiltration: Mammogram – CC **(a)** and MLO **(b)** views reveal an oval nodule (arrows) with mixed fibrous and fatty density. **(c)** Sonography demonstrates an oval gently lobulated solid mass with no significant through transmission or shadowing. The mass parallels the tissue planes and has a thin echogenic capsule. Slight border irregularities in well circumscribed solid lesions can also correspond histologically to fibroadenoma with fat infiltration (arrows) both within **(d)** and at the periphery **(e)** of the lesion.

hamartomas are often encapsulated and contain a mixture of echogenic and hypoechoic tissue in a swirling type pattern. The distinction between the two entities is, in our view, less important than the assessment of the adequacy of the biopsy, i.e., that the targeted lesion was not missed.

A few lesions must be included in this group although they are quite histologically distinct from fibroadenoma/phyllodes tumors. A lactating adenoma is seen in the clinical setting of a palpable mass in a pregnant or lactating patient. Typically benign features seen sonographically include: solid, hypoechoic, round-oval with a circumscribed border, smooth lobulations, long axis parallel to the chest wall, and an echogenic pseudocapsule (Fig. 2.13). Cores reveal breast tissue with lactational change (acinar epithelial cells showing prominent nucleoli, vacuolated cytoplasm, and luminal proteinaceous material); however, these features are identical with those seen in lactating breast tissue, and every attempt should be made to identify the border between the "lesion" and surrounding breast tissue to assure the radiologist that the targeted area has in fact been sampled. In our experi-

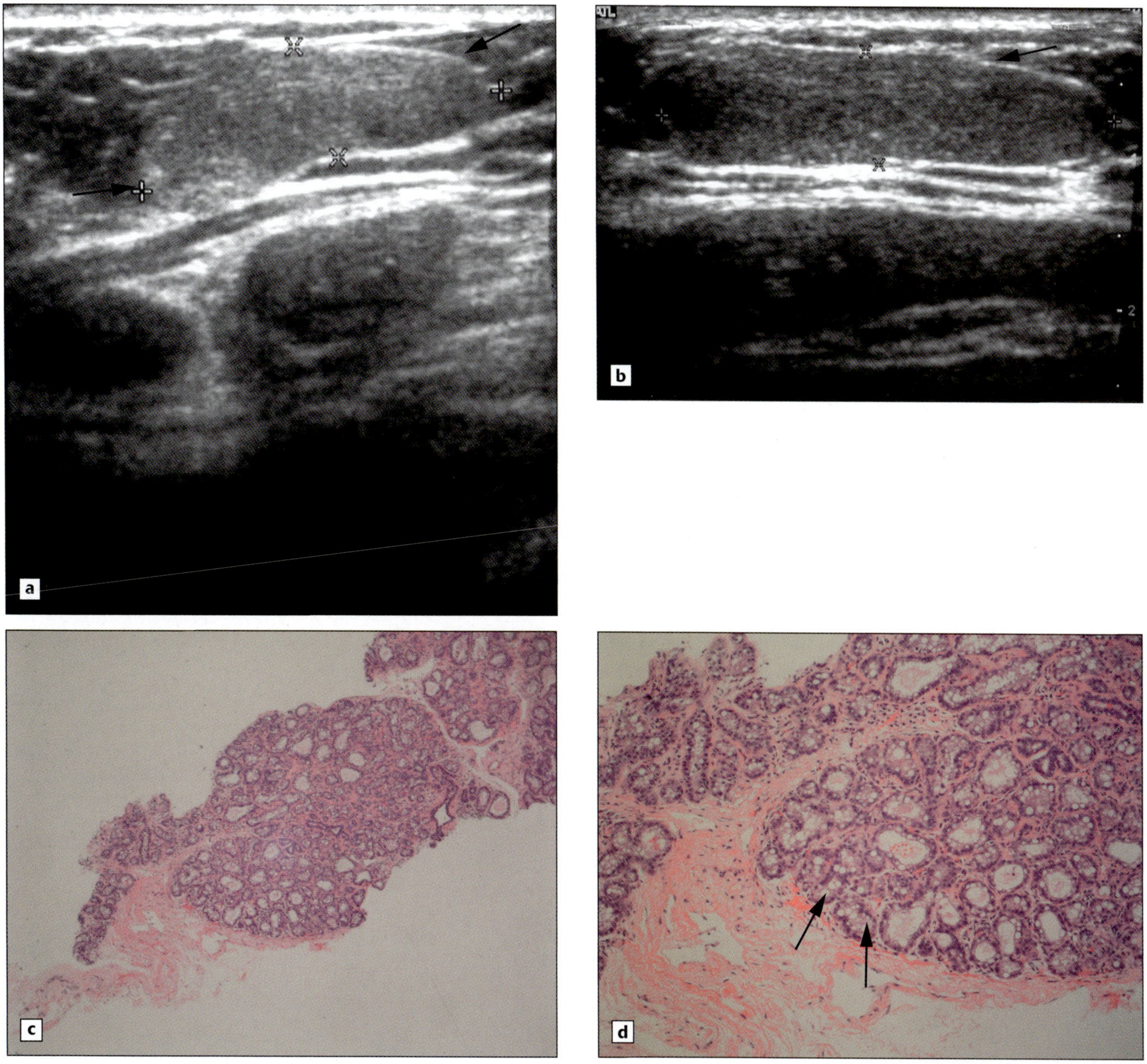

FIGURE 2.13 Lactating adenoma. **(a,b)** Sonography demonstrates a solid oval homogeneous mass with a thin echogenic capsule (arrows). The patient was nursing and noticed a new palpable mass. **(c)** Core biopsies reveal a sharply demarcated area almost entirely composed of well formed glands. **(d)** At higher power the glands show typical lactational changes, i.e., numerous glands composed of cells with vacuolated cytoplasm (arrows) and luminal secretions.

ence this is not always as simple as it would appear, given the young age of the patients with a general relative lack of fatty breast tissue, and the lobular expansion caused by pregnancy. The presence of elongated benign appearing ductular structures would represent tubular adenoma (Fig 2.14), a related diagnosis also associated with pregnancy. Pregnancy can also cause infarction of a fibroadenoma, also to be kept in mind in interpretation of core biopsies.

Finally, one must remember that adenomyoepitheliomata typically are well-circumscribed solid nodules and would therefore lend themselves to core biopsy investigation. We have encountered this entity in core biopsies only once (see Chap. 15), The prominence of a myoepithelial cell layer with clear cytoplasm and close parallel growth with the epithelial cells are hallmarks of the lesion (Fig. 2.15), although this can be a difficult diagnosis even after complete excision. Clearly the differential diagnosis of core biopsies of such lesions would include invasive well differentiated duct carcinoma; however, over diagnosis of malignancy in these instances can be avoided by considering the fact that tubular or invasive well differentiated duct carcinomas typically do not present as well circumscribed masses.

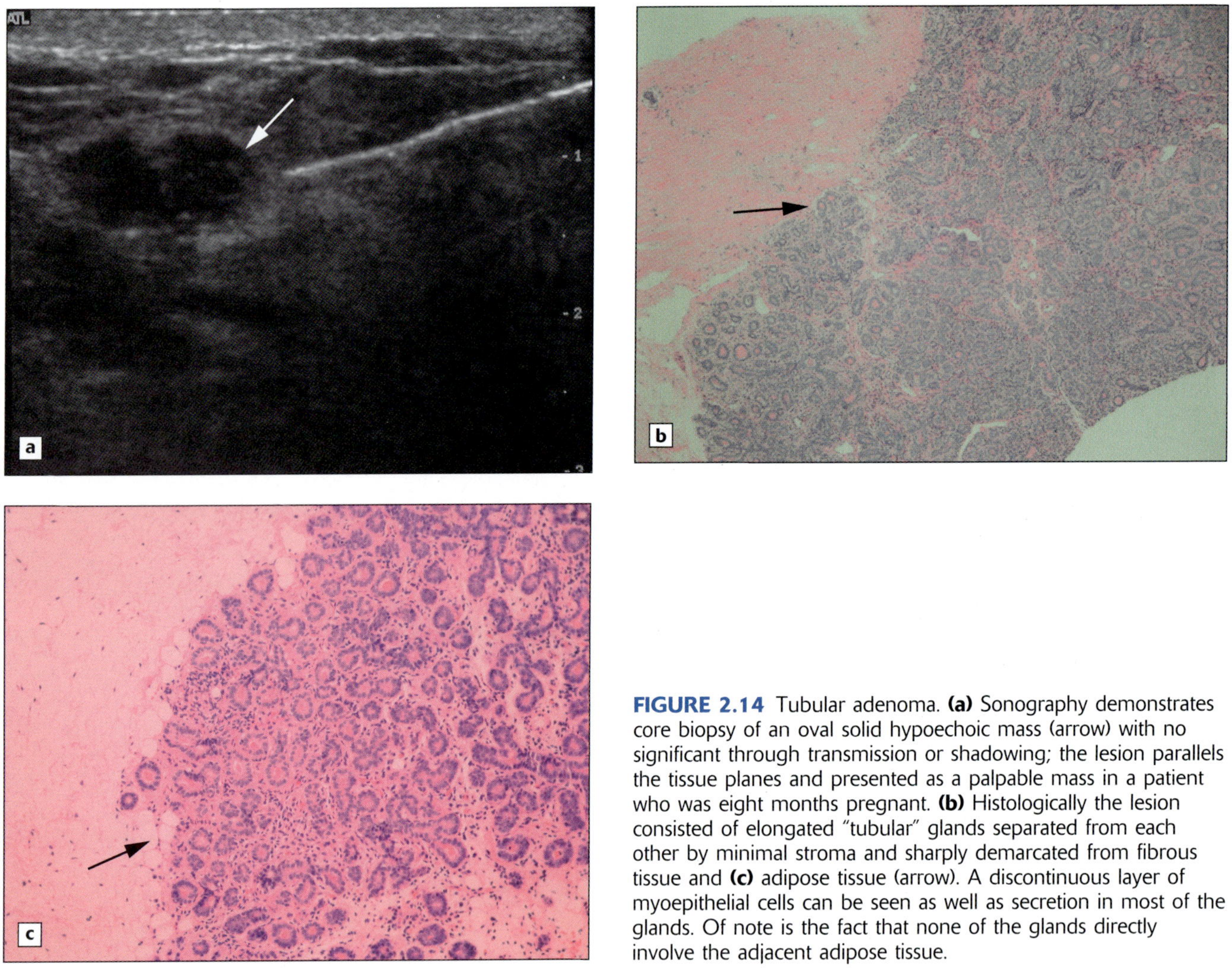

FIGURE 2.14 Tubular adenoma. **(a)** Sonography demonstrates core biopsy of an oval solid hypoechoic mass (arrow) with no significant through transmission or shadowing; the lesion parallels the tissue planes and presented as a palpable mass in a patient who was eight months pregnant. **(b)** Histologically the lesion consisted of elongated "tubular" glands separated from each other by minimal stroma and sharply demarcated from fibrous tissue and **(c)** adipose tissue (arrow). A discontinuous layer of myoepithelial cells can be seen as well as secretion in most of the glands. Of note is the fact that none of the glands directly involve the adjacent adipose tissue.

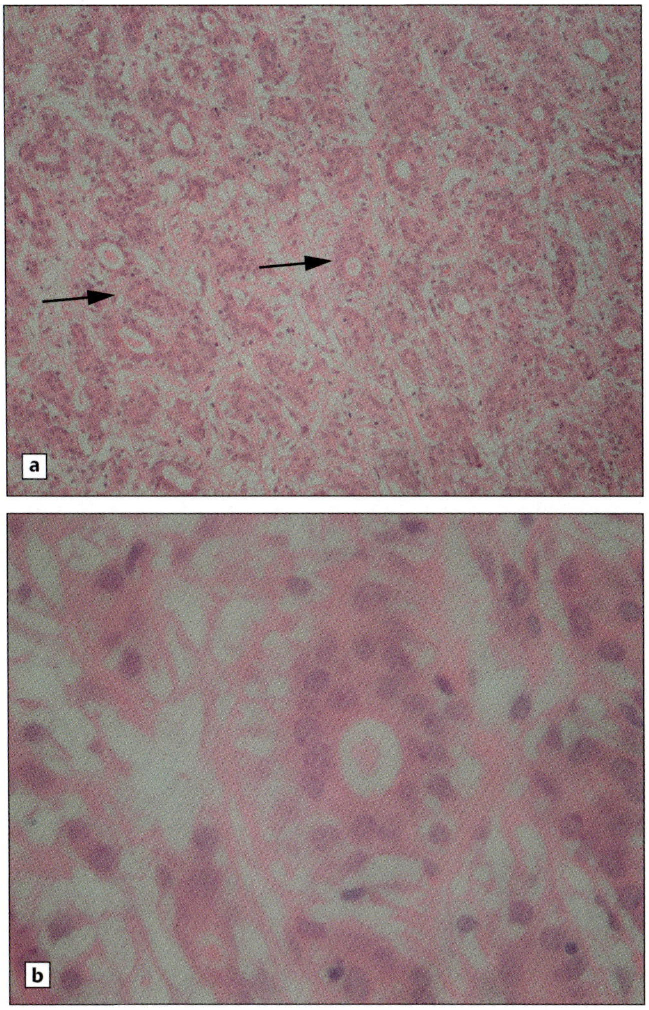

FIGURE 2.15 Adenomyoepithelioma. **(a)** This lesion consists of a proliferation of epithelial elements as well-formed glands accompanied by large myoepithelial cells with clear cytoplasm rimming each gland (arrows). **(b)** Higher power demonstrating the two types of cells.

Differential diagnoses of low radiologic suspicion well-circumscribed solid lesions

- Fibroadenoma
- Complex fibroadenoma
- Cellular fibroadenoma
- Phyllodes tumor
- Nodular fibrocystic change
- Lactating adenoma
- Adenomyoepithelioma
- Hamartoma
- Intraductal papilloma

POINTS TO REMEMBER

- Phyllodes tumor essentially cannot be diagnosed on core biopsy alone.
- Short term clinical follow-up of cellular fibroadenoma on core biopsy is probably safe.
- Fibroadenomata harboring ADH or DCIS should be excised.
- Specific benign diagnoses help to confirm accurate sampling of the lesion.

REFERENCES

1. Carney JA, Toorkey BC. Myxoid fibroadenoma and allied conditions (myxomatosis) of the breast. A heritable disorder with special associations including cardiac and cutaneous myxomas. Am J Surg Pathol 15:713–721,1991.
2. Dupont WD, Page DL, Parl FF, et al. Long-term risk of breast cancer in women with fibroadenoma. N Engl J Med 331:10–15,1994.
3. Yilmaz E, Sal S, Lebe B. Differentiation of phyllodes tumors versus fibroadenomas. Acta Radiol 43:34–39,2002.
4. Foxcroft LM, Evans EB, Porter AJ. Difficulties in the pre-operative diagnosis of phyllodes tumors of the breast: a study of 84 cases. Breast 16:27–37, 2007.
5. Jacobs TW, Chen YY, Guinee DG Jr, et al. Fibroepithelial lesions with cellular stroma on breast core biopsy: are there predictors of outcome on surgical excision? Am J Clin Pathol 124:342–354,2005.
6. Rosen PP, Rosen's Breast Pathology, 1st ed., Lippincott-Raven, New York, 1997 pp. 155–156.
7. Ward RM, Evans HL. Cystosarcoma phyllodes. A clinicopathologic study of 26 cases. Cancer 58:2282–2289,1986.
8. Gill HK, Ioffe OB, Berg WA. When is a diagnosis of sclerosing adenosis acceptable at core biopsy? Radiology 228:50–57,2003.

CHAPTER 3

Well-circumscribed solid lesions with heterogeneous radiodensity

As discussed in the preceding chapter, the avoidance of surgery for benign lesions is one of the advances made possible by core biopsy; however, as will be seen below, the use of core biopsy without careful correlation of imaging and pathologic findings has the potential for the converse, namely unnecessarily sending the patient to surgery or worse.

Hamartoma of the breast (or fibroadenolipoma) is the prototypical well-circumscribed solid nodule that has a heterogeneous radiodensity. It is an encapsulated collection of the major normal constituents of the breast: ducts, lobules, fibrous tissue, and adipose tissue. The lesion is often nonpalpable but at large sizes may correspond to a region of fullness. Its typical mammographic appearance is well recognized: it is sharply marginated and surrounded by a thin capsule with an internal mixture of soft tissue and fat density (Fig. 3.1). The proportion of adipose to parenchymal components varies, and thus the lesion may be relatively radiolucent or dense at mammography (Fig. 3.2). The sonographic features vary from a region of focal mass effect with displacement of surrounding breast tissue by a lesion containing hypoechoic fat and echogenic glandular tissue in a swirling type pattern (Fig. 3.3) to a lack of specific findings. Since the radiologic features of mammary hamartoma are so characteristic, biopsy is not necessary in the vast majority of cases; however, it is reasonable to confirm the diagnosis with core biopsy when the imaging findings are not classical or to appease a patient who is concerned about the finding.

Hamartoma of the breast has, until recently, been a diagnosis almost exclusively the province of radiologists. The entity has such a characteristic mammographic appearance[1] that it was immune to surgical excision and therefore rarely, if ever, seen in routine surgical pathology practice, a long forgotten diagnosis for the average surgical pathologist.[2] The advent of core biopsy technology has changed this situation by providing a relatively noninvasive and accurate mechanism of assuring the patient of the diagnosis. Thus it behooves the pathologist to become reacquainted with the lesion, lest he or she automatically think that a core biopsy yielding benign breast tissue has missed its target.

Essentially hamartoma is a circumscribed, even encapsulated area composed of all the elements of benign breast tissue, appropriately in some circles known as "breast within breast".[3] As such, core biopsies which accurately sample the lesion will simply reveal benign fibrous and fatty breast tissue, and it is difficult to be more diagnostically precise than that, except to suggest that the process may represent a hamartoma (Fig. 3.4). In this scenario only the radiologist can assess with any certainty whether or not the lesion was accurately sampled; however, the suggestion of the diagnosis alone should, in most instances, be confirmatory since the lesion has such distinct imaging characteristics. The pathologist should avoid language such as "non-diagnostic" or "no lesional tissue identified", since this could lead to the incorrect conclusion that the lesion has been missed and theoretically lead to re-biopsy or even surgical excision, especially given the current medicolegal climate. Conversely, if the histology is nonspecific benign fibrous and fatty breast tissue, and the targeted lesion's imaging characteristics are inconsistent with hamartoma, consideration should be made for the possibility that the lesion was indeed missed.

Although by no means specific, we and others[4] have found that many hamartomata contain elements of pseudoangiomatous stromal hyperplasia (PASH); however, this finding can be seen in other entities such as fibrocystic changes and can create a solid well-circumscribed nodule known as nodular PASH,[5,6] a lesion which, in our opinion, can be suggested but not definitively diagnosed on core biopsy (Fig. 3.5).

Occasionally the pathologist will be faced with core biopsies which contain aggregates of bland spindle cells forming tiny fascicles in addition to "normal" breast tissue elements. When these spindle cells are immunohistochemically positive for vimentin, desmin, smooth muscle actin, progesterone receptor protein, often estrogen receptor protein, and negative for cytokeratin (CAM 5.2), consistent with smooth muscle, the appellation "myoid" hamartoma is applied (Fig. 3.6). Smooth muscle is not foreign to the breast, as large bundles are present in the subareolar area and prominently accompanying larger lactiferous ducts. Thus one would expect that myoid hamartomata would occur in regions adjacent to such structures. This, however, turns out to not necessarily be the case. The lesion can be found anywhere in the breast,

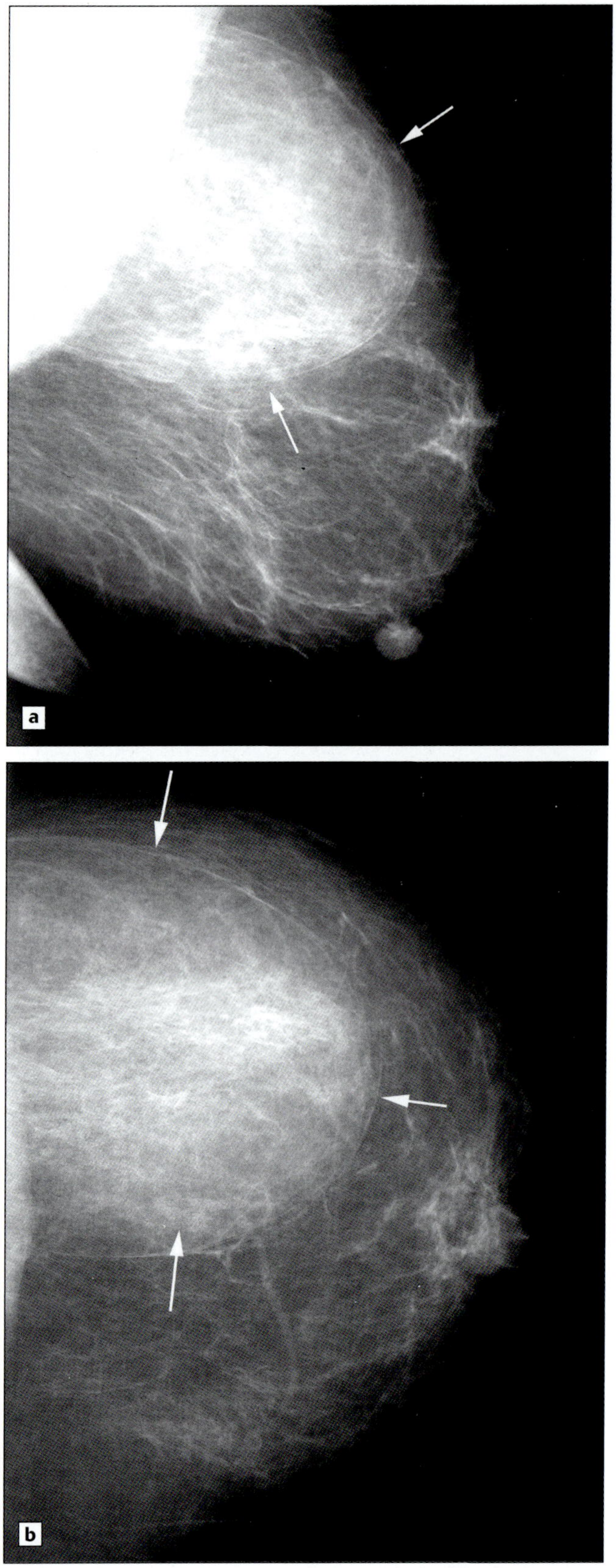

FIGURE 3.1 (a) Left MLO and **(b)** CC views demonstrating a heterogeneous soft tissue mass in the upper outer quadrant (arrows). The lesion has areas of fat and density, surrounded by a thin capsule. This is a classic mammographic appearance of a hamartoma.

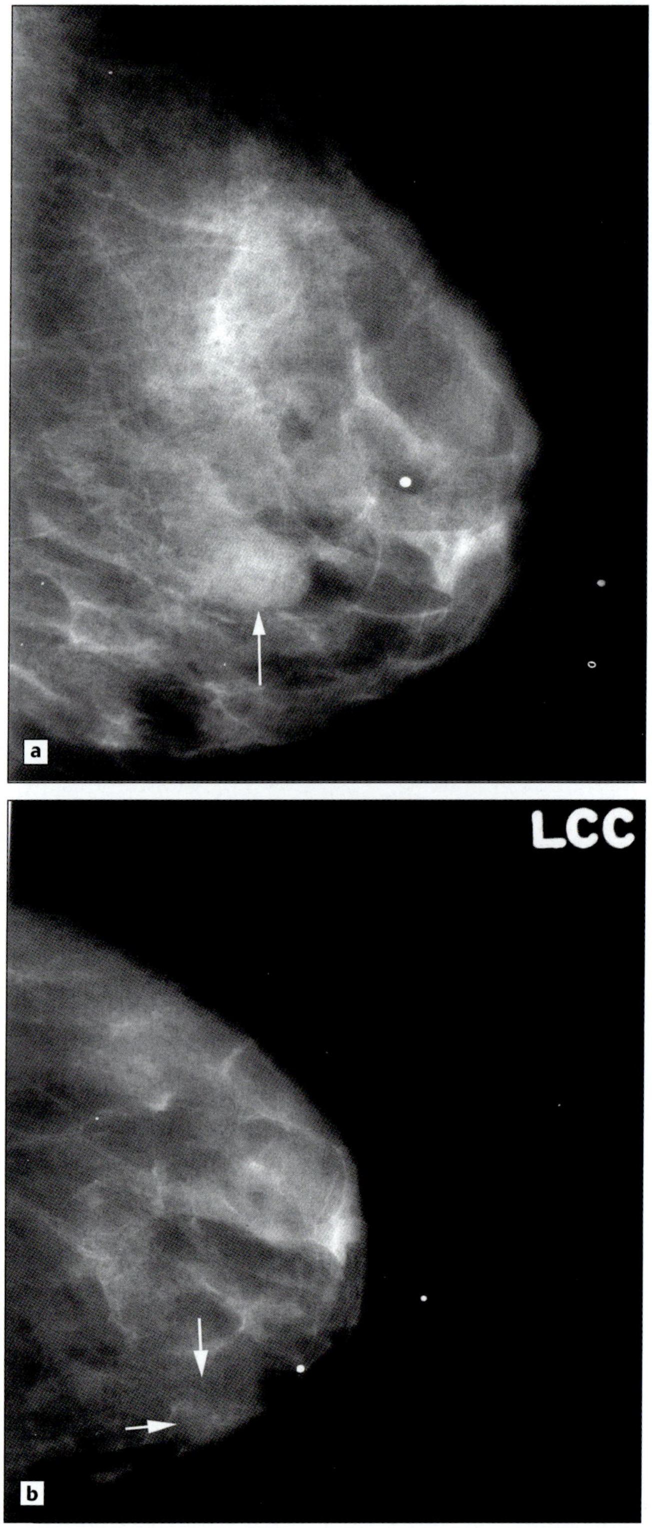

FIGURE 3.2 (a) Left MLO and **(b)** CC views demonstrate a soft tissue mass (arrows) with no definite capsule in the left medial breast. The lesion is palpable and denoted by a radio-opaque BB.

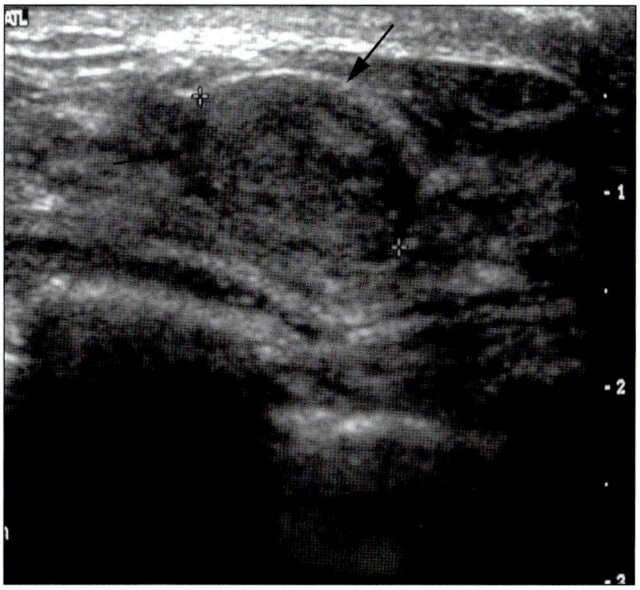

FIGURE 3.3 Sonography demonstrates a heterogeneous hypoechoic and hyperechoic mass with the suggestion of a thin peripheral capsule (arrow). Hamartomas can have varying amounts of soft tissue and fat density.

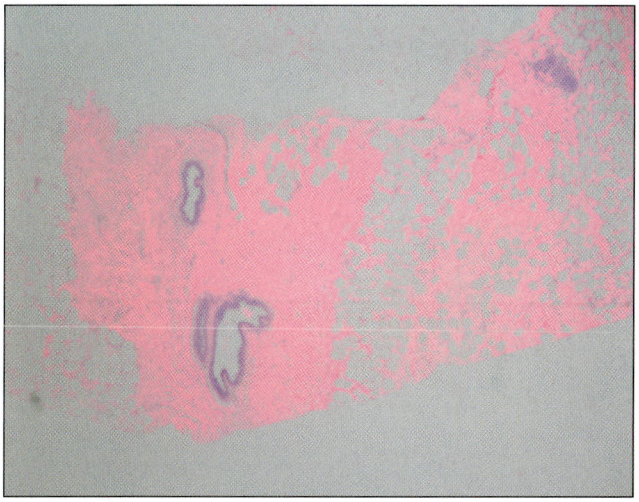

FIGURE 3.4 Core biopsy of hamartoma shows all the normal components of breast tissue-glands, fibrous tissue, and adipose tissue.

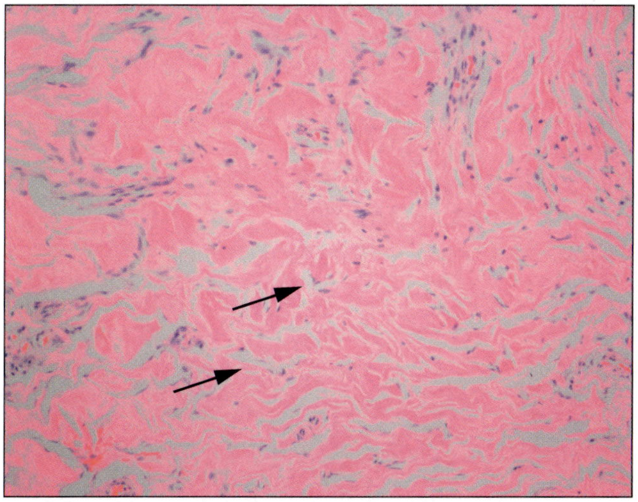

FIGURE 3.5 Pseudoangiomatous stromal hyperplasia (PASH) is a nonspecific histologic pattern, but is frequently found as a component of hamartoma. Fibroblasts form a pattern reminiscent of small blood vessels, interspersed between dense collagen bundles (arrows). In rare instances the pattern forms a mass, so-called nodular PASH.

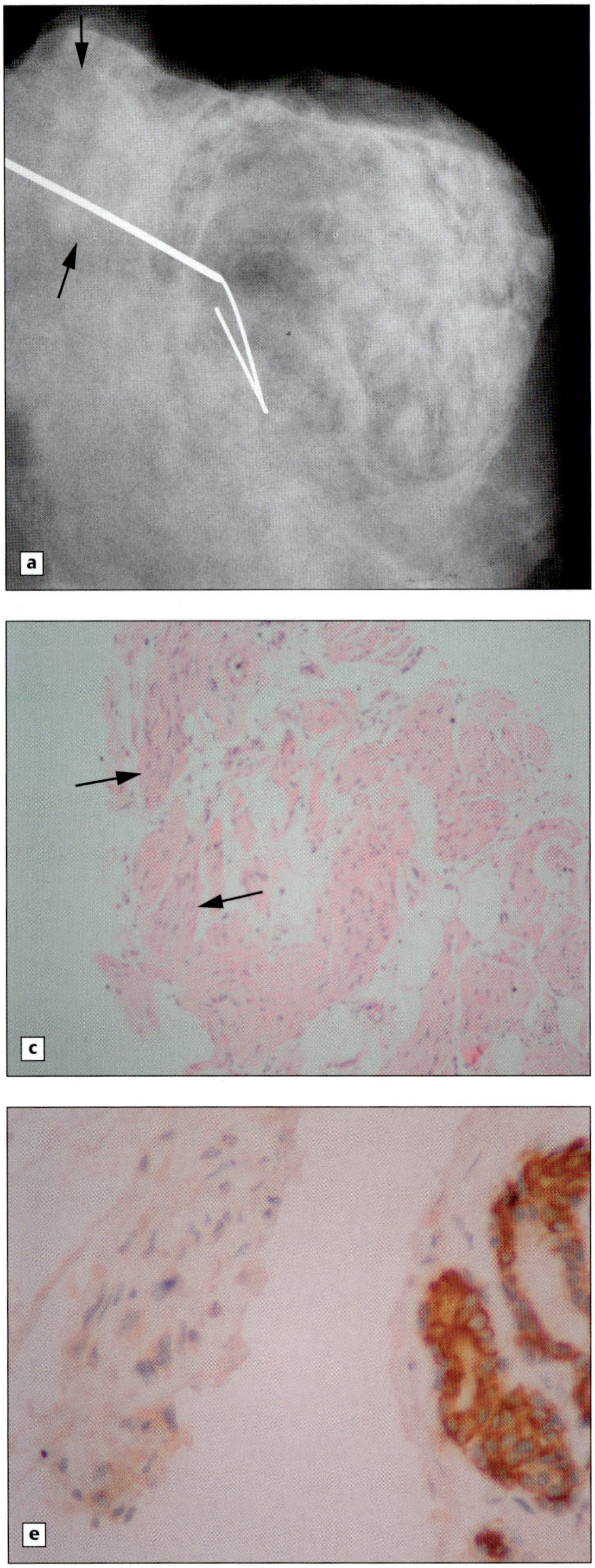

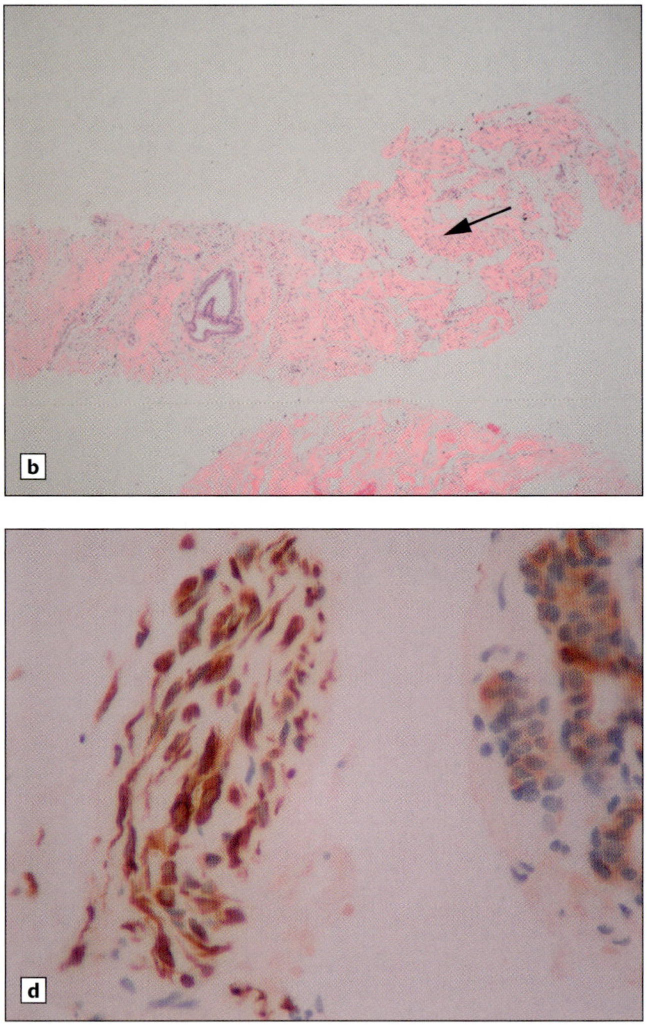

FIGURE 3.6 Myoid hamartoma. **(a)** Specimen radiograph of a wire localized well-circumscribed radiologically heterogeneous mass (arrows). The patient desired removal of the lesion; however, the mass had been previously core biopsied showing **(b)** a mixture of benign glands, spindle cells (arrow) and adipose tissue. **(c)** Closer inspection reveals that the spindle cells are cytologically benign and arranged in small bundles (arrows). Immunohistochemical stains reveal that the spindle cells are positive for desmin **(d),** negative for cytokeratin **(e).**

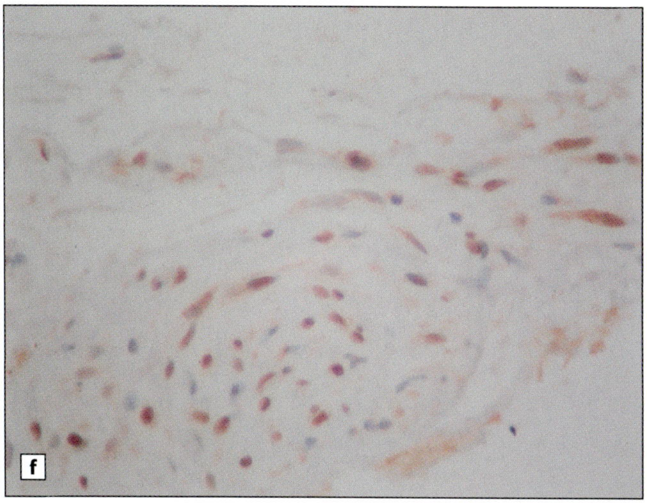

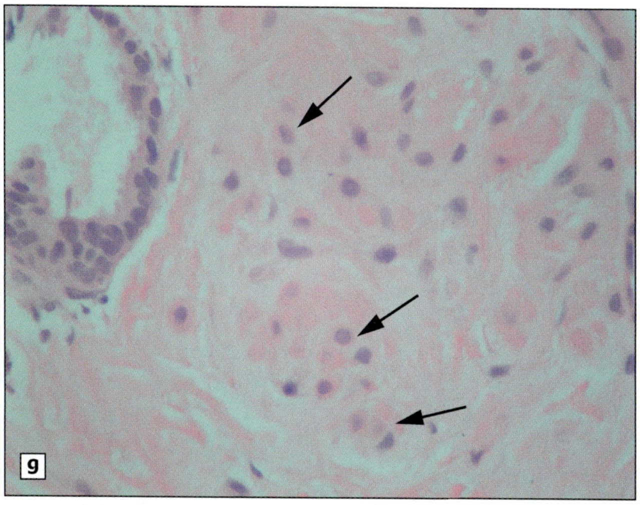

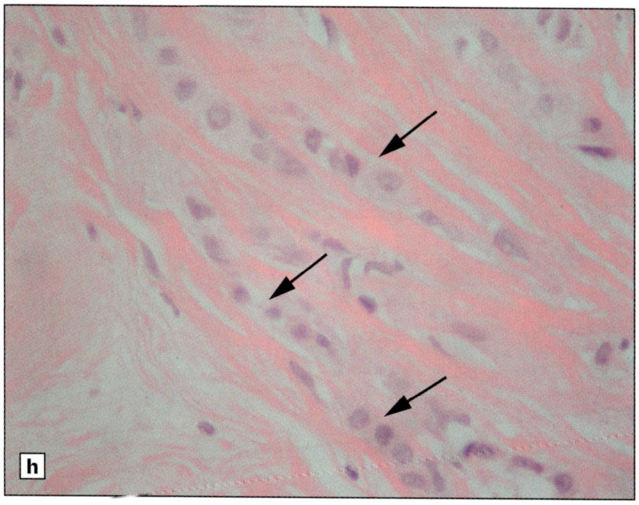

FIGURE 3.6—cont'd and positive for estrogen receptor protein **(f).** These findings classify the spindle cells as smooth muscle. In other areas **(g,h)** the same cells have an epithelioid appearance (arrows) and would easily be mistaken for infiltrating lobular carcinoma without knowledge of the imaging findings.

is typically seen in perimenopausal women, and may be quite large.

It is impossible radiographically or sonographically to distinguish myoid hamartoma from ordinary hamartoma (Fig. 3.6); however, of greater diagnostic importance perhaps is the occasional occurrence of epithelioid differentiation in the muscle cells. We reported this in a large tumor that showed areas in which the epithelioid smooth muscle cells were forming histologic patterns indistinguishable from invasive lobular carcinoma.[7] A core biopsy of such an area could easily be misdiagnosed leading to the consequences of lumpectomy, unnecessary axillary dissection, possibly unnecessary mastectomy, and even perhaps unneeded preoperative chemotherapy. Such a misadventure can be avoided by the knowledge that the core biopsies emanate from a well-circumscribed tumor, a pattern that does not occur with a classical invasive lobular carcinoma. Immunohistochemical stains will confirm the diagnosis, but only if the differential diagnosis is considered; thus, radiographic-pathologic correlation is crucial and has major therapeutic implications.

Also to be considered in the differential diagnosis of this group of lesions is intramammary lymph node, which typically has a well-circumscribed kidney bean shape and is of low to intermediate density on mammography (Fig. 3.7). These have a characteristic sonographic appearance with an oval shape, thin capsule, hypoechoic periphery and echogenic center. Breast fat is isoechoic or of medium echogenicity; however, the fat in the hilum of the node is hyperechoic, likely related to the numerous lymphatic channels within the mediastinum (mid portion) of the lymph node. Intramammary lymph nodes are often found in the upper outer quadrants of the breast and in the mid-axillary line. In thin patients they can be palpable. The majority of lymph nodes can be easily distinguished by their characteristic mammographic and sonographic appearance, and no further

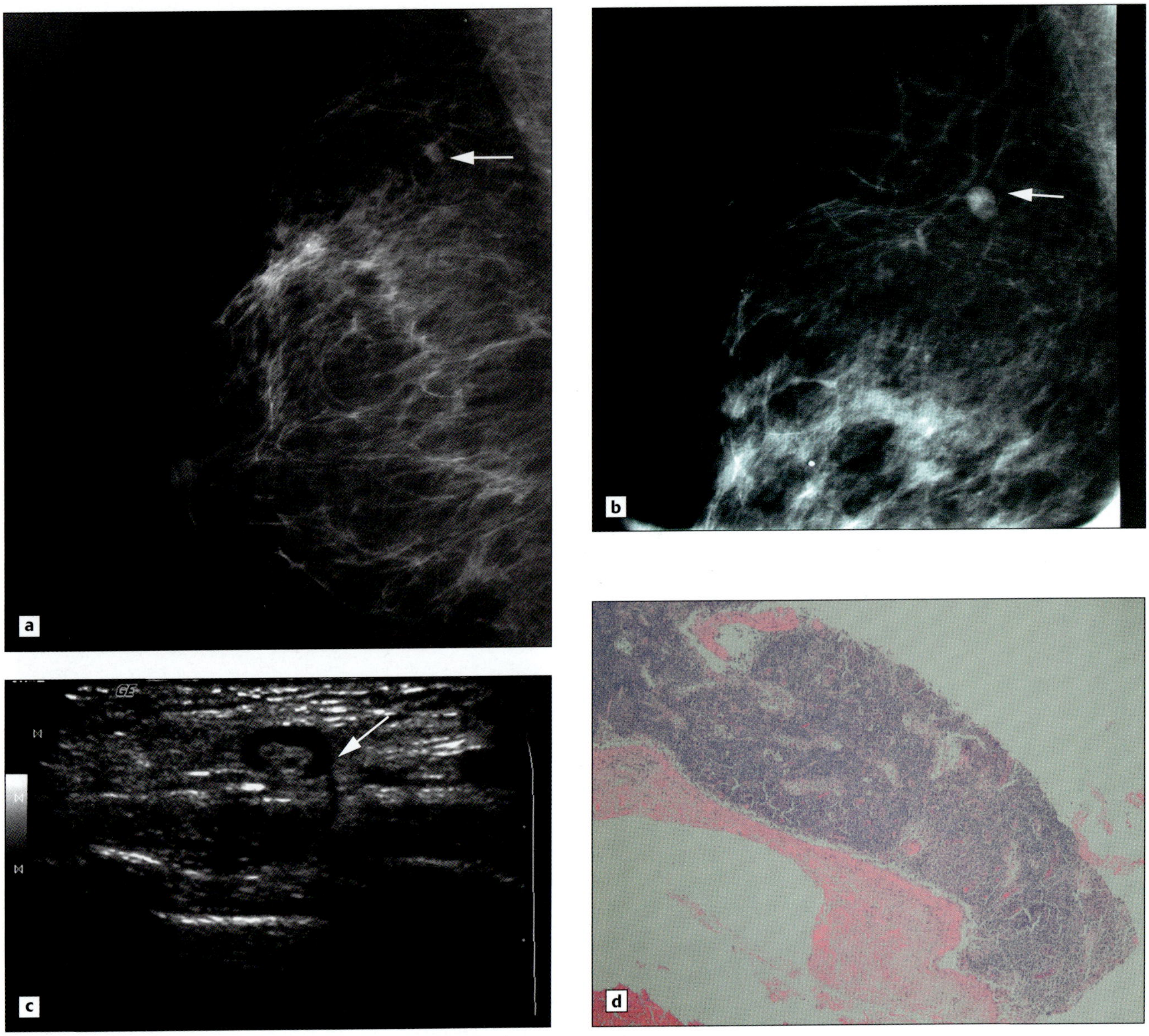

FIGURE 3.7 Intramammary lymph node. **(a)** Mammogram reveals an oval well circumscribed nodule with a fatty cleft (arrow), representing the fatty hilum. **(b)** This is best seen (arrow) on the compression view. **(c)** On sonography the nodule is well circumscribed and oval with a hypoechoic rim (arrow) and an echogenic central fatty hilum. **(d)** Core biopsy reveals normal lymphoid tissue maintained within a fibrous capsule.

intervention is necessary unless they are detected in a patient with a known ipsilateral invasive carcinoma in which case they should be excised because they may represent the "sentinel" lymph nodes and harbor metastatic disease. Core biopsy histology is typically straightforward, although the distinction from malignant lymphoma can be difficult (Fig. 3.8). Low grade malignant lymphoma should be suspected when lymphocytes extend beyond the capsule into surrounding adipose tissue (see also chap. 6). Such cases can be resolved via the use of immunohistochemistry.

Finally, as noted in the previous chapter, fibroadenomata can occasionally contain large amounts of fat and thus may appear radiographically similar to hamartoma. Histologically on core biopsy the typical compressed glandular pattern of fibroadenoma will be retained, albeit amidst a mixture of fibrous and adipose tissue (see Fig. 2.12).

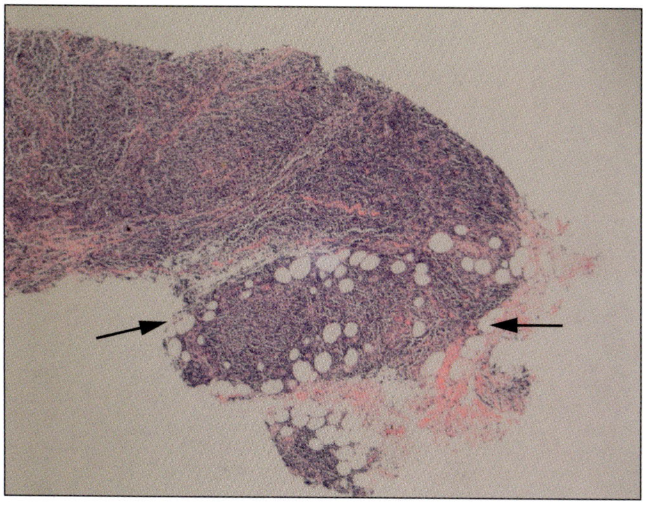

FIGURE 3.8 Malignant lymphoma, follicular small cleaved cell type. Core biopsy reveals a histology similar to that of intramammary lymph node (see Fig. 3.7d) with the exception of lymphocytes directly infiltrating through the fibrous capsule (arrows) into surrounding fatty breast tissue; such an appearance is not specific but should raise the possibility of low grade malignant lymphoma, a diagnosis which can be ruled out via the use of immunohistochemistry.

Differential diagnoses of low radiologic suspicion well-circumscribed solid lesions with heterogeneous radiodensity

- Hamartoma
- Myoid hamartoma
- Benign breast tissue (missed lesion?)
- Fibroadenoma containing fat
- Intramammary lymph node
- Nodular pseudoangiomatous stromal hyperplasia (PASH)

POINTS TO REMEMBER

1. Hamartoma should be suspected with core biopsies showing benign breast tissue.
2. An invasive lobular diagnosis in a well-circumscribed mass should be viewed with great suspicion and may in fact represent epithelioid cells in a myoid hamartoma.
3. Specific benign diagnoses help to confirm accurate sampling of the lesion.

REFERENCES

1. Abbitt PL, de Paredes ES, Sloop FB Jr. Breast hamartoma: a mammographic diagnosis. South Med J 81:167–170,1988.
2. Daya D, Trus T, D'Souza TJ, et al. Hamartoma of the breast, an under recognized breast lesion. A clinicopathologic and radiographic study of 25 cases. Am J Clin Pathol 103:685–689,1995.
3. Paraskevopoulos JA, Hosking SW, Stephenson T. Breast within a breast: A review of breast hamartomas. Br J Clin Pract 44:30–32,1990.
4. Fisher CJ, Hanby AM, Robinson L, Millis RR. Mammary hamartoma-a review of 35 cases. Histopathology 20:99–106,1992.
5. Powell CM, Cranor ML, Rosen PP. Pseudoangiomatous stromal hyperplasia (PASH). A mammary stromal tumor with myofibroblastic differentiation. Am J Surg Pathol 19:270–277,1995.
6. Salvador R, Lirola JL, Dominguez R, et al. Pseudo-angiomatous stromal hyperplasia presenting as a breast mass: imaging findings in three patients. Breast 13:431–435,2004.
7. Garfein CF, Aulicino MR, Leytin A, et al. Epithelioid cells in myoid hamartoma of the breast. A potential diagnostic pitfall for core biopsies. Arch Pathol Lab Med 120:676–680,1996.

CHAPTER

4 Largely cystic lesions

Cysts appear mammographically as well-circumscribed oval to round masses and cannot be distinguished from solid masses on mammography alone. They are often multiple and bilateral, and the definitive diagnosis of a cyst is made on ultrasound when a lesion meets specific criteria:

- round to oval in shape;
- good posterior through transmission of the sound wave;
- thin posterior wall; and
- completely anechoic.

If all of these criteria are met, then the accuracy of the diagnosis is 100%.

When a mass meets the specific criteria of a simple cyst no further intervention is necessary unless the cyst interferes with clinical examination or is the source of a patient's discomfort. If a cyst is not under tension, pressure applied with the ultrasound transducer usually can alter its shape; this is a finding not typically seen with solid masses (Fig. 4.1). When any of the above criteria are not fulfilled, the lesion is termed a complex cyst and aspiration is recommended. If the lesion does not completely collapse upon aspiration, then the procedure is converted to an ultrasound-guided core biopsy. Internal echoes often may be diffuse and low level and may signify old blood or mucus within the lesion. Complex cysts may have irregular anechoic portions, septa, mural nodularity and papillary projections (Fig. 4.2). Aspiration of the lesion and complete collapse support a benign etiology (Fig. 4.3). At present, we submit all cyst aspirates for cytological evaluation. If the cells are atypical or suggest malignancy, large gauge core biopsy or surgical biopsy may be performed. Any bloody cyst aspirate or evacuated material must be analyzed by cytology. Breast cysts are most common in women in the perimenopausal years. After menopause cysts typically decrease in size and disappear; however, they may reaccumulate with hormone replacement therapy.

The percentage of cysts that are seen as "complex" under ultrasound is increasing. This may be related to better resolution with higher frequency transducers with broader bandwidth and higher dynamic range. Those that truly contain internal debris are a result of proteinaceous material, cholesterol crystals, foamy macrophages, sloughed apocrine epithelial cells or white and red blood cells. The radiologist should identify and biopsy those with thick or irregular septations, mural nodules, a central fibrovascular stalk.[1]

Most mural nodules seen sonographically are related to papillary apocrine metaplasia (Fig. 4.4). In rare cases, carcinoma or papillomas are the causes of internal echoes seen with the cyst. Stavros[2] has identified certain sonographic features which raise suspicion, including solid internal echoes that demonstrate angular margins at the point of attachment to the cyst wall. Other worrisome features include the loss of the capsule where there is an attachment to the wall or protrusion beyond the oval-round shape, or a fibrovascular stalk as seen on color Doppler, or non-mobile echoes.

When assessing the histology of a core biopsy of a cystic lesion it is useful to consider the mechanics of what is occurring during the biopsy procedure. When one biopsies a cystic lesion, assuming that the contents of the cyst is fluid, the solid tissue that is removed will by necessity be that which surrounds the cyst. The inner lining of the cyst walls will therefore be represented by the tissue on the edge of the biopsy cylinders, either on their long edges or on either tip of the cylinder (Fig. 4.5). Thus one will typically see apocrine metaplasia or foamy histiocytes lining edges of the cylinders (Fig. 4.6). Along with an awareness of the lesion's clinical shrinkage or disappearance, one can confidently and specifically diagnose a cyst rather than write a nonspecific diagnosis such as fibrocystic changes.

The vast majority of cysts in the breast are benign and are lined by apocrine metaplasia. In fact one of our most specific markers of breast differentiation, gross cystic disease fluid protein-15 (GCDFP-15) is derived from cyst fluid and is expressed strongly and most frequently by apocrine cells.[3] Apocrine metaplasia frequently assumes a papillary configuration and often corresponds to the solid component of a complex cyst (Fig. 4.4). The apocrine cells (or papillae formed by them) line the edge of the individual cores along their length or at their tips. While there is abundant eosinophilic cytoplasm, slight nuclear variability, and prominent nucleoli, the nuclear/

Text continued on p. 42

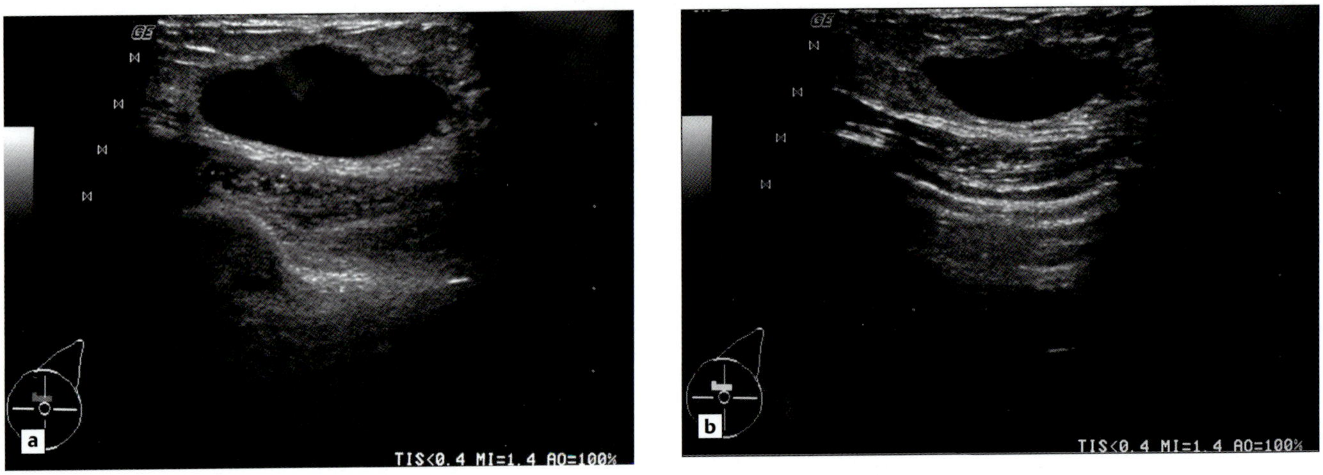

FIGURE 4.1 Sonography showing a simple cyst **(a)** which changes shape with compression **(b)**.

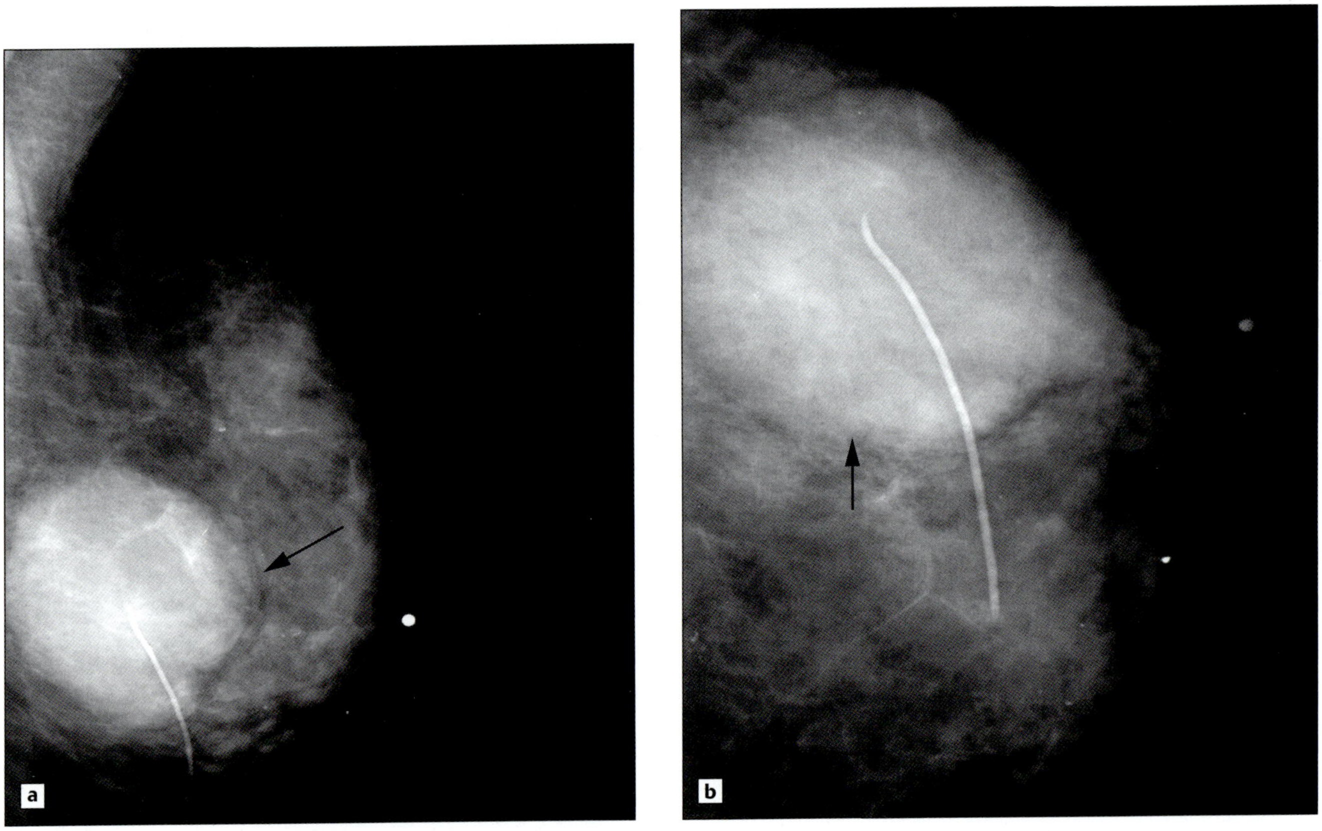

FIGURE 4.2 Complex cyst. **(a,b)** On mammography there is a large intermediate density mass in lateral breast. The lesion is well circumscribed (arrows) and palpable.

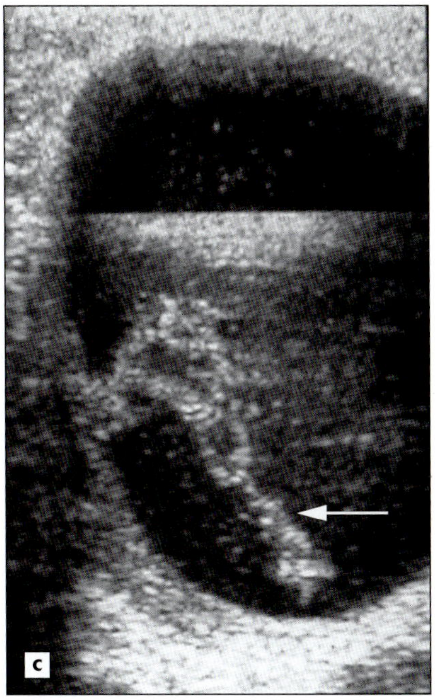

FIGURE 4.2—cont'd (c) Sonography demonstrates a predominantly fluid filled mass with a few thin linear and papillary-like projections (arrow). There is good posterior enhancement.

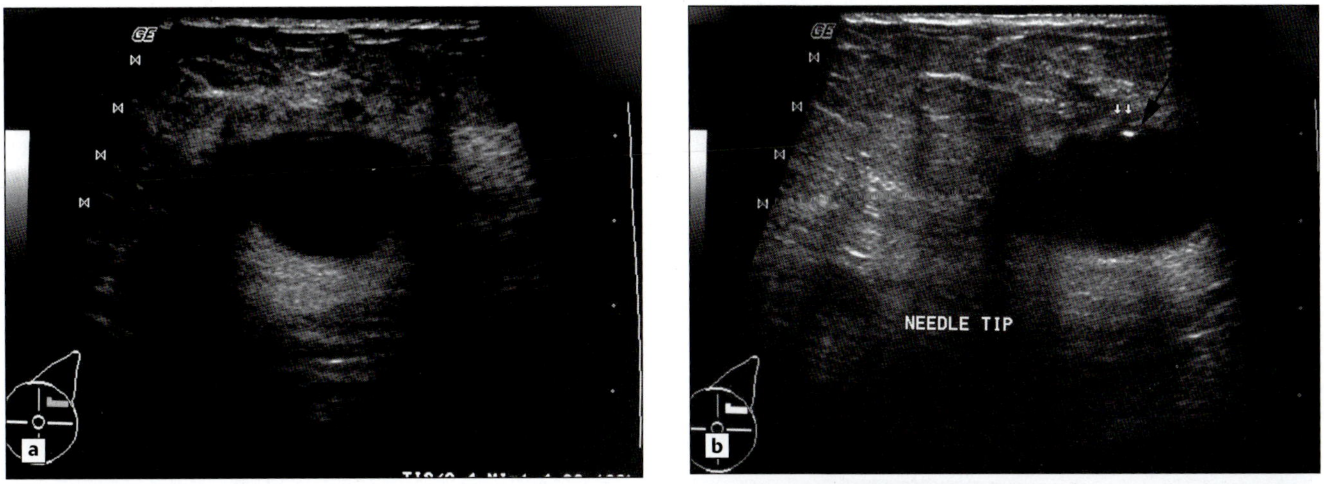

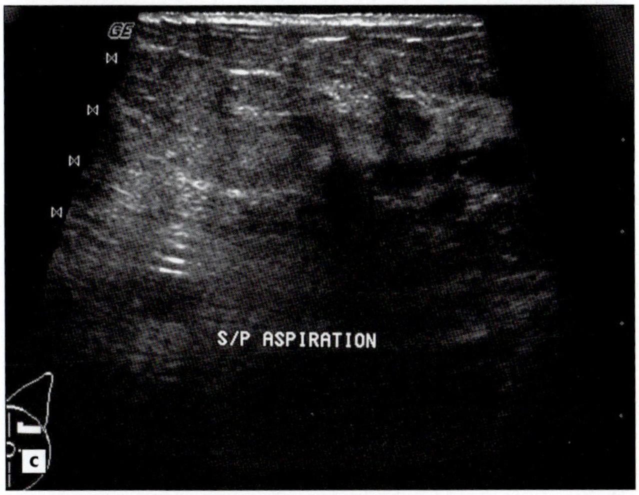

FIGURE 4.3 Aspiration of a cyst. A typical cyst **(a)** is aspirated **(b)** under sonographic control (note the needle tip in the lesion signified by the arrows). **(c)** The cyst has collapsed and is no longer visible after aspiration.

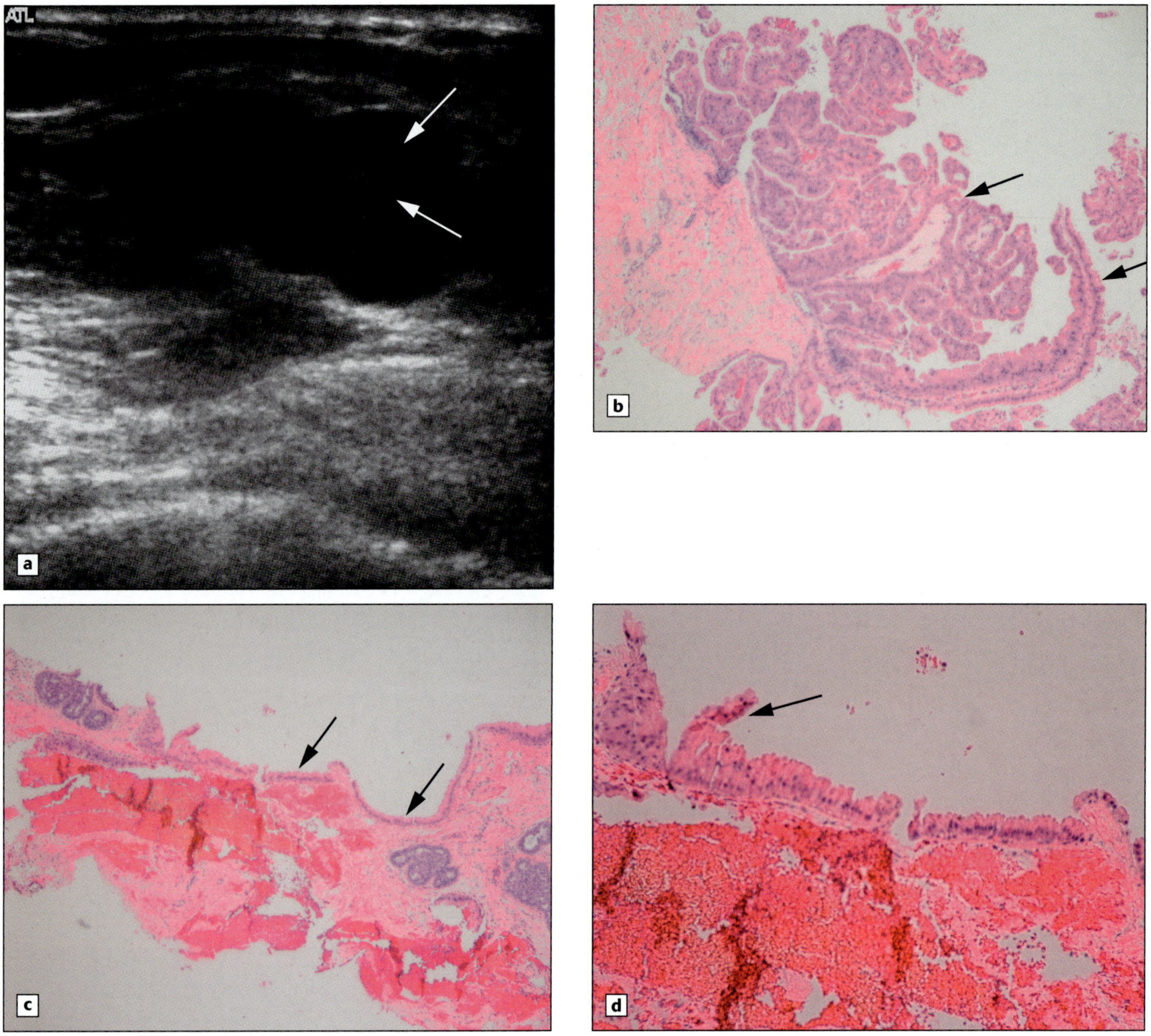

FIGURE 4.4 Cystic papillary apocrine metaplasia. **(a)** Complex cystic and solid, well-circumscribed mass, the anechoic component representing fluid and the hypoechoic component representing the solid portion (arrows). The solid component is nodular and heterogeneous. **(b)** Core biopsy reveals large cells with brightly eosinophilic cytoplasm (apocrine metaplasia) arranged around thin fibrovascular cores (arrows). While this arrangement of cells is papillary by definition, such lesions are unrelated to intraductal papilloma. **(c,d)** Higher power showing apocrine cells lining the core cylinder (arrows) and piling up in micropapillary configurations (arrow) without fibrovascular cores.

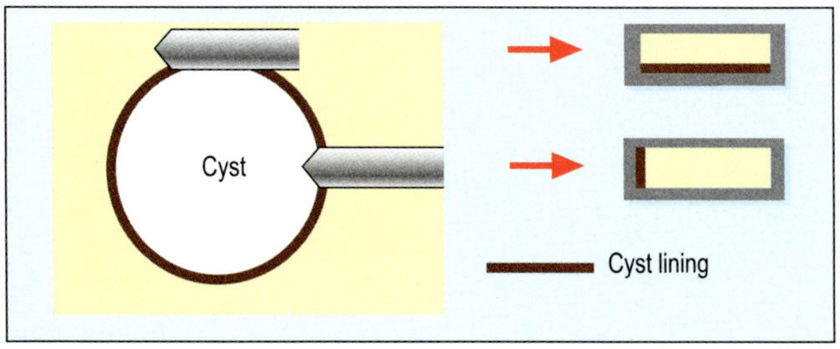

FIGURE 4.5 Cyst wall core biopsy.

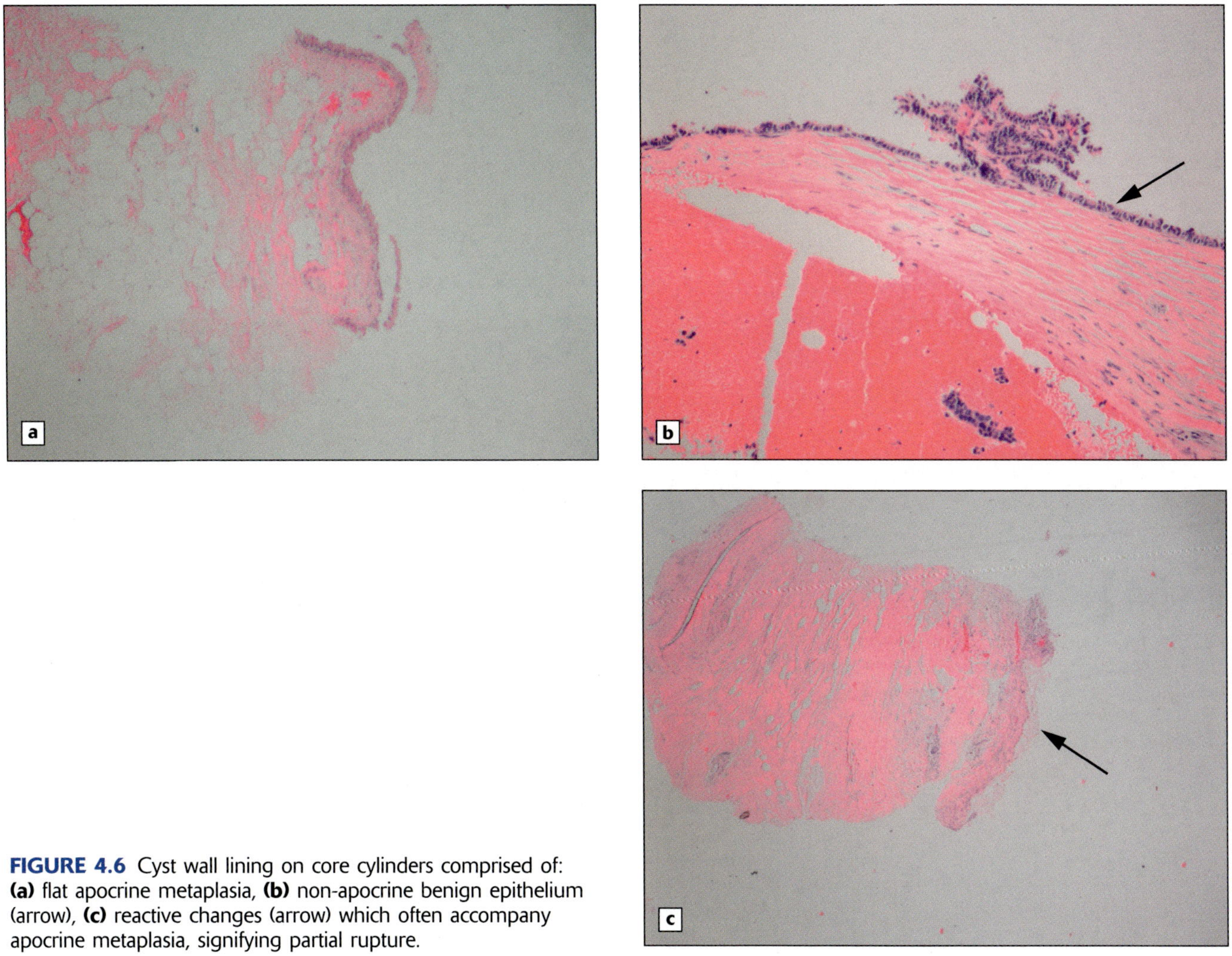

FIGURE 4.6 Cyst wall lining on core cylinders comprised of: **(a)** flat apocrine metaplasia, **(b)** non-apocrine benign epithelium (arrow), **(c)** reactive changes (arrow) which often accompany apocrine metaplasia, signifying partial rupture.

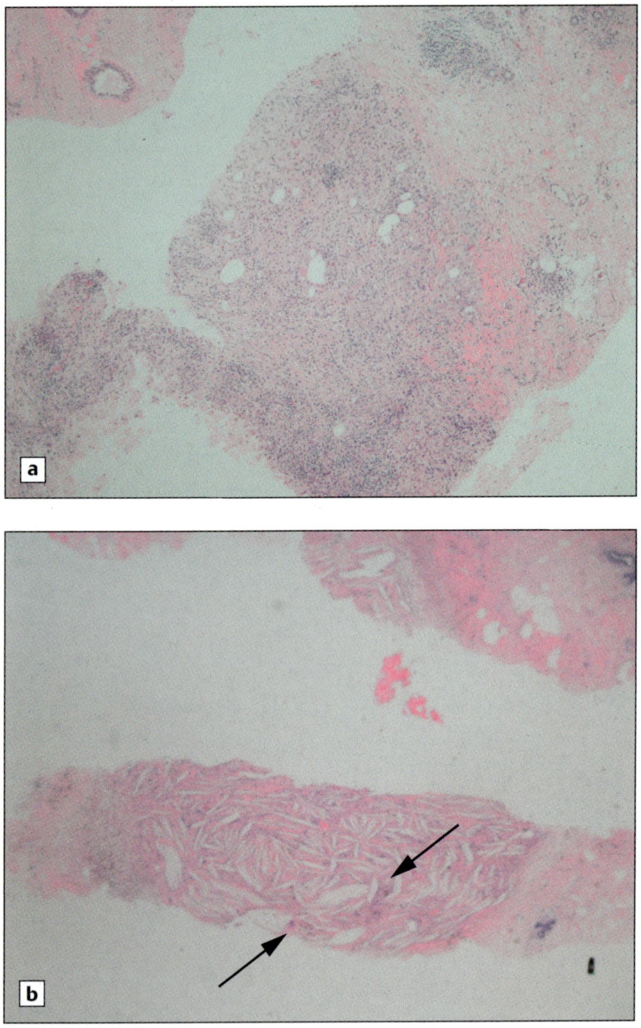

FIGURE 4.7 Cyst wall histology. **(a)** Mixed chronic inflammation: lymphocytes and histiocytes adjacent to a cyst lining (lower aspect) comprised of histiocytes. **(b)** The wall of the cyst may also show solid areas of foreign body reaction (arrows) to lipid appearing histologically as cholesterol clefts.

cytoplasmic ratios are maintained, and there is not nearly the pleomorphism required to consider a malignant diagnosis.

It is not uncommon for cysts to fluctuate in size and to spontaneously rupture, perhaps repeatedly. Thus, it is also not unusual to see reactive changes such as chronic inflammation, a foreign body reaction, and a hyalinized wall (Fig. 4.7a). The solid component of a sonographic cyst may thus also correspond to exuberant reactive changes with a solid foreign body reaction usually containing cholesterol clefts, or simply to cyst contents or debris (Fig. 4.7b). Similarly cysts may be lined by foamy histiocytic appearing cells that also appear in surrounding breast tissue. This histology is caused by leakage of duct contents and may aptly be called cystic duct ectasia (Fig. 4.8). Fat necrosis may also develop a cystic component, often with a hyalinizing and calcifying wall (Fig. 4.9). Finally a tiny intraductal papilloma can form the solid portion of a cyst (see Chap. 5 for a more extensive discussion of papillary lesions).

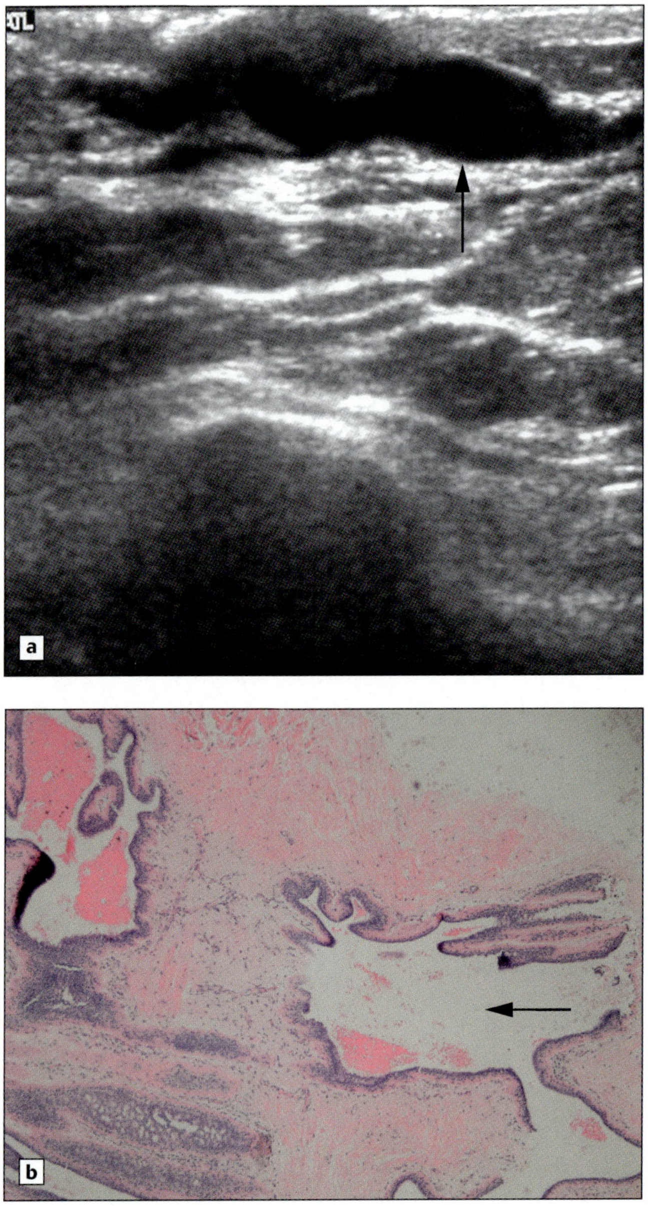

FIGURE 4.8 Cystic duct ectasia. **(a)** Sonography shows dilated ectatic retroareolar ducts (arrow) without an intraductal lesion. **(b)** Core biopsy shows cystically dilated ducts (arrow) which,

The contents of the cysts, if partially solid, will often be evident histologically as separate loose fragments of tissue, sometimes foreign body giant cells with

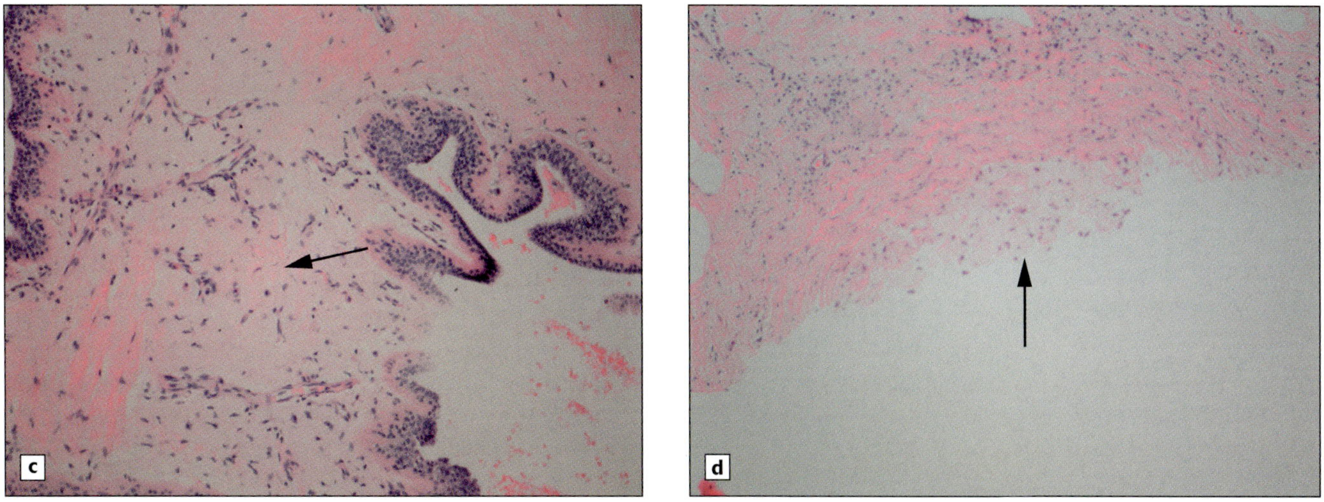

FIGURE 4.8—cont'd (c) at higher power have foamy histiocytes (arrow) in their walls. **(d)** Another area shows foamy histiocytes (arrow) lining the cyst wall at the end of the core cylinder and adjacent chronic inflammation in surrounding breast tissue (ruptured duct).

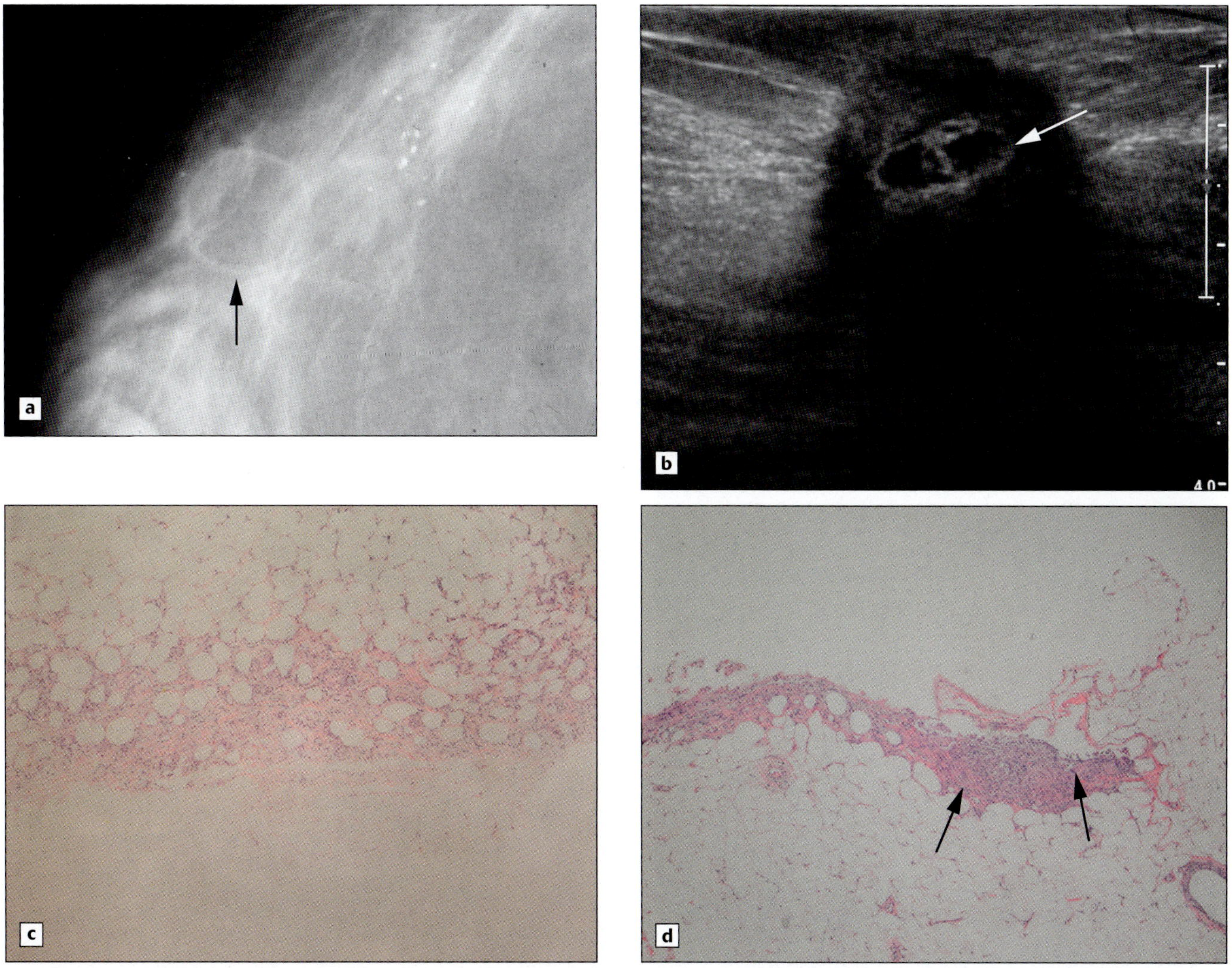

FIGURE 4.9 Cystic fat necrosis. **(a)** Mammography demonstrates a mass with rim-like (eggshell) calcifications (arrow) and a lucent center. This was found adjacent to a prior surgical site. **(b)** Sonography of the lumpectomy bed approximately 3 years post resection of an infiltrating carcinoma demonstrates a ring-like, smoothly marginated mass (arrow) with central cystification. **(c)** Core biopsy reveals a fibrous cyst wall lining and variably sized lipid-laden macrophages in surrounding tissue and **(d)** foreign body giant cells (arrows).

cholesterol clefts. On rare occasions we have also seen squamous metaplasia lining cysts, always accompanying significant reactive changes (Fig. 4.10), often associated with intraductal papilloma. Cystic lesions may also occur during pregnancy or lactation and may represent galactoceles; however, these can be confidently diagnosed on mammography alone by the demonstration of a layering effect between fat and fluid levels on special views.

Malignancy involving a breast cyst[4] is an extremely rare phenomenon and generally may occur in one of three scenarios:

1. intracystic papillary carcinoma;
2. invasive poorly differentiated duct carcinoma with extensive necrosis and cystification; or
3. intraductal carcinoma secondarily involving an adjacent cyst (Fig. 4.11).

The last would be by far the most infrequently encountered situation.

The differential diagnosis in this group of lesions also includes malignant lymphoma and acute or organizing abscesses. Lymphoma can mimic a cyst on ultrasound because of the uniformity of its cell population (Fig. 4.12); lymphoma clearly can be suspected on core biopsy alone, but usually requires surgical excision for definitive diagnosis with immunohistochemically based subtyping. Abscesses, which can have secondary necrosis causing a sonographic cystic appearance, are typically but not exclusively associated with pregnancy (Fig. 4.13).

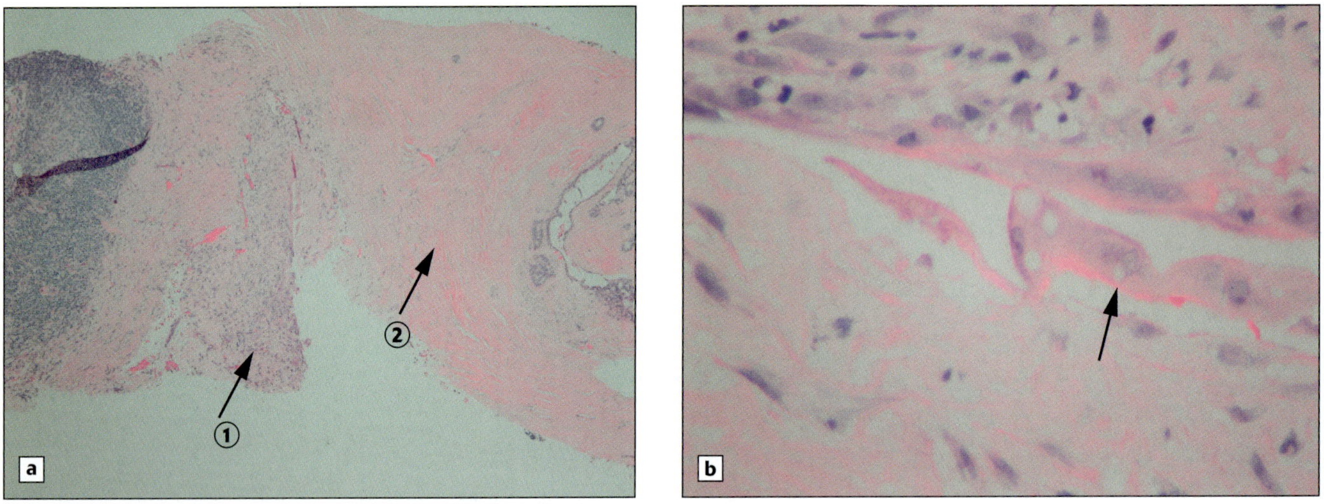

FIGURE 4.10 Reactive cyst wall lining. **(a)** Cyst wall composed of chronic inflammation (arrow 1) and dense fibrosis (arrow 2). A tiny intraductal papilloma is present at the right. **(b)** Higher power reveals that the lining is composed of benign squamous cells (arrow), so-called squamous metaplasia.

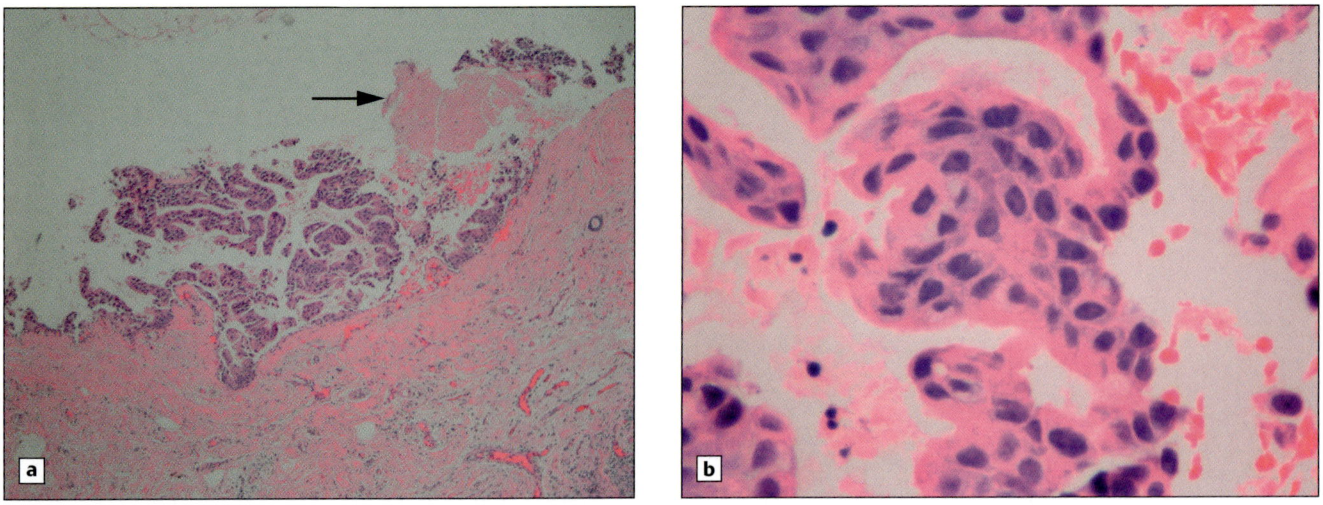

FIGURE 4.11 Malignancy in a cyst. **(a)** A monotonous population of cells lines a cyst wall at the edge of a core, accompanied by necrosis (arrow). **(b)** Higher power view reveals intermediate grade nuclear pleomorphism with prominent nucleoli. Excision of this lesion revealed intraductal carcinoma in tissue surrounding the biopsy site and incomplete involvement of the cyst by tumor.

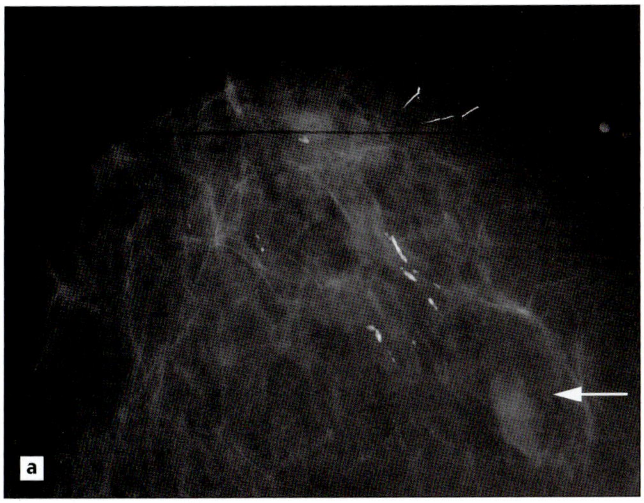

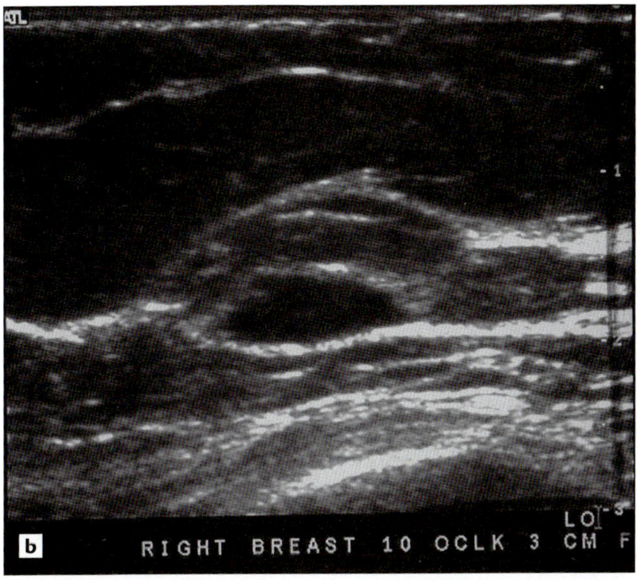

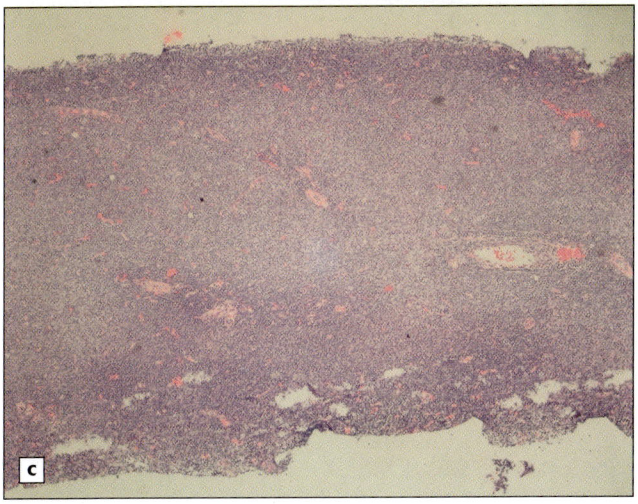

FIGURE 4.12 Malignant lymphoma. **(a)** MLO view demonstrates a new ill defined intermediate density mass (arrow) in the upper outer quadrant. **(b)** Sonography demonstrates an oval markedly hypoechoic-anechoic, homogeneous, smoothly marginated solid mass. No significant shadowing or through transmission. **(c)** Core biopsy reveals a monotonous lymphoid cell population proven to be small lymphocytic lymphoma by immunohistochemical stains. The patient was subsequently found to have chronic lymphocytic leukemia.

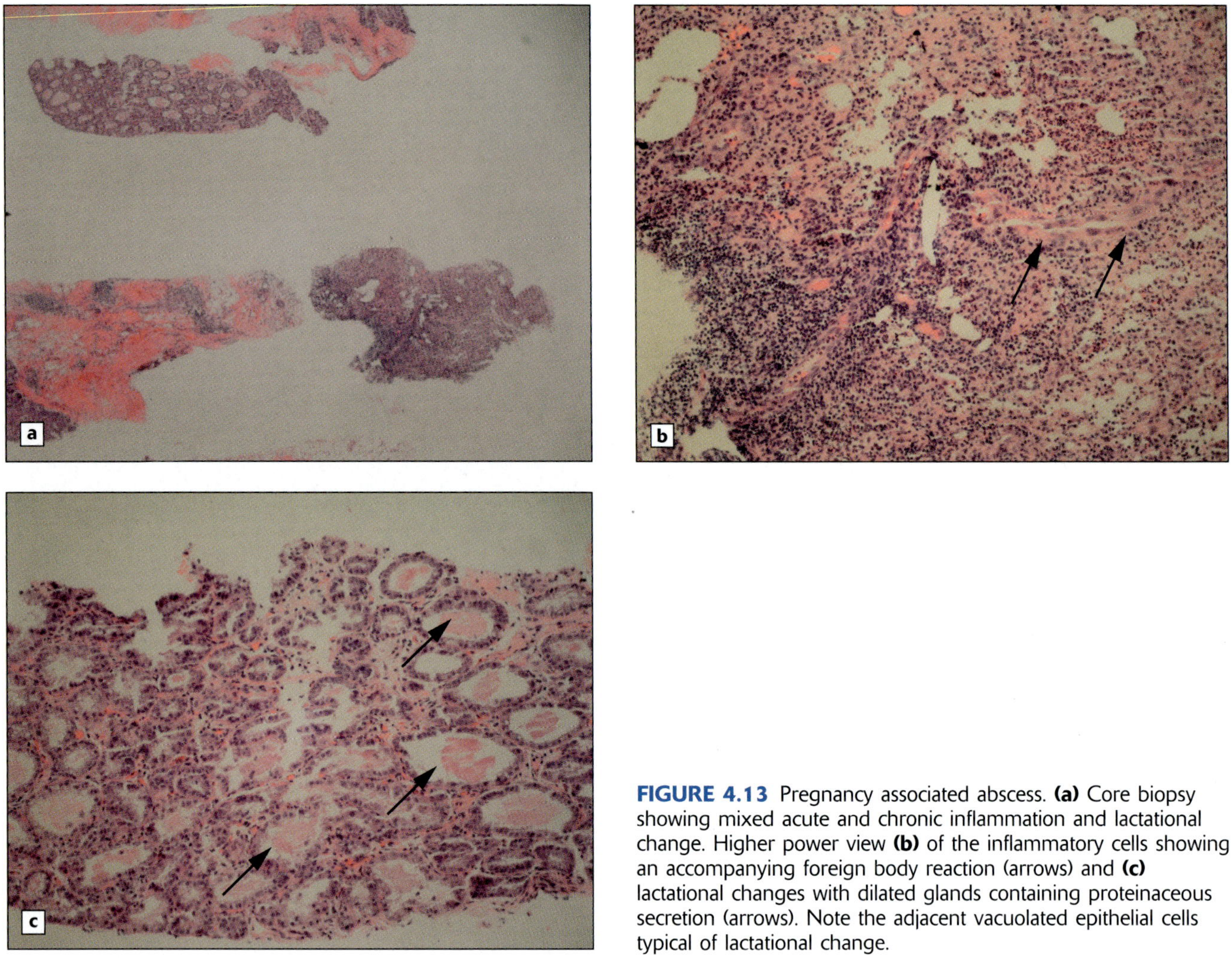

FIGURE 4.13 Pregnancy associated abscess. **(a)** Core biopsy showing mixed acute and chronic inflammation and lactational change. Higher power view **(b)** of the inflammatory cells showing an accompanying foreign body reaction (arrows) and **(c)** lactational changes with dilated glands containing proteinaceous secretion (arrows). Note the adjacent vacuolated epithelial cells typical of lactational change.

Differential diagnosis of largely cystic lesions

- Apocrine metaplasia lined cyst
- Cystic duct ectasia
- Cyst with tiny intraductal papilloma
- Galactocele

POINTS TO REMEMBER

1. Cysts that disappear and do not recur are benign.
2. Cyst wall linings will be apparent on the edges of core cylinders and usually show apocrine metaplasia or duct ectasia.
3. Solid components may be debris, reactive changes, or papillary apocrine metaplasia.
4. Malignancy involving a cyst is possible but rare.

REFERENCES

1. Berg WA, Campassi CI, Ioffe OB. Cystic lesions of the breast: sonographic-pathologic correlation. Radiology 227:183–191,2003.
2. Stavros AT. Unpublished data.
3. Wick MR, Lillemoe TJ, Copland GT, et al. Gross cystic disease fluid protein-15 as a marker for breast cancer: immunohistochemical analysis of 690 human neoplasms and comparison with alpha-lactalbumin. Hum Pathol 20:281–287,1989.
4. Bleiweiss IJ, Schwartz IS, Mizrachy B, Kaneko M. Infiltrating cystic carcinoma of the breast: An unusual variant of breast cancer. Breast Dis 2:87–89,1989.

CHAPTER 5

Partially solid, partially cystic lesions

Spontaneous, unilateral bloody or serous discharge from a single duct orifice should be investigated and is most commonly caused by an intraductal papilloma or carcinoma. Traditionally galactography has been utilized in the workup; however, sonography is often used and is extremely helpful if an intraductal mass is identified. Sonography may guide the core biopsy and /or wire localization of the intraductal lesion. It has become an excellent adjunct in the workup of nipple discharge. Papillomata tend to secrete fluid into the ducts, leading to distention of the distal duct orifice and thus nipple secretions. Because papillomata are soft and friable, they may fragment or even partially infarct, either of which can result in a bloody nipple discharge. Occasionally a papilloma will obstruct the distal duct and continue to secrete, causing secondary cyst formation or intracystic papilloma. When a papillary carcinoma or intraductal carcinoma involving a papilloma is the cause of bloody nipple discharge, but the lesion is small and confined to the duct, it is impossible to differentiate a true papilloma from carcinoma on imaging unless malignant calcifications are present. Likewise, intracystic papillary carcinomas are not easily distinguishable from benign intracystic papillomas. Invasive papillary carcinoma may be suspected if there is a bulky solid papillary-like mass within the duct which demonstrates calcifications, micro- or macrolobulation, or duct extension. An interval change from prior studies should also arouse suspicion; examples would be growth, development of irregular margins, and development of calcifications. Lobulation and duct extension, however, can also be seen in papillomas. Papillary lesions are often highly vascular and tend to demonstrate abnormal amounts of bleeding as the friable components and fibrovascular stalk are sampled.

Intraductal papilloma usually occurs in the retroareolar region and is the most common cause of a serous or serosanguineous nipple discharge. Usually the lesion is no greater than a few millimeters and may show slight bulging of the retroareolar ducts on mammography. Papillomas appear mammographically as well-circumscribed, solid, round to oval masses that may cause dilatation of the adjacent duct or ductal system (Fig. 5.1). Mammography cannot reliably distinguish benign from malignant papillary breast lesions,[1] but the need for intervention may be indicated by an interval increase in size of the lesion between screening exams or development of focal border irregularity (Fig. 5.2) or development of associated calcifications within the lesion (Fig. 5.3). This may indicate the development of carcinoma with the lesion. Many papillomas will be suspected on the basis of ultrasound alone. Solitary papillomas are often central in location, mammographically occult, and associated with nipple discharge. Ultrasound may show a complex mass within a duct or with mural thickening and nodularity and internal and/or cystic areas.[2]

An uncomplicated intraductal papilloma can be readily diagnosed on core biopsies in which two types of cells line a variably densely fibrotic papillary structure (Fig. 5.4). In our experience other secondary histologic features associated with intraductal papilloma can also be appreciated on core biopsies and may be helpful in the diagnosis:

- Since papillary lesions commonly cause secondary cystic duct dilatation, the edges of the core cylinders will typically be lined by epithelial and myoepithelial cells in a manner analogous to that of core biopsy of simple cysts (Figs 5.1h and 5.5a).
- Since intraductal papilloma may present clinically as bloody nipple discharge, the histologic correlate of this is resorbing hemorrhage in the cyst wall and surrounding otherwise nonspecific reactive changes (Fig. 5.5b,c); significant amounts of fresh blood may also accompany the cores (Fig. 5.1i).
- Papillary lesions are friable whether they are benign or harbor malignancy; thus, detached fragments of the lesion frequently are present along with the main cores and may be seen within areas of hemorrhage (Fig. 5.1j).
- Since intraductal papillomata can spontaneously infarct, finding necrotic "ghosts" of papillary structures on core biopsies should not automatically trigger a diagnosis of malignancy (Fig. 5.5d,e).
- Collagenous spherulosis is a well-described lesion[3,4] composed of secretion of myofibrillar material in a central area surrounded by bland uniform cells in a pattern which must be distinguished from low

Text continued on p. 55

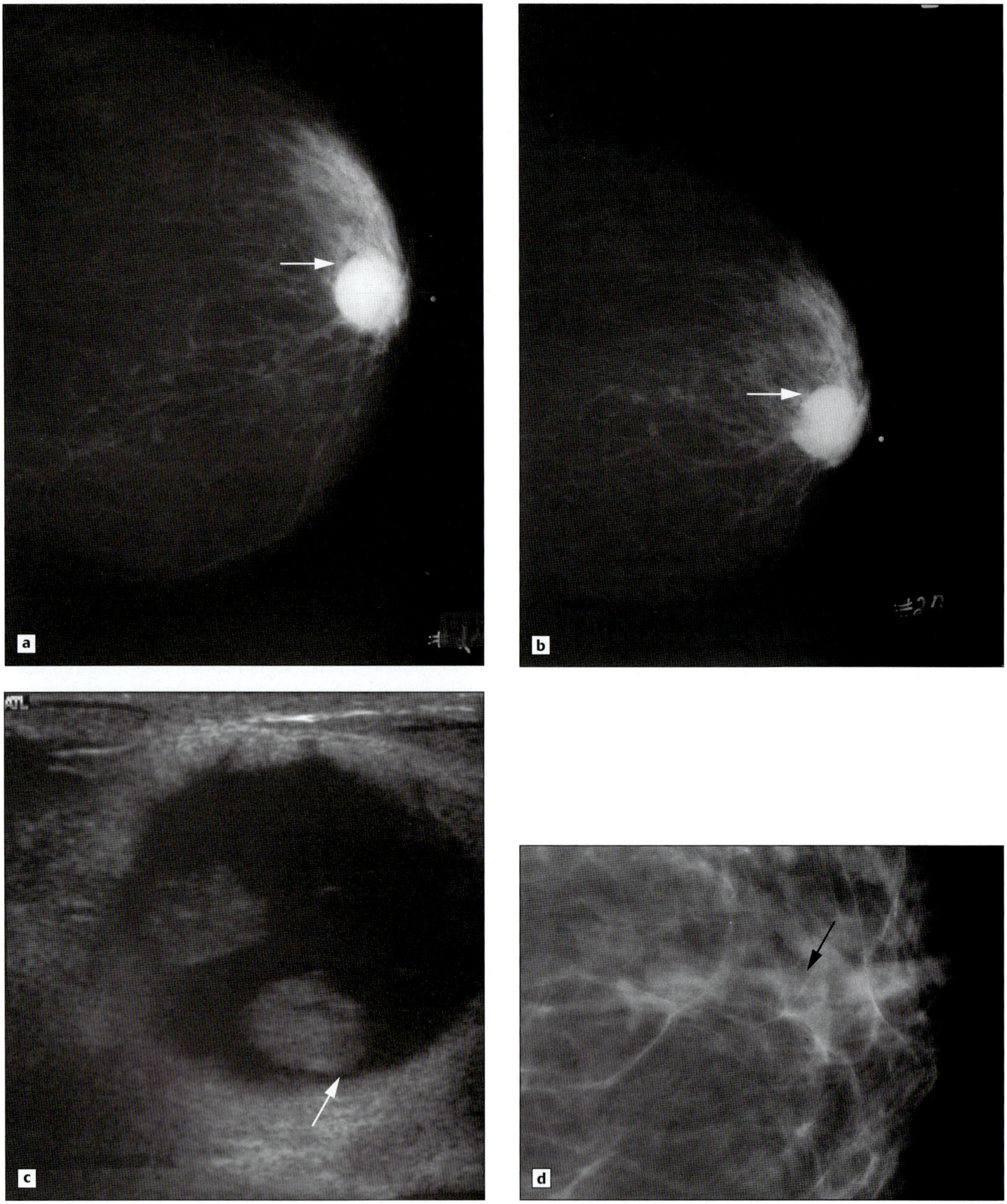

FIGURE 5.1 Two examples of imaging findings of intraductal papilloma: Case 1: **(a,b)** There has been interval development of a dense lobulated retroareolar (arrows) mass in this patient with a history of bloody nipple discharge. **(c)** Sonography demonstrates a complex cystic solid mass. There is a dilated retroareolar duct with multiple papillary internal components (arrow) adherent to the wall. Case 2: **(d)** Low magnification view of a craniocaudal mammogram demonstrates a solitary dilated, ectatic (arrow) duct in the retroareolar location.

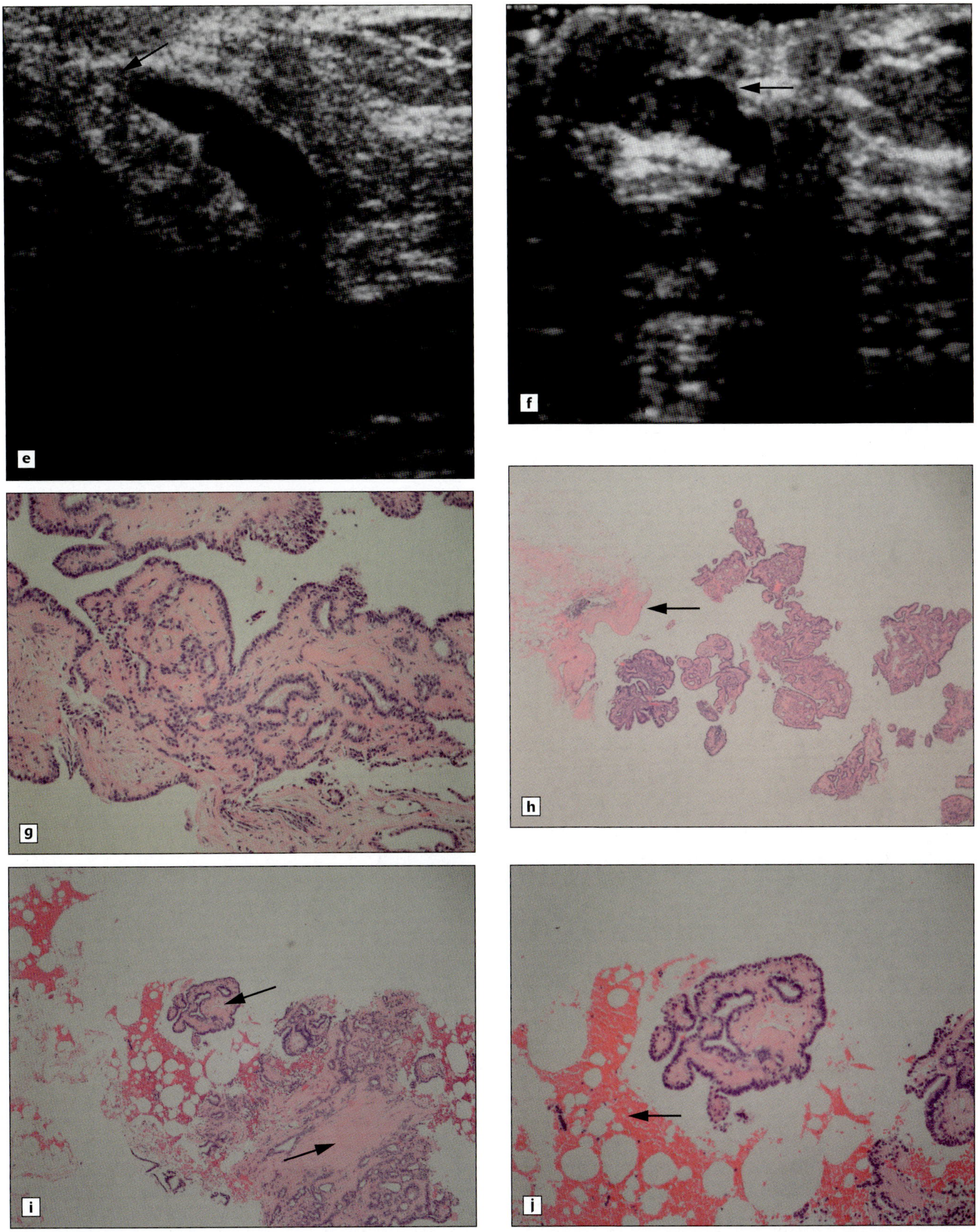

FIGURE 5.1—cont'd (e) Ultrasound demonstrates a dilated retroareolar duct with a solitary echogenic intraluminal mass (arrow). **(f)** Scanning with a standoff pad demonstrates an intraluminal echogenic mass (arrow) with a dilated, ectatic duct behind the nipple. Core biopsy of both cases showed nearly identical findings. **(g)** Benign epithelial and myoepithelial cells lining densely fibrous cores. **(h)** Note the fragmentation evident at low power and that the fragments appear to fall off the end of the core cylinder which shows a cyst wall lining (arrow). **(i)** Various degrees of hyalinization are typical of intraductal papilloma; core biopsies tend to be not only fragmented but also hemorrhagic **(j)** with loose epithelial clusters in blood (arrow) adjacent to the fragments of papilloma.

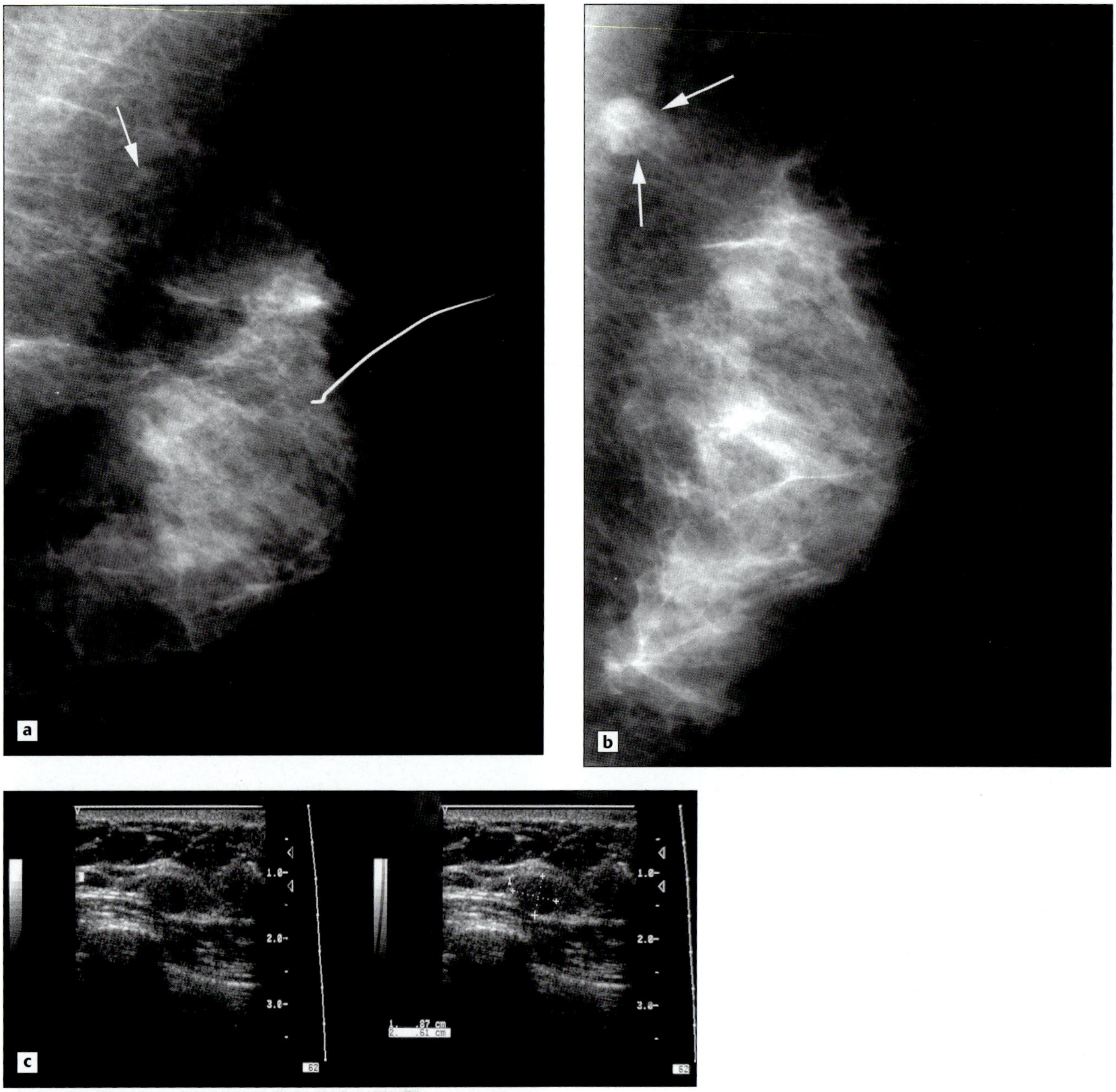

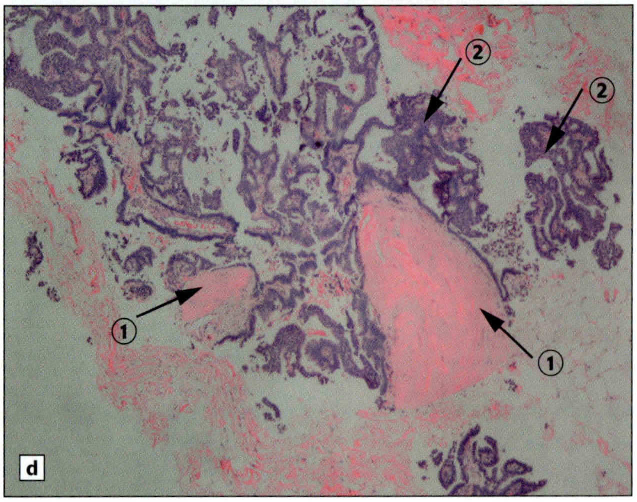

FIGURE 5.2 Intraductal carcinoma arising in intraductal papilloma. **(a)** There is a small well-circumscribed mass (arrow) in the upper outer breast that has a likely benign appearance. This was being followed at short term six month intervals. **(b)** After one year, however, this demonstrated interval increase in size and density (arrows). **(c)** Sonography demonstrates a well-circumscribed solid oval mass. **(d)** Core biopsy shows densely fibrotic papillary structures (arrows 1) lined in some areas by benign cells but additionally having a uniform epithelial proliferation with cribriform (back to back glands) architecture (arrows 2); this pattern is diagnostic for intraductal carcinoma.

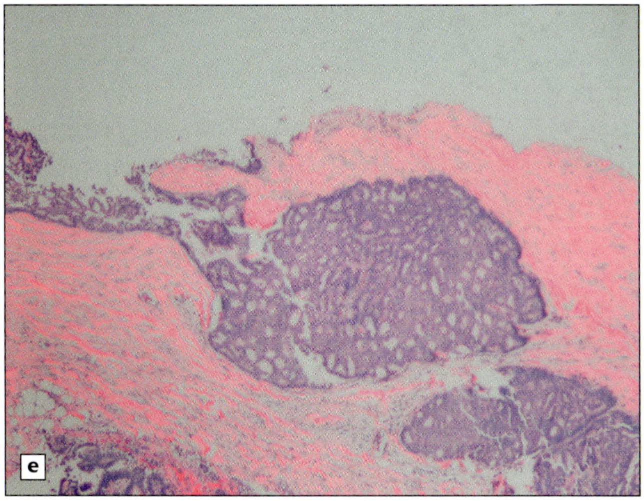

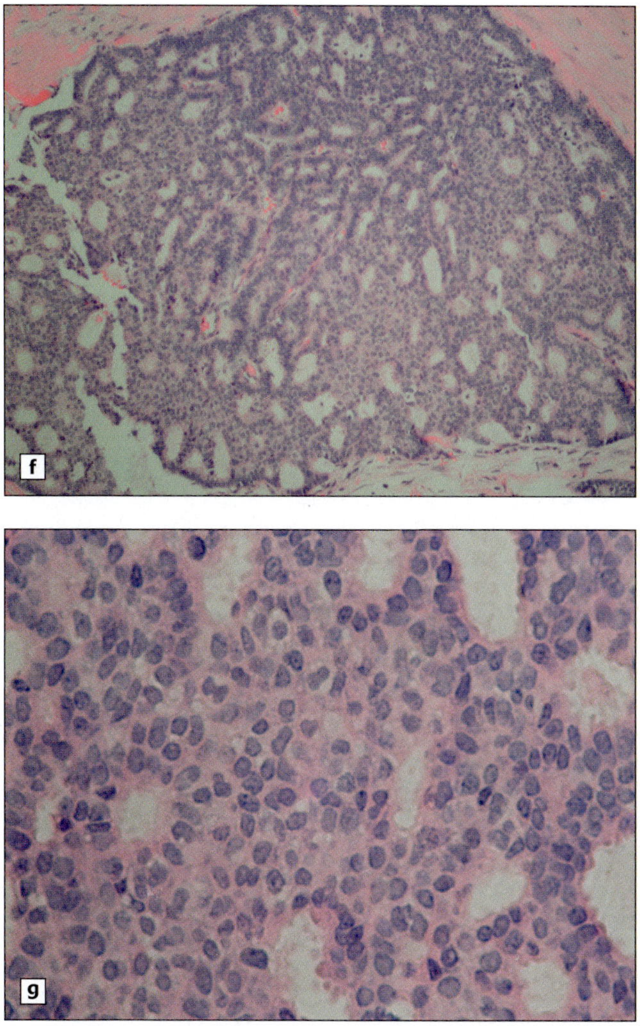

FIGURE 5.2—cont'd (e) The cribriform proliferation involves the lining of a cyst and forms round spaces which should not be misinterpreted as invasion. **(f)** At higher power the cribriform spaces are rigid, similar in size and shape, and spread rather evenly across the duct space, while **(g)** the cells show minimal nuclear pleomorphism, consistent with low grade intraductal carcinoma.

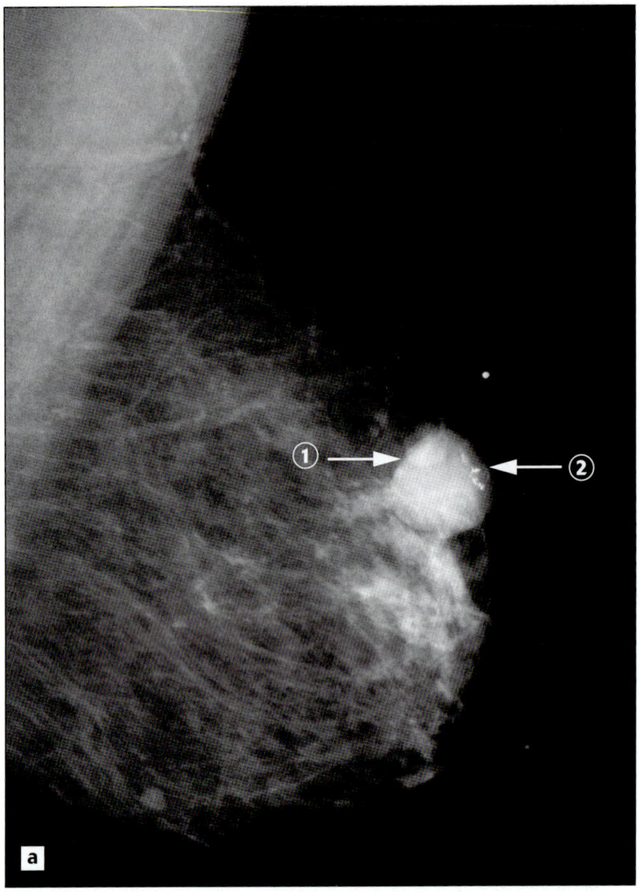

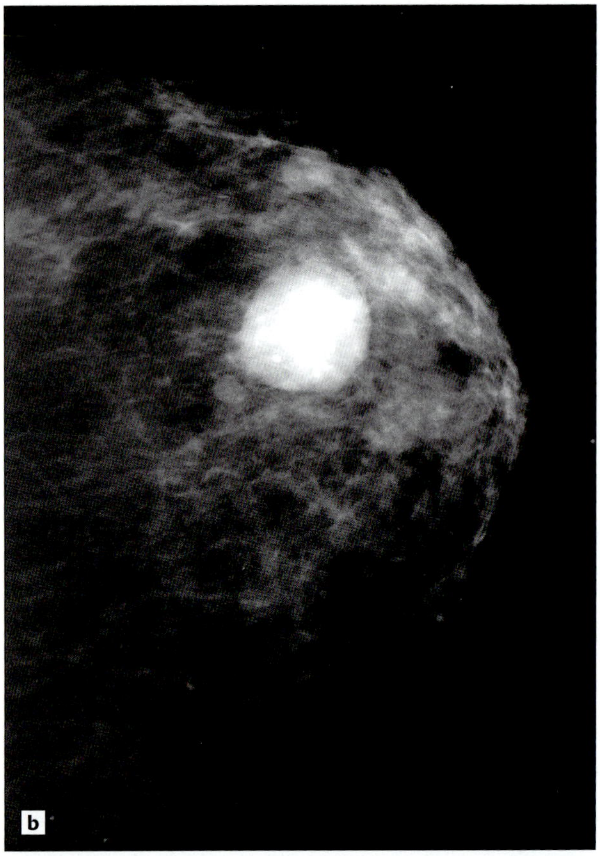

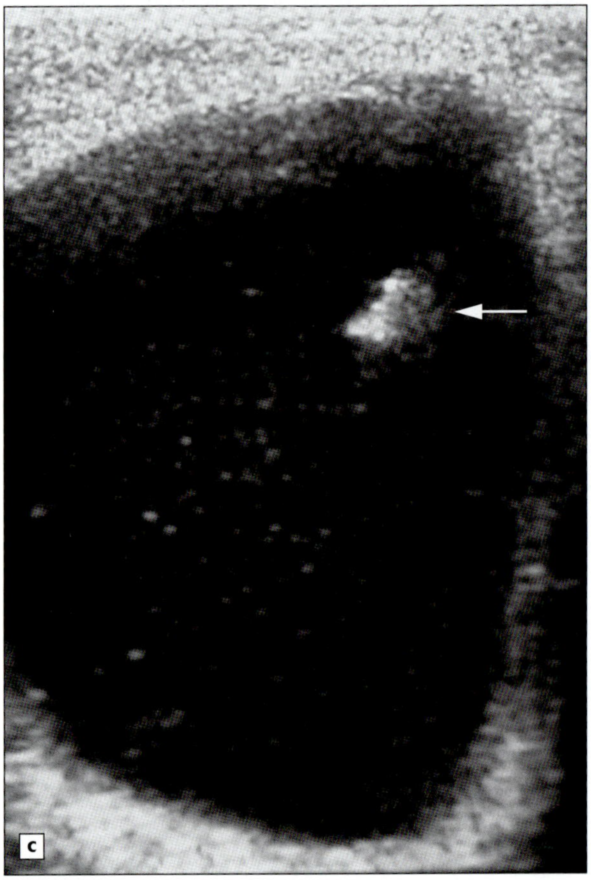

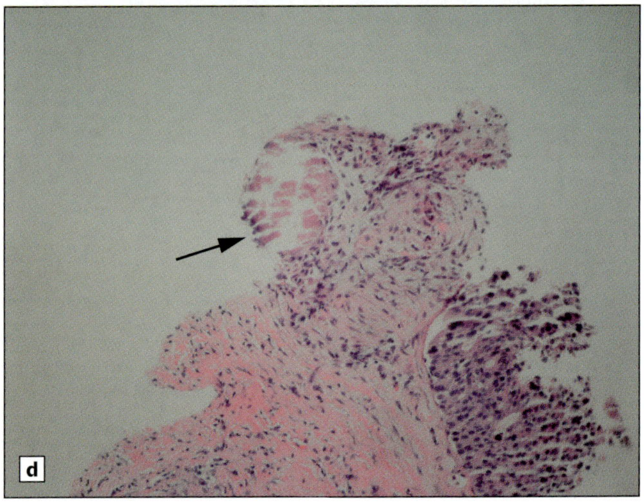

FIGURE 5.3 Intraductal carcinoma arising in intraductal papilloma. **(a,b)** Medial lateral oblique and craniocaudal views demonstrate a round dense mass (arrow 1) with associated coarse and faint calcifications (arrow 2). The need for intervention was related to the interval development of calcifications. **(c)** Sonography demonstrates a partially cystic mass with central echogenic calcification (arrow) and good posterior enhancement. **(d)** Core biopsy shows intraductal carcinoma with calcifications (arrow), lining a cyst wall at the end of the core cylinder

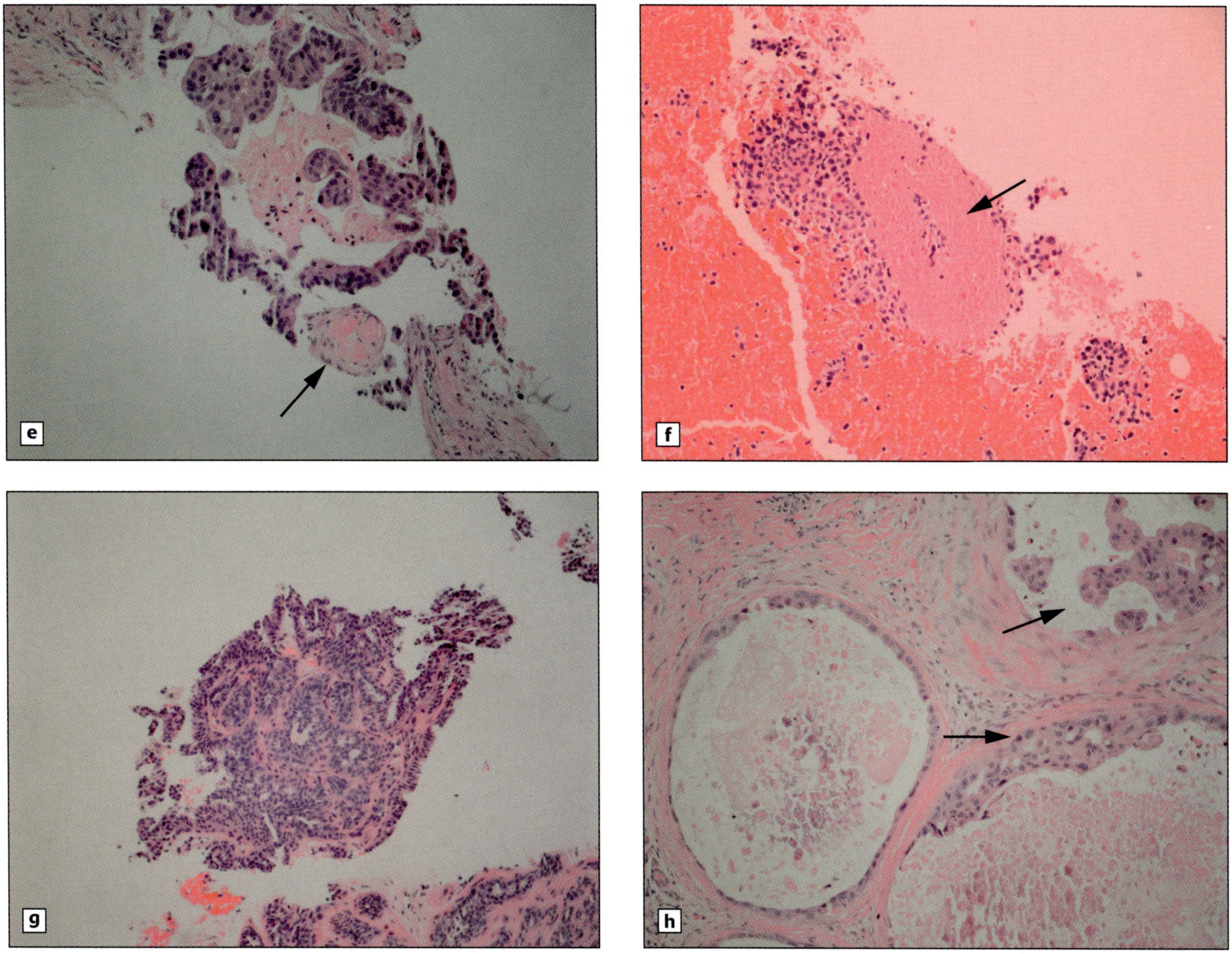

FIGURE 5.3—cont'd (e) high nuclear grade intraductal carcinoma adjacent to a tiny hyalinized focus (arrow), suggesting old intraductal papilloma. While calcification in such cases is typically associated with the carcinoma, the malignancy is often more extensive than the calcifications would mammographically suggest. Note the necrosis which, in this field, is not calcifying. **(f)** In such cases, tumor and associated calcifications with necrosis (arrow) are frequently found as loose fragments in fresh blood, an effect of the biopsy procedure. **(g)** Separate core fragments of the same lesion reveal fragments of papilloma uninvolved by carcinoma. **(h)** Excision of the lesion revealed intraductal carcinoma (arrows) in breast tissue surrounding the mass lesion, a finding which may occur, in our experience, even in excision of uncomplicated papillomas.

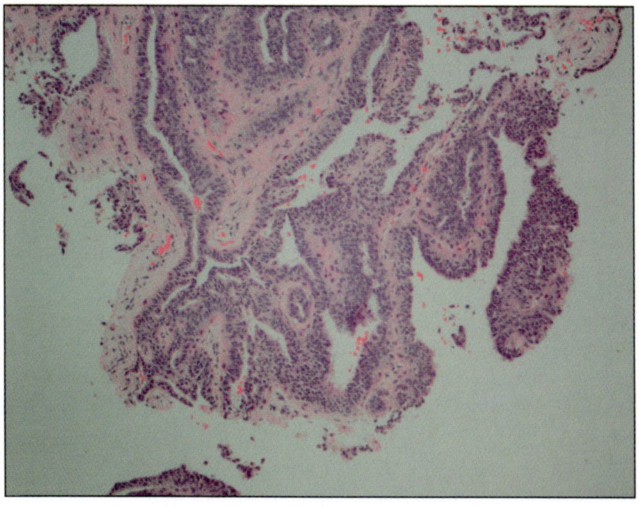

FIGURE 5.4 Uncomplicated intraductal papilloma. Intraductal papilloma is classically composed of two cell layers lining hyalinizing vascular cores.

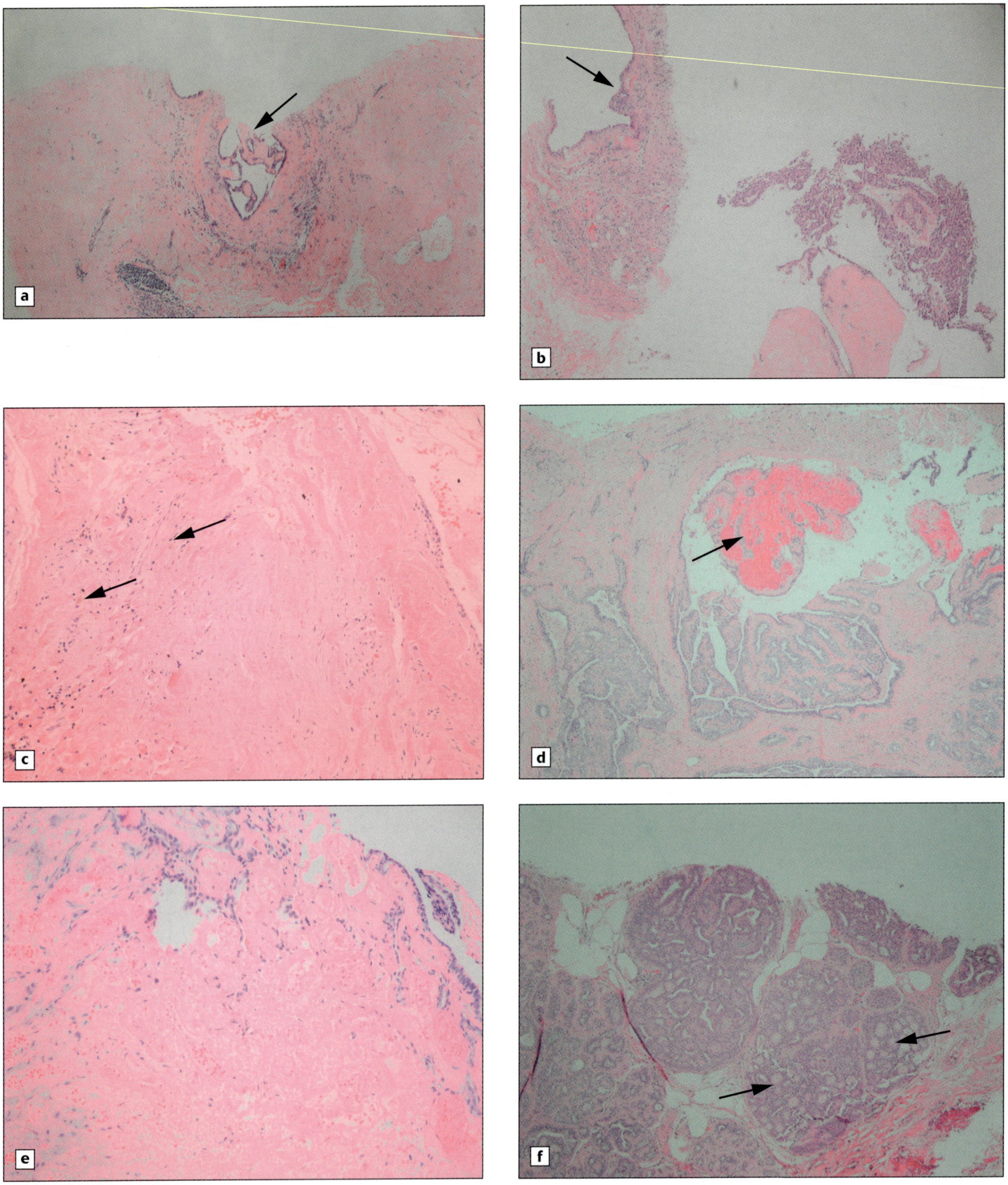

FIGURE 5.5 Additional histologic features of intraductal papilloma on core biopsy. **(a)** Note that a tiny area of papilloma (arrow) is present at the edge of the core cylinder. **(b)** While the papilloma is present at the end of this core cylinder, the adjacent core shows a cyst lining (arrow) with a histiocytic reaction in its wall. **(c)** The wall of this cystically dilated duct shows hemosiderin-laden macrophages (arrow), indicating old hemorrhage. **(d)** Hemorrhagic infarction (arrow) of part of an intraductal papilloma shows **(e)** nearly total loss of cytologic detail but maintenance of the architectural pattern. **(f)** Collagenous spherulosis is characterized by pseudocribriform spaces (arrows) which at higher power

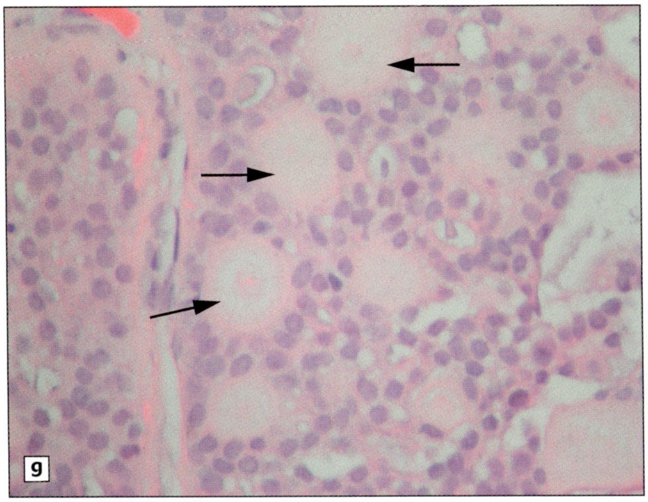

FIGURE 5.5—cont'd (g) are formed by secretions (arrows), probably myofibrillary in nature.

nuclear grade intraductal carcinoma. The secreted material often assumes a radial pattern with spokes arrayed towards a central concentration (Fig. 5.5f,g). In our experience the vast majority of instances of collagenous spherulosis are associated with intraductal papilloma.

The above five features should be regarded as supportive evidence of papilloma rather than diagnostic criteria for it.

Intraductal papillomas very frequently develop areas of sclerosis both centrally and peripherally to the extent that the lesion can histologically closely mimic an invasive carcinoma (Fig. 5.6). In such instances it is important to keep in mind that papillomas tend to be well-circumscribed lesions, whereas invasive duct carcinomas are usually ill-defined, stellate areas on imaging studies.

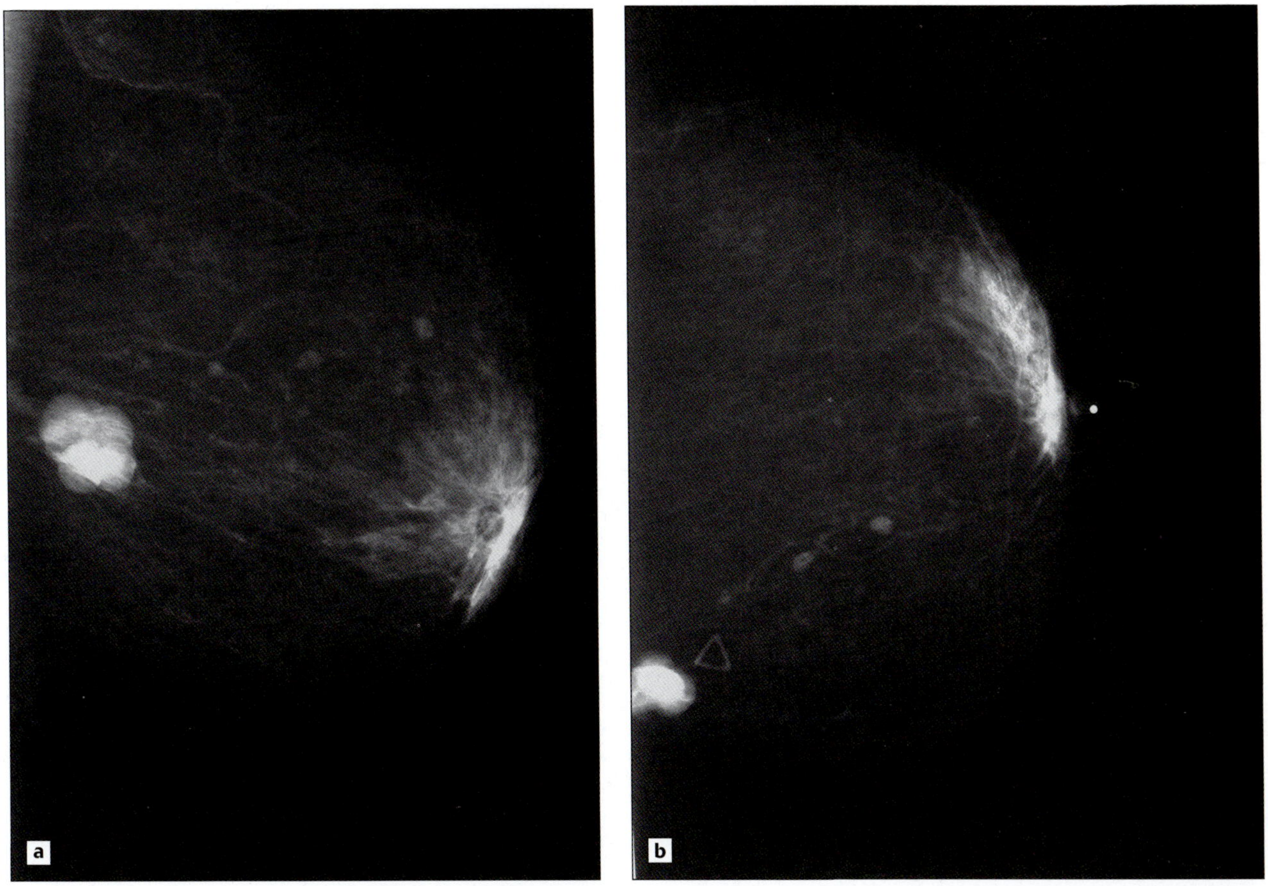

FIGURE 5.6 Sclerosing duct papilloma. **(a,b)** Mammogram of a dense lobulated, well-circumscribed new mass in the left medial breast. There are no associated calcifications.

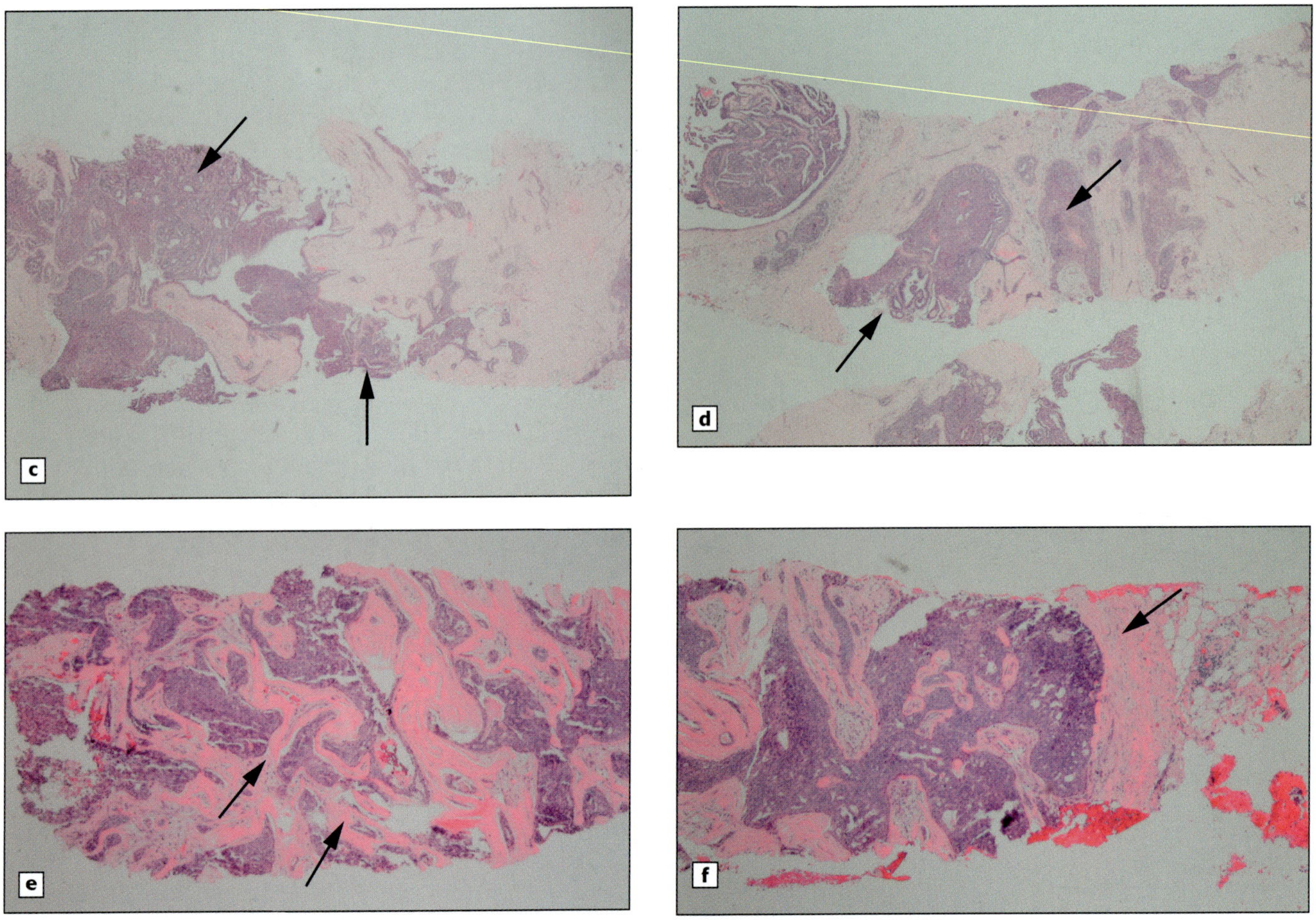

FIGURE 5.6—cont'd (c,d) Core biopsies reveal a clearly papillary proliferation with florid duct hyperplasia and dense fibrosis in which the epithelial proliferation is enveloped (so-called pseudoinvasion). This sclerotic process can become quite pronounced **(e),** particularly at the center of the cores (arrows); however, the periphery **(f)** of the same core cylinder reveals the sharp circumscription (arrow) and florid duct hyperplasia around fibrous cores, rather than an infiltrative periphery.

The peripheral areas of such cores should be carefully examined for true papillary foci. It is well known that epithelial foci become entrapped by fibrosis in such lesions and do not represent invasion. This pattern of proliferation in the context of a well-circumscribed lesion should make a malignant diagnosis extremely questionable, and invasion should be diagnosed only on the basis of direct infiltration of fat or breast tissue clearly beyond the edge of the papilloma. The distinction can occasionally be difficult even after radiologic correlation and is sometimes best made on surgical excision.

The entire spectrum of duct hyperplasia from usual to florid to atypical can be seen within intraductal papillomata and may be problematic on core biopsy (Fig. 5.7). Apocrine metaplasia may be seen intimately admixed within duct hyperplasia and is considered good evidence that the lesion is in fact benign (Fig. 5.8). The same criteria of growth pattern and cytology for classification of duct hyperplasia apply here as do in non-papillomatous breast tissue.

True papillary carcinoma differs sonographically from intraductal papilloma by the ability to visualize the for-

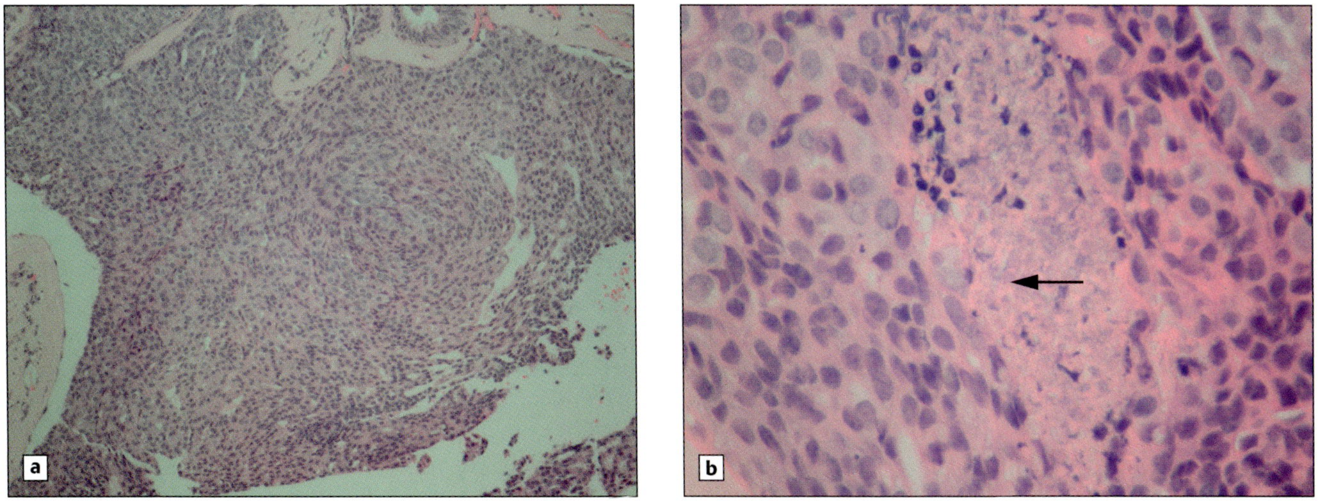

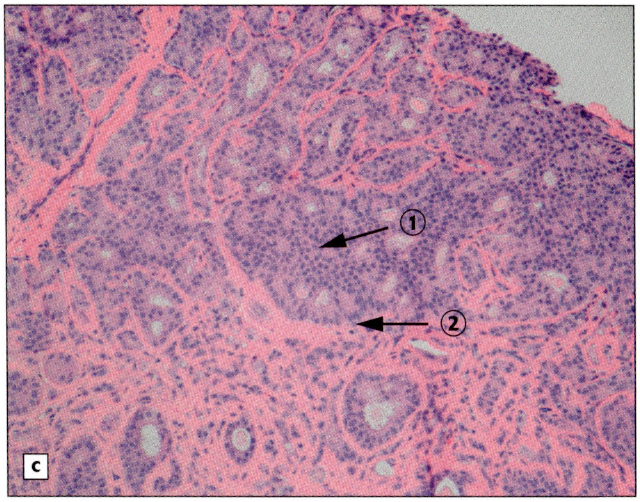

FIGURE 5.7 Epithelial hyperplasia within intraductal papilloma. **(a)** This area of an intraductal papilloma shows a typical pattern of florid duct hyperplasia with streaming epithelial cells, variably sized and shaped cribriform spaces, and interspersed myoepithelial cells. **(b)** Although worrisome, necrosis (arrow) can occur within florid duct hyperplasia, usually in the context of an intraductal papilloma, and does not necessarily imply malignancy. **(c)** Atypical duct hyperplasia within a papilloma is characterized by more rigid, uniform cribriform spaces with a monotonous low grade epithelial proliferation (arrow 1). The basal cells have nuclei which are oriented perpendicular to the basement membrane (arrow 2), a feature of atypical duct hyperplasia, and the area lacks complete involvement of two duct spaces, thereby, not fulfilling minimum criteria for intraductal carcinoma.

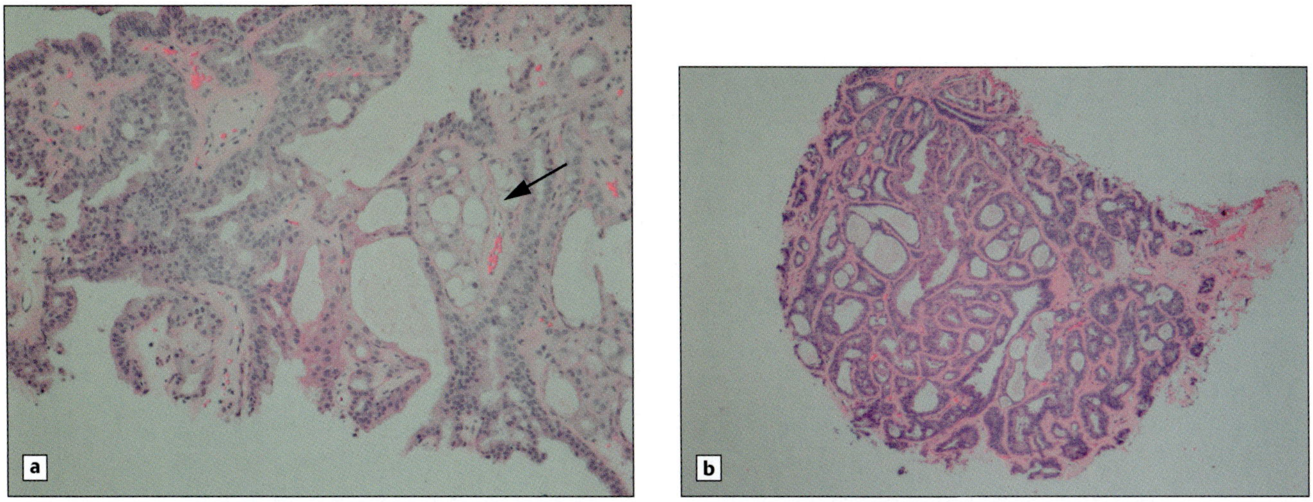

FIGURE 5.8 Varying degrees of apocrine metaplasia in intraductal papilloma. **(a)** Apocrine metaplasia (arrow) blending imperceptibly with florid duct hyperplasia, **(b)** adjacent to duct hyperplasia both within an intraductal papilloma, and

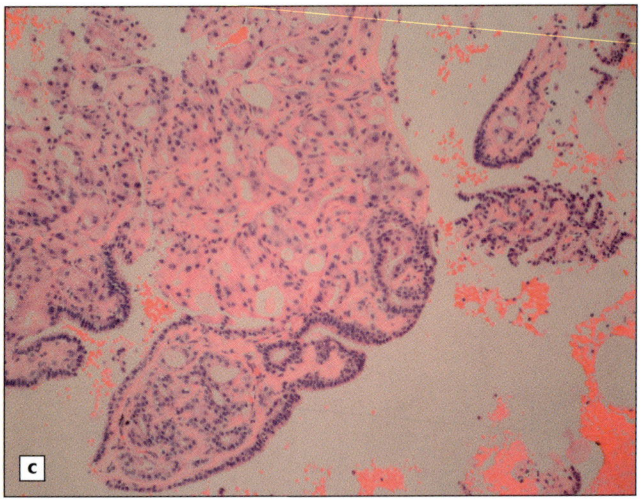

FIGURE 5.8—cont'd (c) more extensive in nature in the papilloma with somewhat larger cells and variable nuclei, but maintenance of normal nuclear/cytoplasmic ratios.

mer's frond-like papillary projections with an associated cyst (Fig. 5.9). Histologically the lesion is composed of a single population of columnar cells lining thin papillae containing a delicate vasculature. Cytologically the tumor cells typically have low to intermediate grade nuclear pleomorphism. The above secondary features of old and new hemorrhage, partial cystic characteristics, and detached fragments also may be seen in core biopsies of papillary carcinoma (in some cases known as intracystic papillary carcinoma). We believe that true papillary carcinomas are distinct lesions which should be differentiated histologically from the more frequent occurrence of intraductal carcinoma involving intraductal papilloma (Fig. 5.10) and that, in the latter, the DCIS should be typed and graded by criteria identical to those for more routinely encountered DCIS. As with intraductal papilloma, a core biopsy diagnosis of invasive carcinoma accompanying DCIS in a papilloma should be made with great trepidation; we reserve such a diagnosis for instances

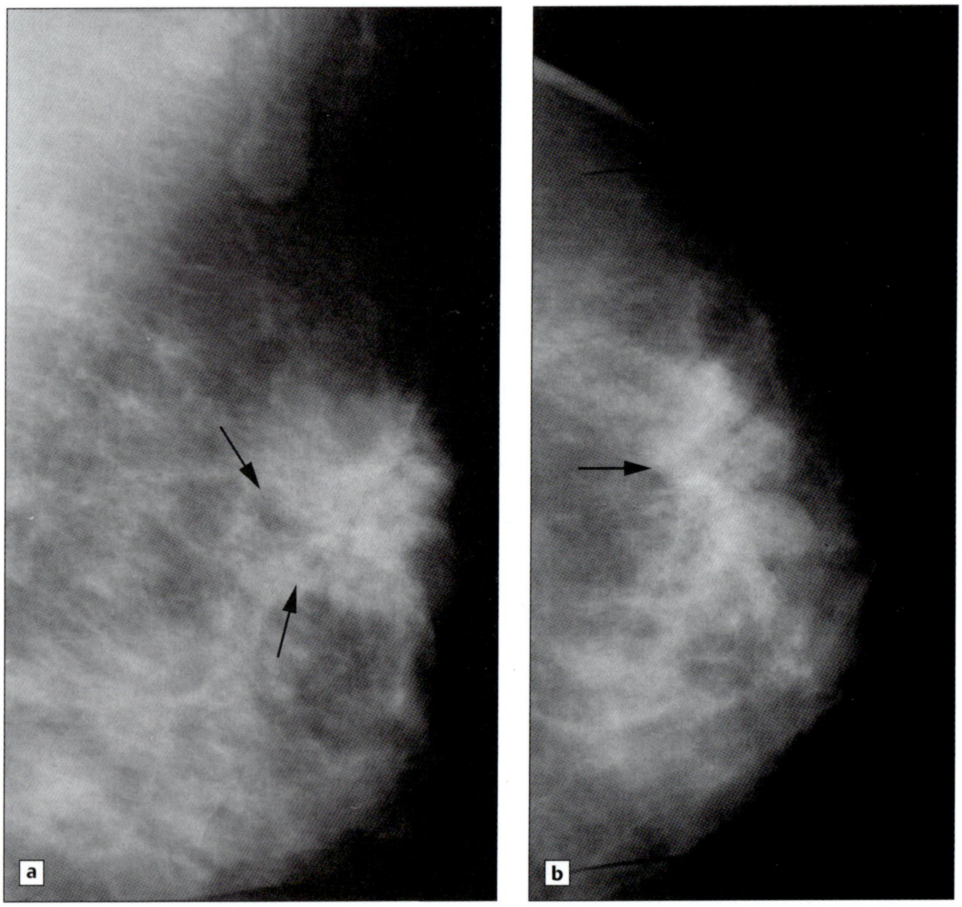

FIGURE 5.9 True papillary carcinoma. **(a,b)** Mammography demonstrated a macrolobulated mass (arrows) in the upper outer quadrant without associated calcifications.

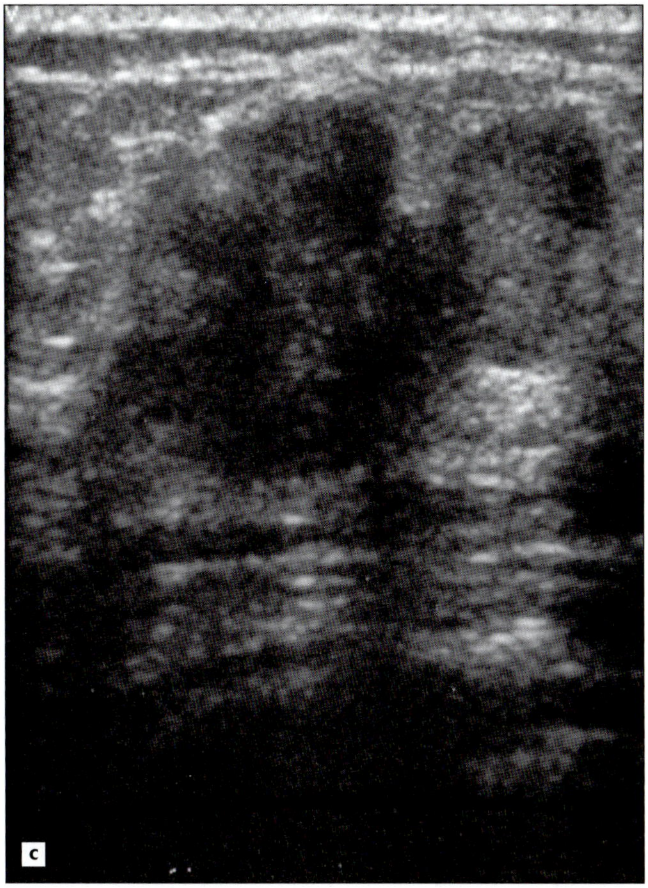

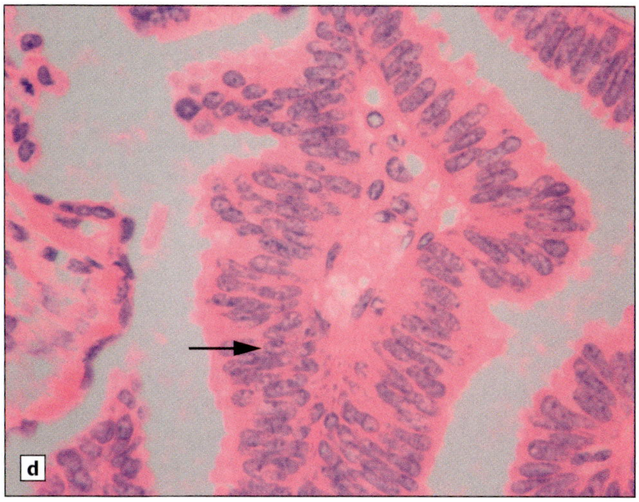

FIGURE 5.9—cont'd (c) Sonography demonstrates a cystic and solid mass with macrolobulated borders and internal frond like papillary nodules. **(d)** Core biopsy reveals true papillary carcinoma composed of columnar cells (arrow) with uniform, low grade nuclei surrounding papillary structures that contain delicate blood vessels.

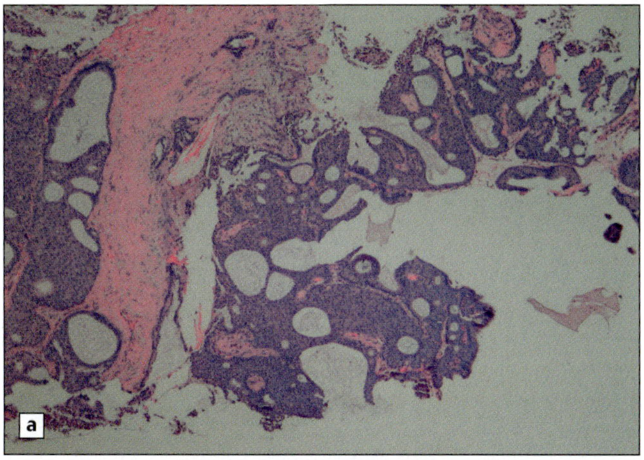

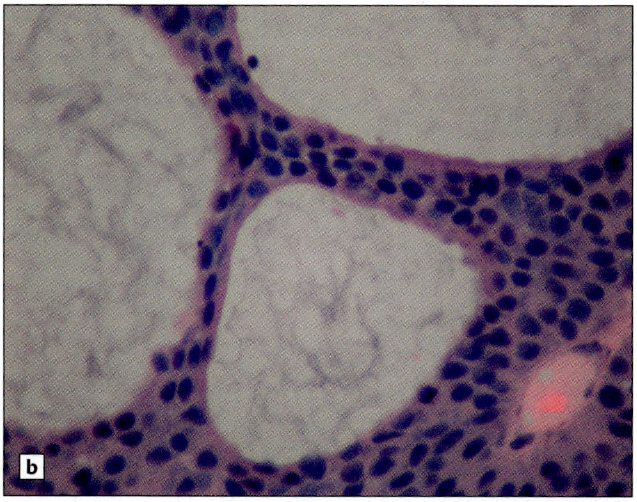

FIGURE 5.10 Intraductal carcinoma involving intraductal papilloma. **(a)** Low grade cribriform intraductal carcinoma growing in an intraductal papilloma. Note the thick fibrous cores (top). **(b)** Higher power view shows uniform low grade nuclei and a rigid cribriform architecture. In our view, such lesions should be regarded as separate entities from true papillary carcinomas.

of tumor infiltrating adipose tissue or breast tissue clearly external to the papilloma (Fig. 5.11).

The idea that surgical excision is necessary for all core biopsies of intraductal papilloma is currently a very controversial question. The literature[5–17] shows a variable small but not insignificant incidence of intraductal carcinoma and, less frequently, invasive carcinoma on subsequent surgical excision. We have noted a 16% incidence of disease upstaging upon excision[14] approximately half of which occurred in cases diagnosed on core biopsy as uncomplicated papilloma, i.e., lacking ADH or DCIS. Some authors[9,14–17] feel that the diagnosis of papilloma on core biopsy, regardless of the degree of duct hyperplasia or sclerosis, should be a trigger for surgical excision in order to exclude intraductal carcinoma and invasive carcinoma (in sclerotic lesions). We would add to this reasoning the possibility that removal of intraductal papilloma may, in at least some patients, be preventive. The question of whether intraductal papilloma represents a premalignant lesion is not a new one, especially when the lesion is a central one. There is some supportive molecular evidence to this view in that intraductal papillomata have been found to be clonal.[18] Additionally, in the early years of our experience with core biopsies, we encountered many cases of well-circumscribed lesions which had been stable for years and then developed interval changes of growth, change in shape, or new calcifications, all features previously shown to be suspicious findings.[19] These lesions typically showed intraductal carcinoma involving intraductal papillomata (Figs 5.2 and 5.3). The original lesions were presumably of such low radiologic suspicion that they were not excised; the technology of core biopsy did not exist at the time to allow sampling. Thus, there is somewhat peripheral and anecdotal evidence that intraductal papillomata may represent the seed from which a carcinoma may arise, and, by recommending surgical excision, we may actually be practicing preventive medicine. The downside of this is, by doing so, it becomes impossible to verify the lesion's malignant potential. An alternative to surgical excision may be the removal[20,21] of intraductal papillomas with an 8-gauge vacuum-assisted core biopsy device, i.e., a core biopsy based re-excision (Fig. 5.12). We have performed this successfully in several patients, and we believe that this technique should be reserved for patients whose initial core biopsies reveal uncomplicated papillomas, these being less likely to be upstaged on excision, and for which definitive margin evaluation would not be necessary. Longer term follow-up is needed to consider the issues of recurrence rate of percutaneously removed

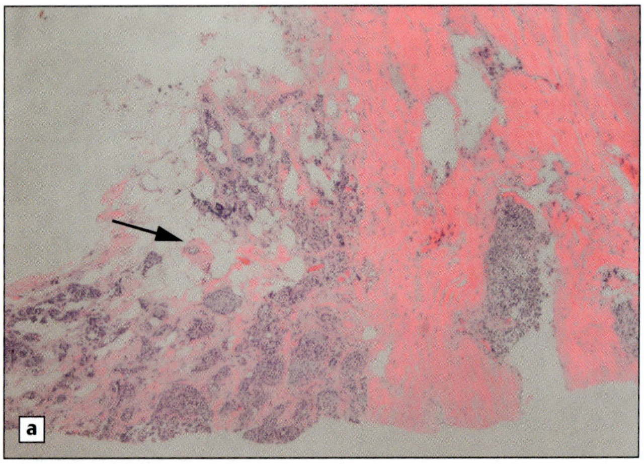

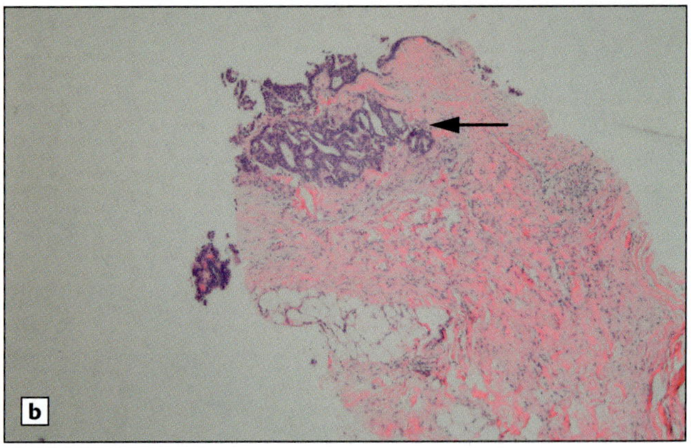

FIGURE 5.11 Invasive carcinoma associated with carcinoma in papilloma. **(a)** We require clear-cut tumor involvement of tissue external to the papilloma, usually adipose tissue (arrow) to diagnose invasive carcinoma in the context of intraductal carcinoma involving a papilloma. Loss of the circumscribed round nature of the nests of carcinoma is also a useful feature. **(b)** In contrast, cribriform intraductal carcinoma lines the periphery of a core cylinder and displaying entrapment (arrow) of circumscribed tumor nests in fibrous tissue (pseudoinvasion).

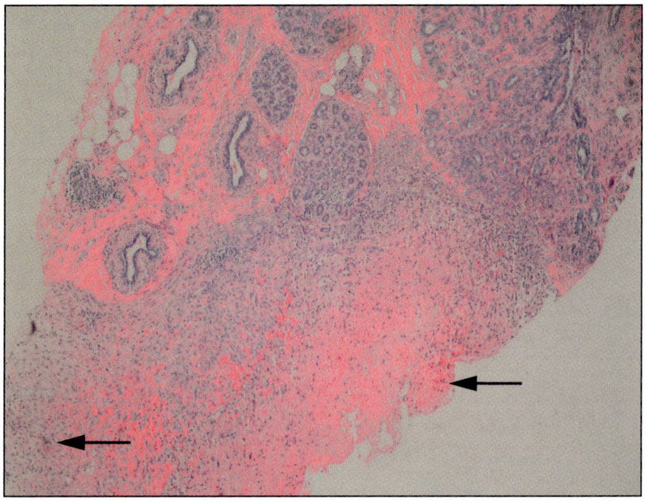

FIGURE 5.12 Core biopsy reexcision of intraductal papilloma. Core biopsies showing intraductal papilloma and granulation tissue with foreign body reaction (arrow), signifying prior core biopsy.

lesions and the possibility that surrounding ducts may form additional papillomata.

Finally, an issue that needs to be considered in this context is the occurrence of epithelial cell (both benign and malignant) displacement into stroma, vessels, and even axillary lymph nodes as a complication of needling procedures (see also Chap. 16). The majority of such cases have been reported as a result of core biopsy.[22] We have noted this situation almost exclusively in papillary lesions.[23] This probably occurs at least in part because of the inherent friability of papillary areas.[24] The physical trauma induced by core biopsy is probably greater with sonographically directed procedures than with stereotactic (vacuum) techniques, and it will be interesting to see if the advent of vacuum assisted sonography-directed biopsy will decrease this occurrence. Until that time, it may be prudent to avoid core biopsy of lesions suspected to be papillary based on imaging characteristics, especially since the majority of such lesions will probably be surgically excised anyway. Clearly epithelial cell displacement seen on excision of core biopsy sites should be evaluated with great caution, as should the presence of epithelial cells in lymph nodes in patients without proven invasive carcinoma.[25,26]

Differential diagnoses of partially solid, partially cystic lesions

- Intraductal papilloma
- Papillary carcinoma
- Intraductal carcinoma involving intraductal papilloma

POINTS TO REMEMBER

1. Intraductal carcinoma may involve intraductal papilloma.
2. Papillary lesions contain friable tissue which can be displaced into stroma by biopsy procedures.
3. Invasive carcinoma should be diagnosed with great caution in papillary lesions.
4. Intraductal papillomas diagnosed on core biopsy should be excised in order to exclude (and possibly prevent) malignancy.

REFERENCES

1. Lam WW, Chu WC, Tang AP, et al. Role of radiologic features in the management of papillary lesions of the breast. AJR Am J Roentgenol 186:1322–1327,2006.
2. Ganesan S, Karthik G, Joshi M, Damodaran V. Ultrasound spectrum in intraductal papillary neoplasms of breast. Br J Radiol 79:843–849,2006.
3. Clement PB, Young RH, Azzopardi JG. Collagenous spherulosis of the breast. Am J Surg Pathol 11:411–417,1987.
4. Resetkova E, Albarracin C, Sneige N. Collagenous spherulosis of breast: morphologic study of 59 cases and review of the literature. Am J Surg Pathol 30:20–27,2006.
*5. Philpotts LE, Shaheen NA, Jain KS, et al. Uncommon high-risk lesions of the breast diagnosed at stereotactic core-needle biopsy: Clinical importance. Radiology 216:831–837,2000.
*6. Irfan K, Brem RF. Surgical and mammographic follow-up of papillary lesions and atypical lobular hyperplasia diagnosed with stereotactic vacuum-assisted biopsy. Breast J 8:230–233,2002.
7. Liberman L, Bracero N, Vuola MA, et al. Percutaneous large-core biopsy of papillary breast lesions. AJR Am J Roentgenol 172:331–337,1999.
8. Rosen EL, Bentley RC, Baker JA, Soo M. Imaging-guided core needle biopsy of papillary lesions of the breast. AJR Am J Roentgenol 179:1185–1192, 2002.
9. Liberman L, Tornos C, Huzjan R, et al. Is surgical excision warranted after benign, concordant diagnosis of papilloma at percutaneous breast biopsy? AJR Am J Roentgenol 186:1328–1334,2006.
10. Shah VI, Flowers CI, Douglas-Jones AG, et al. Immunohistochemistry increases the accuracy of diagnosis of benign papillary lesions in breast core needle biopsy specimens. Histopathol 48:683–691,2006.
11. Agoff SN, Lawton TJ. Papillary lesions of the breast with and without atypical duct hyperplasia: Can we accurately predict benign behavior from core needle biopsy? Am J Clin Pathol 122:440–443,2004.
12. Renshaw AA, Derhagopian RP, Tizol-Bianco DM, Gould EW. Papillomas and atypical papillomas in breast core needle biopsy specimens: risk of carcinoma in subsequent excision. Am J Clin Pathol 122:217–221,2004.
13. Ivan D, Selinko V, Sahin AA, et al. Accuracy of core needle biopsy diagnosis in assessing papillary breast lesions: histologic predictors of malignancy. Mod Pathol 17:165–171,2004.
14. Jaffer S, Nagi CS, Bleiweiss IJ. Should intraductal papilloma diagnosed on core needle biopsy be excised? Mod Pathol 18(Suppl 1):37A,2005.
15. Valdes EK, Tartter PI, Genelus-Dominique E, et al. Significance of papillary lesions at percutaneous breast biopsy. Ann Surg Oncol 13:480–482,2006.
16. Mercado CL, Hamele-Bena D, Oken SM, et al. Papillary lesions of the breast at percutaneous core-needle biopsy. Radiology 238:801–808,2006.
17. Puglisi F, Zuiani C, Bazzocchi M, et al. Role of mammography, ultrasound, and large core biopsy in the diagnostic evaluation of papillary breast lesions. Oncology 65:311–315,2003.
18. Noguchi S, Motomura K, Inaji H, et al. Clonal analysis of solitary intraductal papilloma of the breast by means of polymerase chain reaction. Am J Pathol 144:1320–1325,1994.
19. Hermann G, Keller RJ, Tartter P, et al. Interval changes in nonpalpable breast lesions as an indication of malignancy. Can Assoc Radiol J 46:105–110,1995.
20. Vargas HI, Vargas MP, Gonzalez K, et al. Percutaneous excisional biopsy of palpable breast masses under ultrasound visualization. Breast J 12(Suppl 2):S218–222,2006.
21. Baez E, Huber A, Vetter M, Hackeloer BJ. Minimal invasive complete excision of benign breast tumors using a three-dimensional ultrasound-guided mammotome vacuum device. Ultrasound Obstet Gynecol 21:267–272,2003.
22. Youngson BJ, Cranor M, Rosen PP. Epithelial displacement in surgical breast specimens following needling procedures. Am J Surg Pathol 18:896–903,1994.
23. Nagi C, Bleiweiss IJ, Jaffer S. Epithelial displacement: a papillary phenomenon. Arch Pathol Lab Med 129:1465–1469,2005.
24. Douglas-Jones AG, Verghese A. Diagnostic difficulty arising from displaced epithelium after core biopsy in intracystic papillary lesions of the breast. J Clin Pathol 55:780–783,2002.
25. Carter BA, Jensen RA, Simpson JF, Page DL, Benign transport of breast epithelium into axillary lymph nodes after biopsy. Am J Clin Pathol 113:259–265,2000.
26. Bleiweiss IJ, Nagi CS, Jaffer S. Axillary sentinel lymph nodes can be falsely positive due to iatrogenic displacement and transport of benign epithelial cells in patients with breast carcinoma. J Clin Oncol 24:2013–2018,2006.

CHAPTER 6

Well-circumscribed solid malignancies

Well-circumscribed masses are typically benign (see Chap. 2). Although some invasive breast cancers exhibit circumscribed margins on routine mammography, cone compression magnification views often demonstrate some border irregularity, and careful ultrasound often demonstrates areas of microlobulation and heterogeneity. The classic well-circumscribed malignancies are medullary, colloid (mucinous), and intracystic papillary (intraductal); however, these are relatively unusual in pure form.

While most conventional invasive duct carcinomas are ill-defined, a subset are well circumscribed.[1] In our experience poorly differentiated tumors form the majority of well-circumscribed invasive breast carcinomas (Fig. 6.1). These lesions are often extremely cellular, having grown very rapidly with little time to incite a host desmoplastic response. Their rapid growth is histologically evidenced by extensive mitotic activity and necrosis. On sonography the tumors are heterogeneous with hypoechoic and anechoic components but highly vascular, demonstrating marked Doppler flow secondary to tumor angiogenesis and inflammatory hyperemia. In addition, the rapid growth of these tumors may outstrip their blood supply, accounting for central necrosis and secondary cystification which appears as posterior through transmission on ultrasound. These lesions are histologically distinct from other well-circumscribed invasive malignancies such as medullary carcinoma, colloid carcinoma, and metaplastic carcinoma.

Many such tumors have probably been in the past classified as atypical medullary carcinoma or invasive poorly differentiated duct carcinoma with medullary features. Interestingly, the majority of BRCA-1 mutation-associated invasive carcinomas whose pathology has been reported have fallen into this general category, as have some newly molecularly characterized "basal-like" subtypes or so-called triple negative (ER, PR, and Her2neu) carcinomas.[2,3] Medullary (or atypical medullary) carcinoma (Fig. 6.2), however, is a diagnosis dependent on histologic examination of the entire tumor with particular attention to the syncytial or sheet-like growth pattern of the tumor cells, lack of fibrosis, and sharply demarcated periphery.[4,5] Thus, a definitive diagnosis of medullary carcinoma should not be made on core biopsy alone. Pure, good prognosis, colloid carcinoma (Fig. 6.3) may be suspected when core biopsy reveals tumor cells of low nuclear grade surrounded by pools of mucin; however, it should be kept in mind that excision may reveal higher grade areas, particularly in lesions whose sonograms show slight border irregularities (Fig. 6.4).

Metaplastic carcinoma is the conventional term for a lesion that is essentially carcinosarcoma of the breast with the exception that the combination of squamous cell carcinoma with ordinary invasive duct carcinoma also suffices for the diagnosis. The diagnosis on core biopsy requires the presence of both the epithelial and stromal (or squamous) components (Fig. 6.5). Cores containing only malignant stroma should yield a descriptive rather than definitive diagnosis, since sampling issues could preclude correct classification. An overdiagnosis of metaplastic carcinoma would lead to unnecessary axillary dissection, while the alternative incorrect diagnosis of malignant phyllodes tumor or pure sarcoma (so rare as to be essentially a diagnosis of exclusion) could lead to a lack of node sampling. All three lesions are typically well circumscribed.

The exact subclassification of invasive carcinoma as ductal or medullary or metaplastic in this scenario is probably not crucial, however, since the next treatment steps (surgery or preoperative chemotherapy) will be based on primarily on the clinical and/or radiologic size of the invasive tumor. Thus, surgery will follow core biopsy for most such patients, while neoadjuvant chemotherapy is primarily utilized for invasive carcinomas large enough that biopsy would not require imaging guidance, i.e., they are palpable masses.

The adequate core biopsy of such lesions will be typically readily diagnosable as invasive carcinoma, keeping in mind that, although the circumscribed periphery of the tumor will usually be apparent towards the ends of the cylinders (Fig. 6.6), this circumscription is not due to a duct wall as one might see in a high grade intraductal carcinoma involving an intraductal papilloma or a cyst. In the face of a palpable mass, core biopsy has the distinct advantage over fine needle aspirate in that the former allows a ready definitive diagnosis of invasion, whereas very few pathologists

Text continued on p. 71

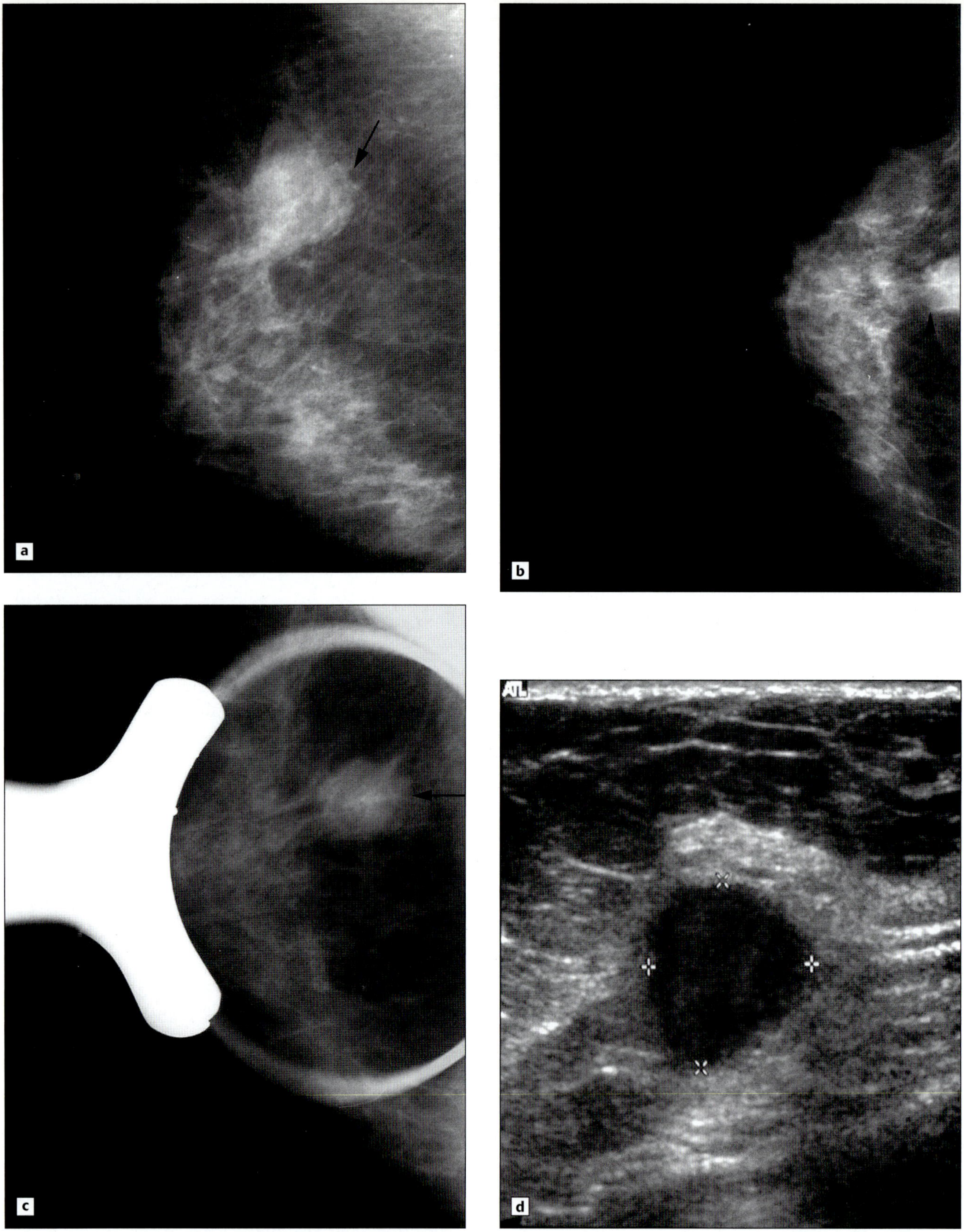

FIGURE 6.1 Well-circumscribed infiltrating poorly differentiated duct carcinoma. **(a)** MLO and **(b)** CC views demonstrate a dense mass in the upper outer quadrant with an indistinct posterior margin (arrows). **(c)** Cone compression demonstrates a tail along the posterior aspect of the mass (arrow). The borders are indistinct in areas. **(d)** Sonography demonstrates a well-defined hypoechoic mass with irregular margins and some posterior enhancement. The lesion contains some central anechoic areas which likely represent central necrosis. These lesions can grow so rapidly that they outstrip their blood supply, leading to secondary cystification and inciting less desmoplastic reaction in the adjacent breast tissue.

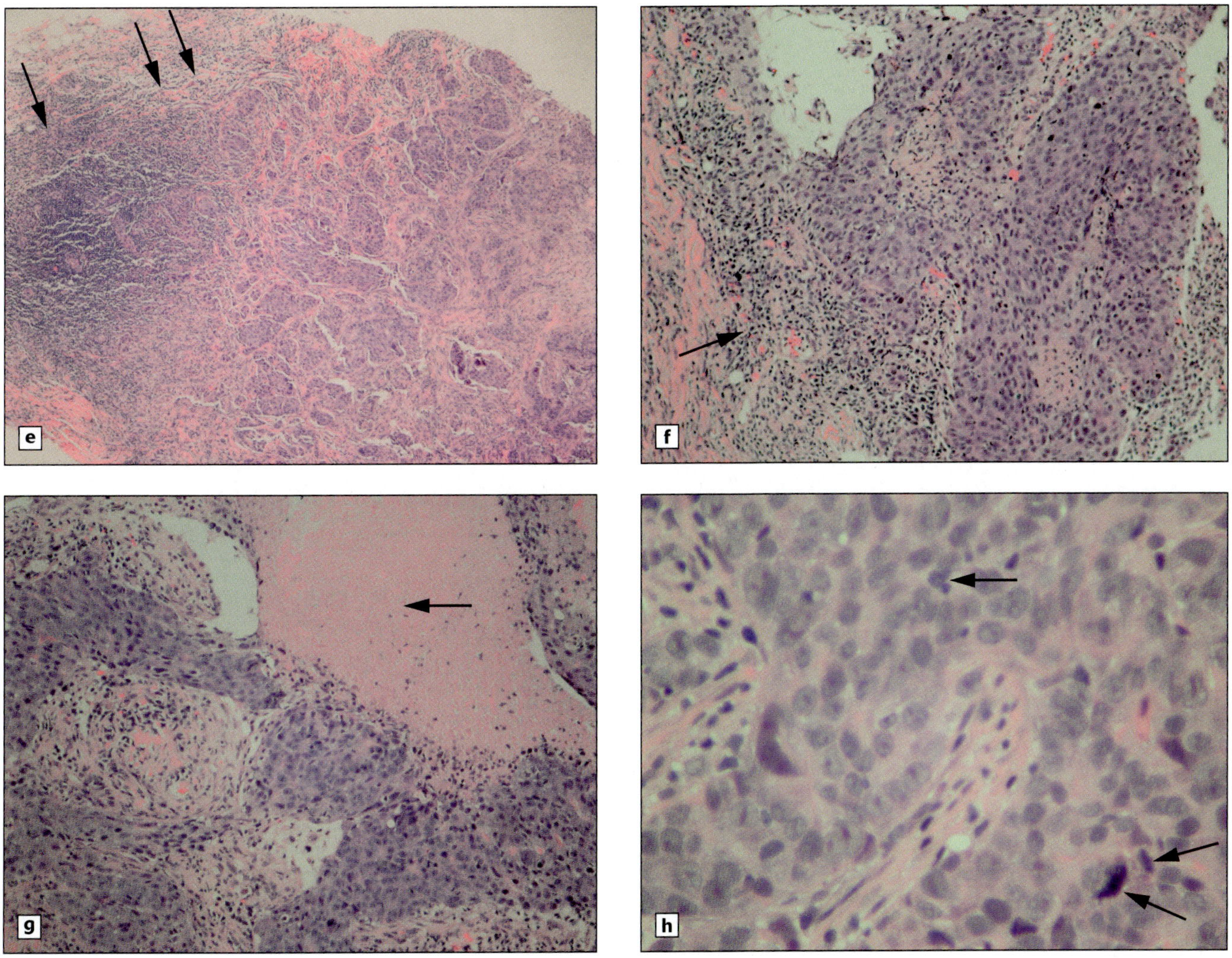

FIGURE 6.1—cont'd (e) Core biopsy reveals nests of invasive poorly differentiated duct carcinoma with a sharply defined border (arrows). Other areas **(f)** show a more solid tumor proliferation with intense inflammatory infiltrate (arrow). **(g)** Necrosis (arrow) is present towards the center of the lesion, and **(h)** higher power reveals marked nuclear variability and frequent mitoses (arrows).

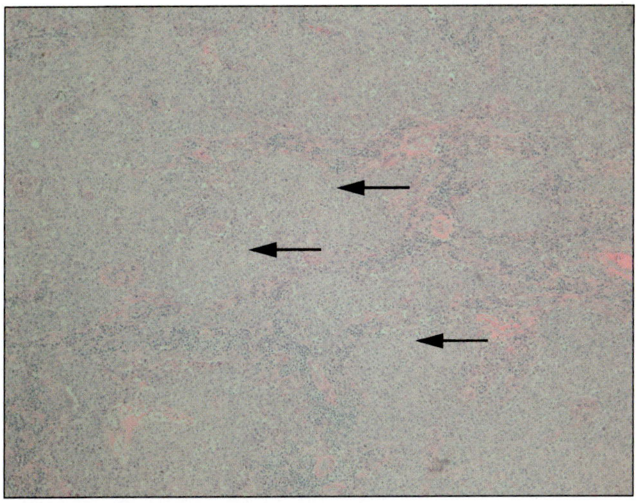

FIGURE 6.2 Medullary carcinoma, excision. The classical picture of medullary carcinoma is that of sheets or syncytia of pleomorphic tumor cells (arrows) and reactive inflammatory cells forming a well-circumscribed mass.

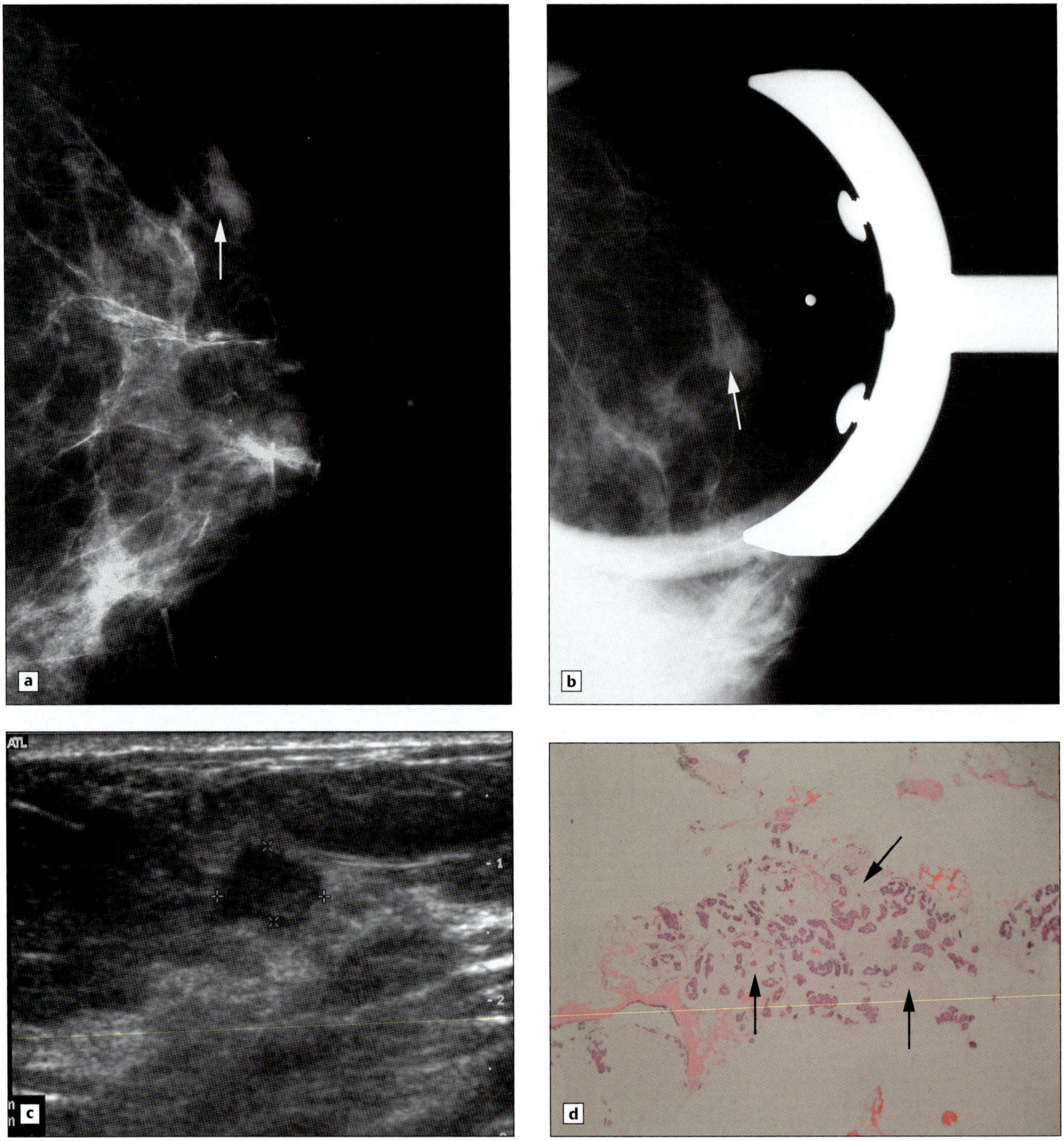

FIGURE 6.3 Colloid carcinoma. **(a)** CC view showing an asymmetric new nodular mass (arrow) in the right medial breast. **(b)** The lesion persists on spot tangential view (arrow). A BB denotes that the nodule is vaguely palpable. **(c)** Sonography shows a lobulated hypoechoic well-defined 8 mm × 6 mm mass with no significant posterior shadowing or through transmission. **(d)** Core biopsies reveal colloid carcinoma composed of nests and gland forming tumor cells embedded in pools of extracellular mucin (arrows).

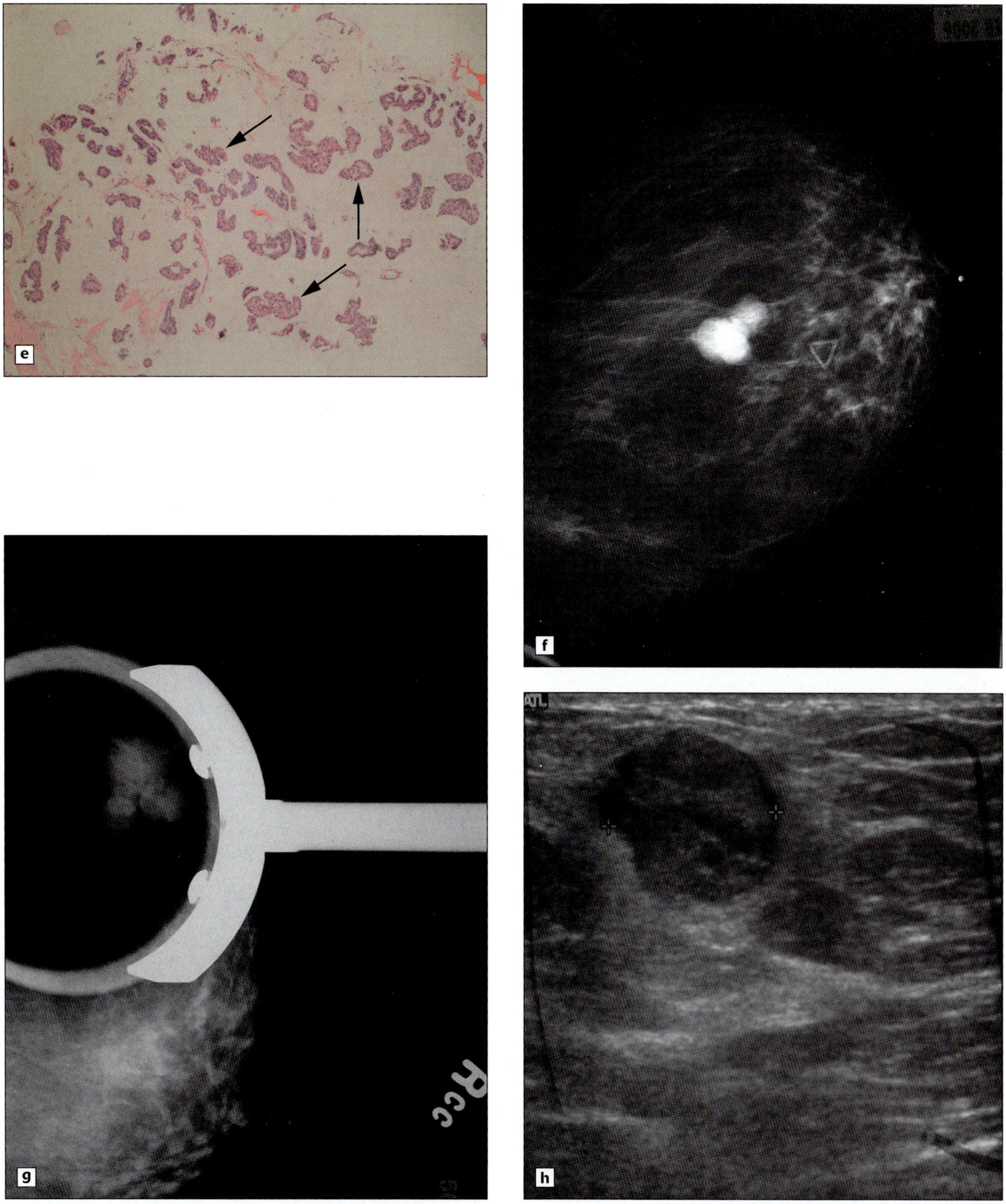

FIGURE 6.3—cont'd (e) On higher power the tumor cells have low grade, relatively uniform nuclei (arrows). **(f)** Colloid carcinoma can also be multilobed. This example is represented on mammographic CC view as a bilobed dense smoothly marginated mass corresponding to the patient's palpable finding. **(g)** Cone compression view demonstrates some border irregularity, and **(h)** sonography demonstrates a bilobed, lobulated solid hypoechoic mass with homogeneous internal echoes and some posterior through transmission.

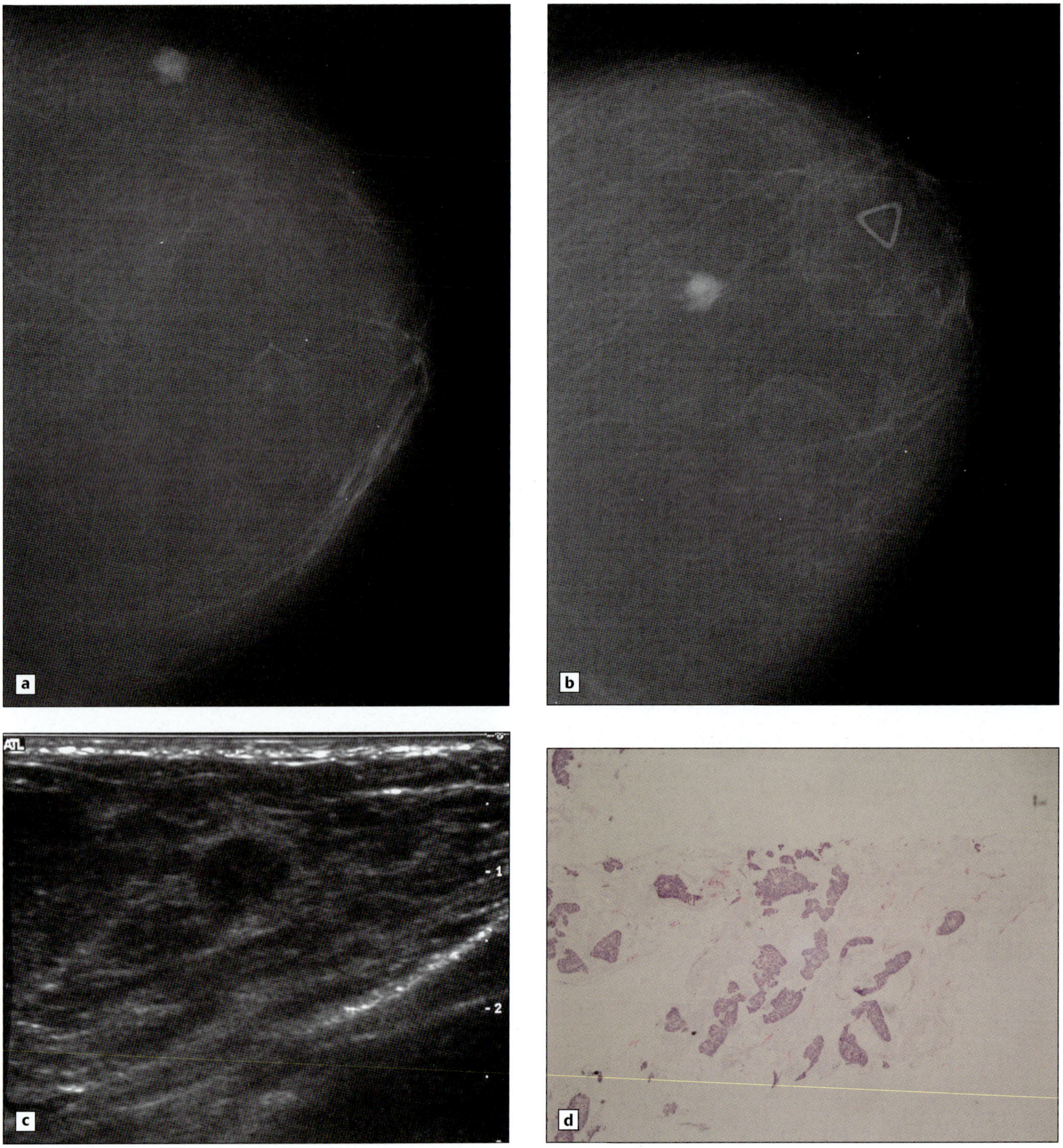

FIGURE 6.4 Partial colloid carcinoma. **(a)** MLO and **(b)** CC views demonstrate a dense lobulated mass. Margins in some areas are smooth while other margins show subtle spiculation. **(c)** Sonography, however, demonstrates a solid markedly hypoechoic mass which has well defined margins along some of its periphery and some areas that are microlobulated. There is some posterior through transmission. **(d)** Core biopsy shows pools of mucin surrounding clusters of tumor cells forming glands.

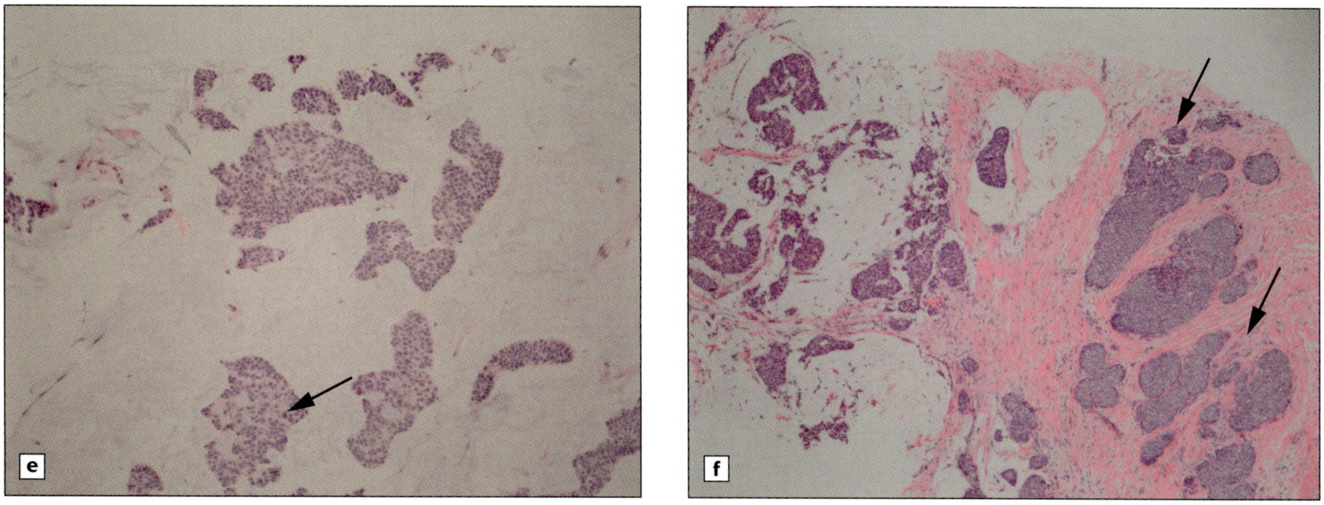

FIGURE 6.4—cont'd (e) On higher power the cells form larger nests which are still surrounded by mucin; however, there is more nuclear pleomorphism (arrow) than that seen in Fig 6.3f, and other areas **(f)** reveal invasive moderately differentiated duct carcinoma (arrow) adjacent to mucinous carcinoma.

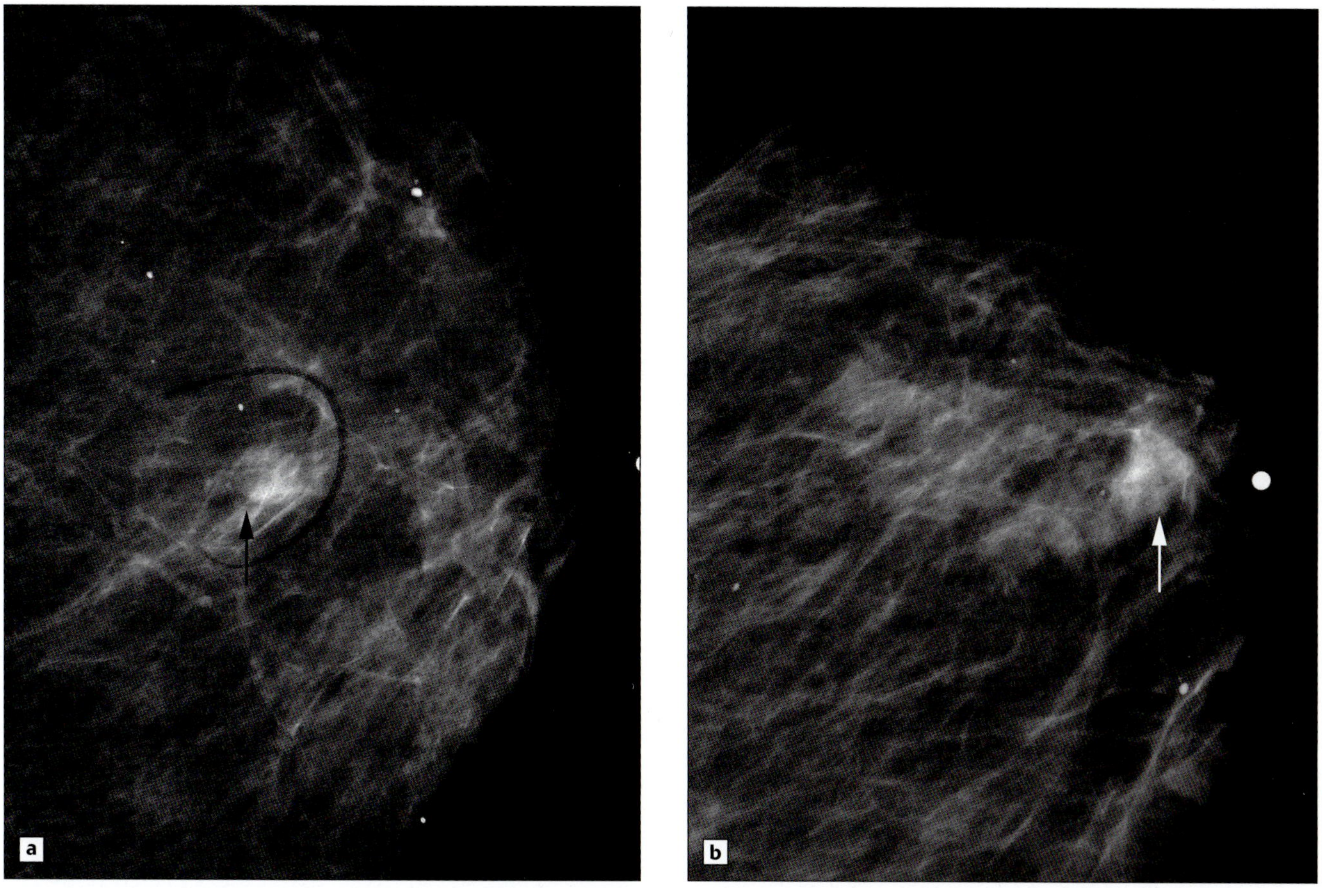

FIGURE 6.5 Metaplastic carcinoma. **(a,b)** Mammography demonstrates a new gently lobulated, smoothly marginated right retroareolar mass (arrows).

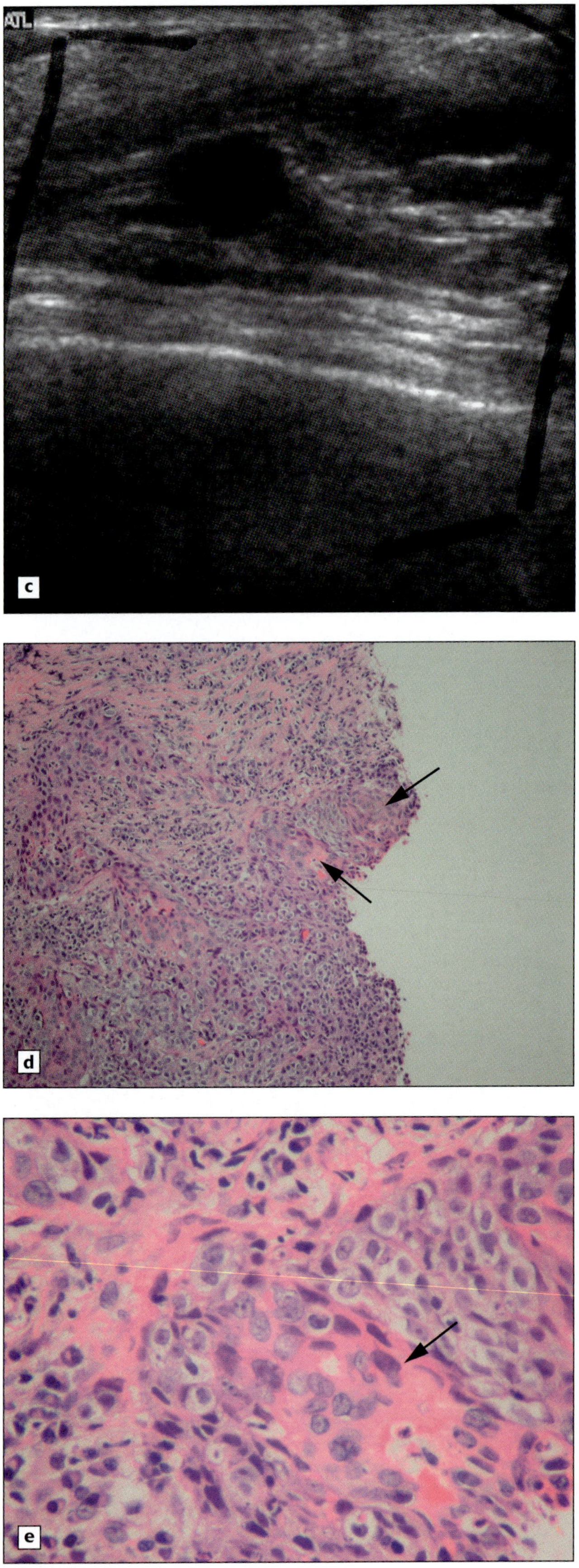

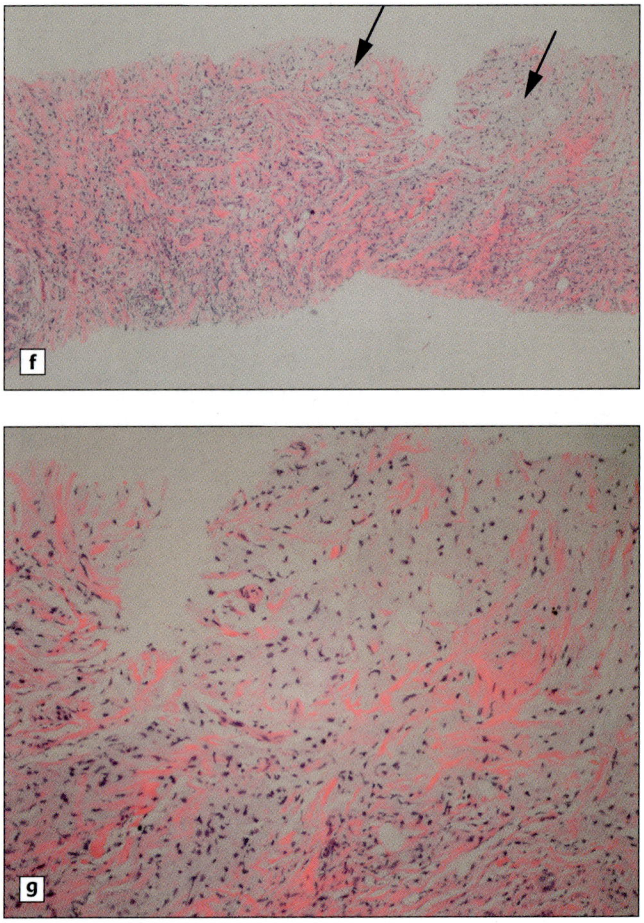

FIGURE 6.5—cont'd **(c)** Sonography of the right breast: 6 o'clock axis demonstrates a predominantly well-circumscribed solid mass. **(d)** Core biopsy shows a tumor composed of conventional invasive poorly differentiated duct carcinoma admixed with squamous cell carcinoma (arrow). **(e)** Higher power view showing squamous differentiation in the tumor cells (arrow). **(f)** Core biopsy of a different case of metaplastic carcinoma which is composed of both invasive duct carcinoma and myxo-chondroid sarcomatous differentiation (arrows), seen best on high power **(g)**.

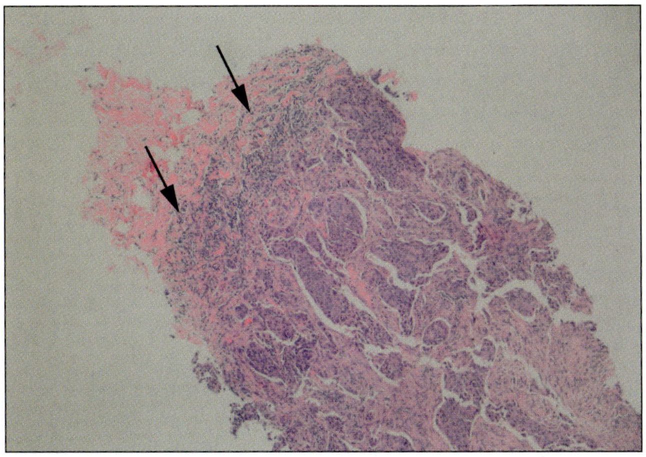

FIGURE 6.6 Well-circumscribed infiltrating poorly differentiated duct carcinoma. Note that the sharp demarcation of the tumor is evident at the end of the core cylinder (arrows).

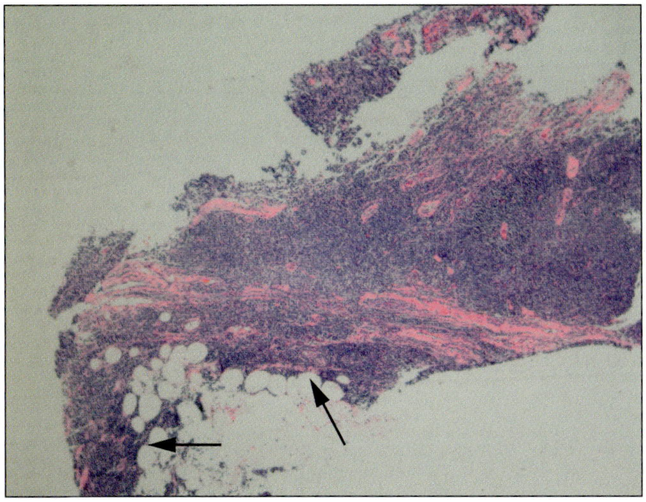

FIGURE 6.7 Malignant lymphoma, low grade. In this core biopsy, the lymphocytes look rather benign, yet infiltration of fat (arrows) calls suspicion to the true diagnosis of lymphoma.

will readily admit that they are able to differentiate in situ from invasive carcinoma simply on the basis of fine needle aspiration.

The differential diagnosis of well-circumscribed solid malignancies also includes malignant lymphoma. Such lesions show a variable sonographic appearance, may be lobulated in shape, and may demonstrate uniform hypoanechoic appearance with some through transmission. Unless careful sonographic criteria are adhered to, lymphoma can sometimes mimic a cystic lesion (see Chap. 3). Histologically, the diagnosis can be challenging on core biopsy alone unless tumor cells diffusely infiltrate fat (Fig. 6.7). Immunohistochemistry can be very helpful, but often the diagnosis is best made on surgical excision of the lesion. Occasional cases are difficult to distinguish from invasive lobular carcinoma (Fig. 6.8). In such

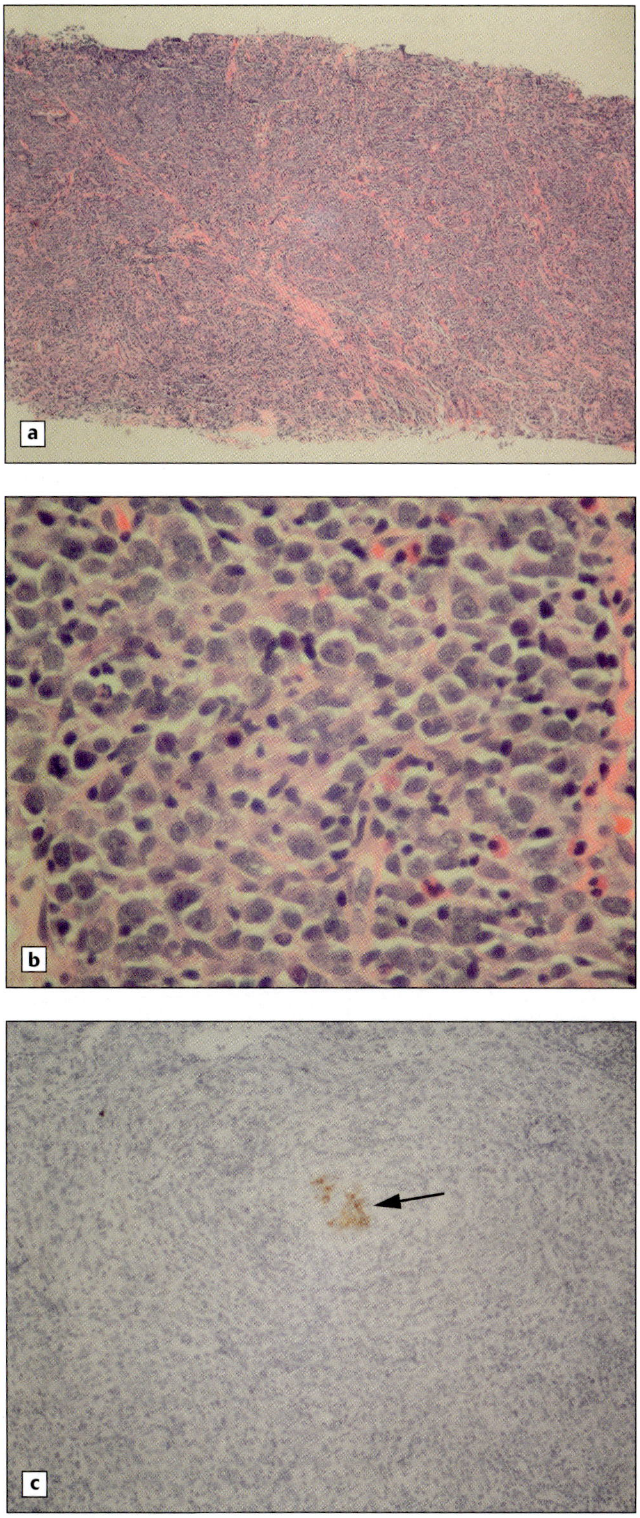

FIGURE 6.8 Malignant lymphoma, diffuse large cell type. **(a)** This core biopsy of a well-circumscribed lesion shows a monotonous populations of cells which on higher power **(b)** are pleomorphic and cytologically malignant but the distinction between lymphoma and carcinoma is difficult. Immunohistochemical stains show that the tumor cells are **(c)** negative for cytokeratin (note the epithelial cells of a benign entrapped terminal duct are staining-arrow) and

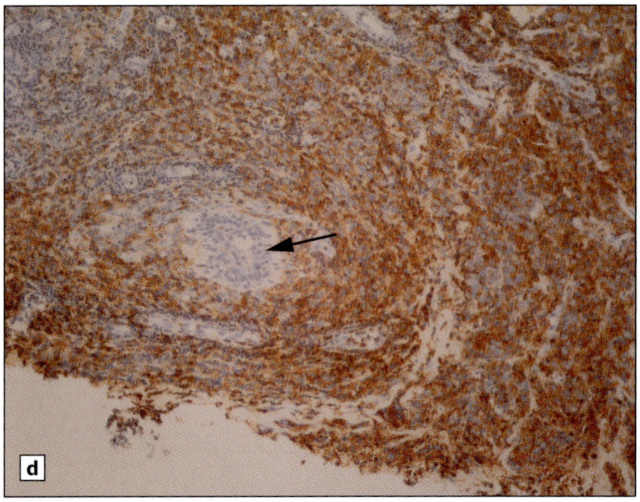

FIGURE 6.8—cont'd (d) strongly and uniformly positive for leukocyte common antigen (note the negative staining breast ductule-arrow). Other markers revealed a B-cell phenotype.

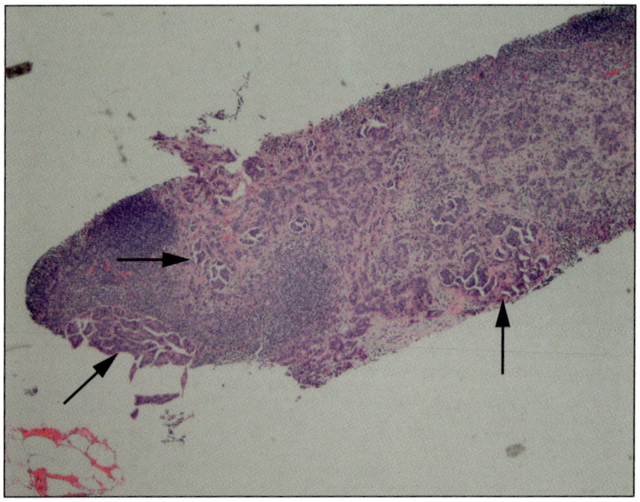

FIGURE 6.9 Metastatic carcinoma in an intramammary lymph node. Core biopsy of a lymph node containing extensive metastatic carcinoma (arrows).

instances immunohistochemical stains for keratins are quite valuable.

Finally intramammary lymph nodes may harbor or be replaced by metastatic carcinoma (Fig. 6.9). In fact they may represent the sentinel lymph nodes.[6] Core biopsies may or may not be adequate to correctly differentiate these rare instances from medullary carcinoma because both may show germinal center formation and a circumscribed border. Therefore excision is warranted. Furthermore, in a patient with a known invasive mammary carcinoma, the radiologic discovery of a lesion suspected to be an intramammary lymph node should lead to excision of the lesion since it may be the sentinel node, and core biopsy may be falsely negative due to sampling error.

Differential diagnoses of well circumscribed solid malignancies

- Invasive poorly differentiated duct carcinoma
- Medullary carcinoma
- Atypical medullary carcinoma
- Colloid carcinoma
- Metaplastic carcinoma
- Intramammary lymph node with metastasis

POINTS TO REMEMBER

1. Invasive carcinomas can be well circumscribed and develop very quickly.
2. Medullary carcinoma cannot and need not be diagnosed on core biopsy alone.
3. Intramammary lymph nodes should be excised in patients with ipsilateral invasive carcinoma.

REFERENCES

1. Jimenez RE, Wallis T, Visscher DW. Centrally necrotizing carcinomas of the breast: A distinct histologic subtype with aggressive clinical behavior. Am J Surg Pathol 25:331–337,2001.
2. Nielsen TO, Hsu FD, Jensen K, et al. Immunohistochemical and clinical characterization of the basal-like subtype of invasive breast carcinoma. Clin Cancer Res 2004;10:5367–5374.
3. Foulkes WD, Stefansson IM, Chappuis PO, et al. Germline BRCA1 mutations and a basal epithelial phenotype in breast cancer. J Natl Cancer Inst 95:1482–1485,2003.
4. Ridolfi RL, Rosen PP, Port A, et al. Medullary carcinoma of the breast: A clinicopathologic study with 10 year follow-up. Cancer 40:1365–1385, 1977.
5. Wargotz ES, Silverberg SG. Medullary carcinoma of the breast: A clinicopathologic study with appraisal of current diagnostic criteria. Hum Pathol 19:1340–1346,1988.
6. Gajdos C, Bleiweiss IJ, Drossman S, Tartter PI. Breast cancer in an intramammary sentinel node. The Breast Journal 7:260–262,2001.

CHAPTER 7

Irregular densities

Irregular masses can range from subtle microlobulations to frank spiculations, the most common mammographic appearance of invasive carcinoma (Fig 7.1). These lesions typically incite a host response, a desmoplastic reaction, as they extend into the surrounding breast tissue. While it can be easily identified on mammography of a fatty breast, when a tumor is surrounded by dense fibroglandular tissue its invasive spiculated margin becomes difficult to delineate; ultrasound is invaluable in these cases. The most common sonographic appearance of an infiltrating carcinoma is that of a markedly hypoechoic or heterogeneous, taller than wide mass with angular, ill-defined, or spiculated margins and posterior acoustic shadowing (Fig 7.2). Sonographic spiculation is similar to mammographic spiculation. Lesions which are taller than wide suggest growth across normal tissue planes, and these lesions, unlike cysts, are incompressible. Posterior shadowing is common with scirrhous carcinomas or tumors that have been present long enough to incite an intense host desmoplastic response (Fig 7.2b–d).

Most invasive duct carcinomas will not present a great diagnostic challenge on core biopsy, yet the diagnosis obviously must not be taken lightly, as further surgery, possibly mastectomy, will ensue. In our consultation practice, however, we have occasionally encountered overdiagnosis of malignancy with unfortunate results. A repeating pattern has been the overdiagnosis of infiltrating well differentiated duct carcinoma in the context of core biopsy of a well circumscribed mass. This diagnostic pairing is discordant (see Chap. 6 for a discussion of well-circumscribed malignancies) and should raise the possibility of alternative (benign) histologic diagnoses. As with other lesions, to be most accurate an individual core cylinder should traverse the entire lesion so that both peripheral edges of the tumor are evaluable (Figs 7.2b and 7.3). This is usually not problematic, since the likely candidates for image-guided core biopsy are small carcinomas. Careful evaluation of the periphery of the lesion combined with knowledge of the lesion's imaging characteristics should result in diagnostic accuracy in the vast majority of cases.

While most invasive carcinomas diagnosed by core biopsy will be surgically treated in identical fashion regardless of the tumor subtype, proper classification of the carcinoma on core biopsy may influence the extent of local surgery performed. A specific case in point is that of invasive micropapillary carcinoma (see also below). An unusual subtype of infiltrating duct carcinoma,[1] its imaging features are similar to other tumors; however, it has a distinct tendency for multifocality (Fig 7.4). In addition, although these tumors may be discovered at a small size, they are aggressive and demonstrate a propensity to invade the lymphatic system and metastasize to axillary lymph nodes,[2] and they tend to co-express estrogen and progesterone receptors as well as Her2-neu. Paradoxically these lesions have a similar clinical outcome to other invasive carcinomas when matched by stage; however, the majority present with positive lymph nodes.[3] Thus a diagnosis of this entity on core biopsy should prompt an imaging search for additional ipsilateral tumors in order to evaluate the feasibility of breast conservation versus the necessity for mastectomy.

Pleomorphic calcifications within a spiculated mass are virtually diagnostic of carcinoma (Fig 7.5). The presence of suspicious calcifications both within a carcinoma and in surrounding breast tissue is characteristic of an invasive carcinoma with an extensive intraductal component, a lesion that may require a more extensive lumpectomy to achieve negative margins. Invasive carcinomas have been defined as having extensive intraductal components if (1) greater than 25% of a tumor mass is histologically DCIS, and DCIS is present in breast tissue clearly outside the mass; or (2) if a tumor is composed of DCIS with microinvasion.[4,5] The presence of an extensive intraductal component (EIC) has been used by some surgeons as justification for mastectomy; however, in reality it signifies that a more extensive lumpectomy would be needed to achieve negative margins. Some authors have assessed the predictability of EIC based on finding DCIS in core biopsies;[6] however, we feel, as do others,[7] that this is not very feasible since probably the more clinically relevant aspect of EIC (the presence of DCIS in tissue outside the mass) cannot be adequately assessed on core biopsies of invasive tumor masses, the goal of the procedure obviously being the evaluation of the target density, not its surrounding breast tissue.

Most studies have shown reasonably good correlation between tumor type diagnosed on core biopsy compared

Text continued on p. 79

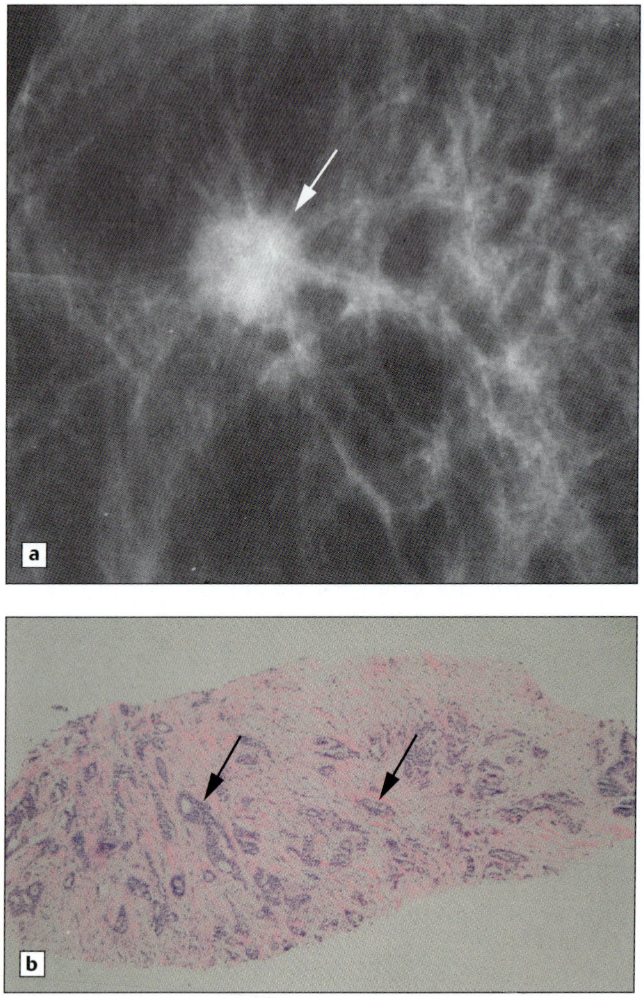

FIGURE 7.1 Typical mammogram of invasive duct carcinoma. **(a)** Mammography demonstrates a spiculated mass, irregularly marginated, infiltrating into surrounding breast tissue (arrow). **(b)** Core biopsy reveals an irregular pattern of partially gland forming carcinoma, invasive moderately differentiated duct carcinoma (arrows). Despite the absence of the lesion's periphery in this field, invasion can be confidently diagnosed based on the irregular growth patterns, variability of the epithelial nests, and early desmoplastic reaction.

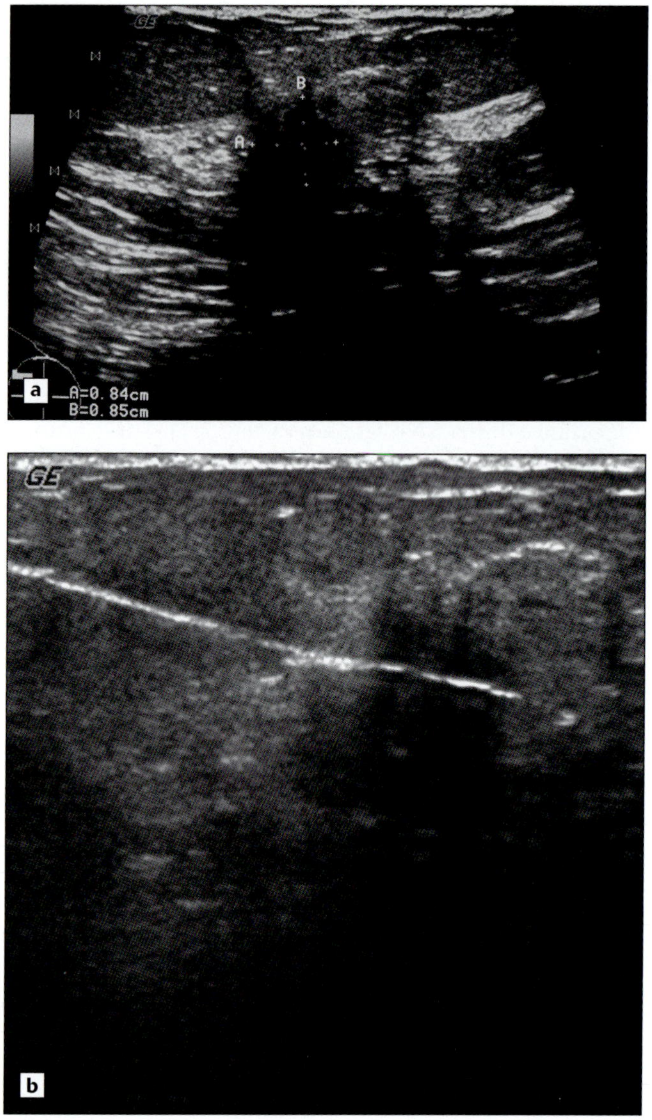

FIGURE 7.2 Typical sonogram of invasive duct carcinoma. **(a)** Sonography shows an irregular, hypoechoic mass which is taller (dotted line "B") than wide (dotted line "A") with posterior acoustical shadowing. **(b)** Sonography showing accurate sampling with the core biopsy needle passing through the mass.

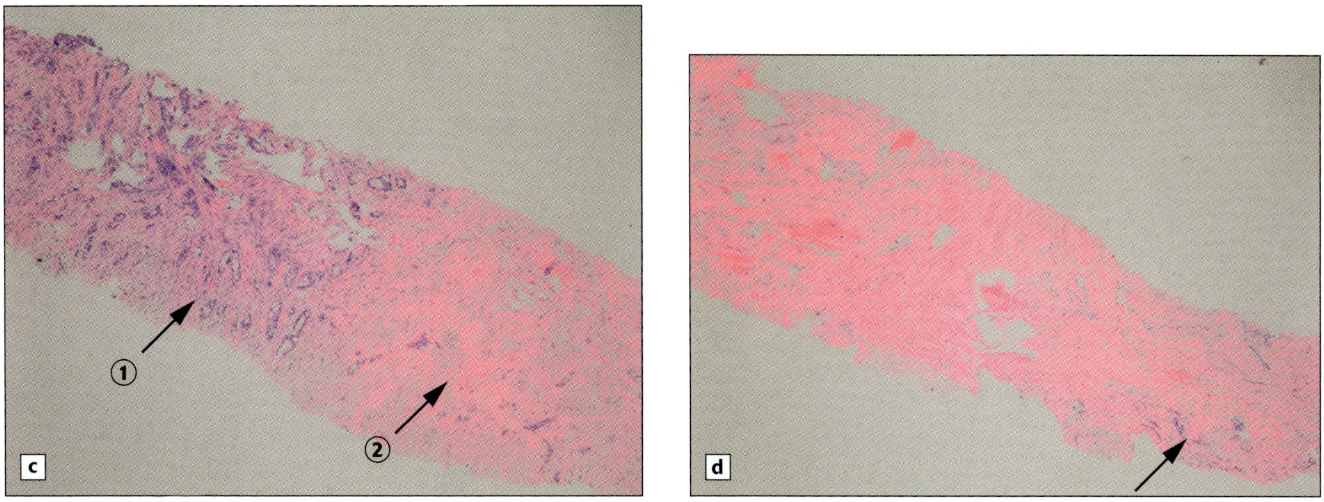

FIGURE 7.2—cont'd (c) Core biopsy shows infiltrating moderately differentiated duct carcinoma at the periphery (arrow 1) but dense fibrosis nearly devoid of tumor cells centrally (arrow 2), so-called scirrhous carcinoma. **(d)** The central portion of the same core is completely fibrotic. Without proper sampling of and careful attention to the peripheral end of the lesion, such a core would be nondiagnostic because of the paucity of tumor cells (a few are present at one end – arrow).

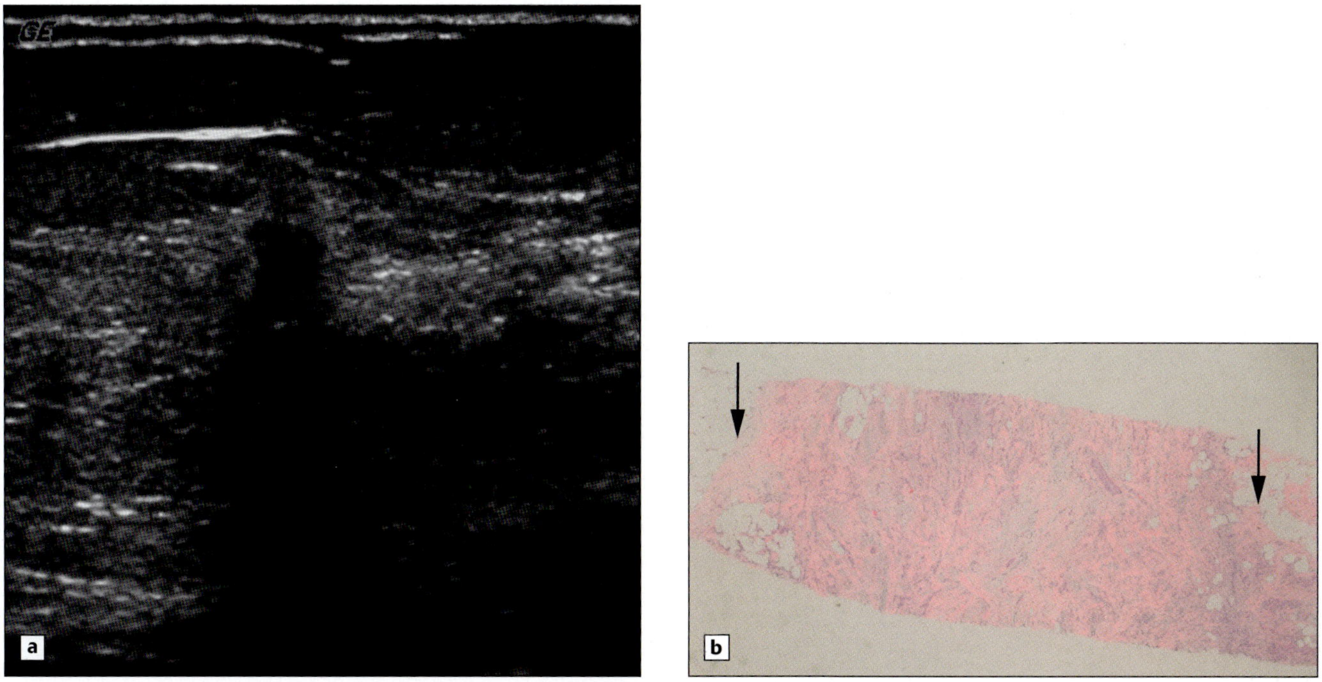

FIGURE 7.3 Invasive carcinoma sampling. **(a)** Sonography shows a small irregular, solid mass. **(b)** This core biopsy cylinder represents a sample taken through the lesion with both edges (arrows) of the invasive carcinoma as well as the center evident on the same core.

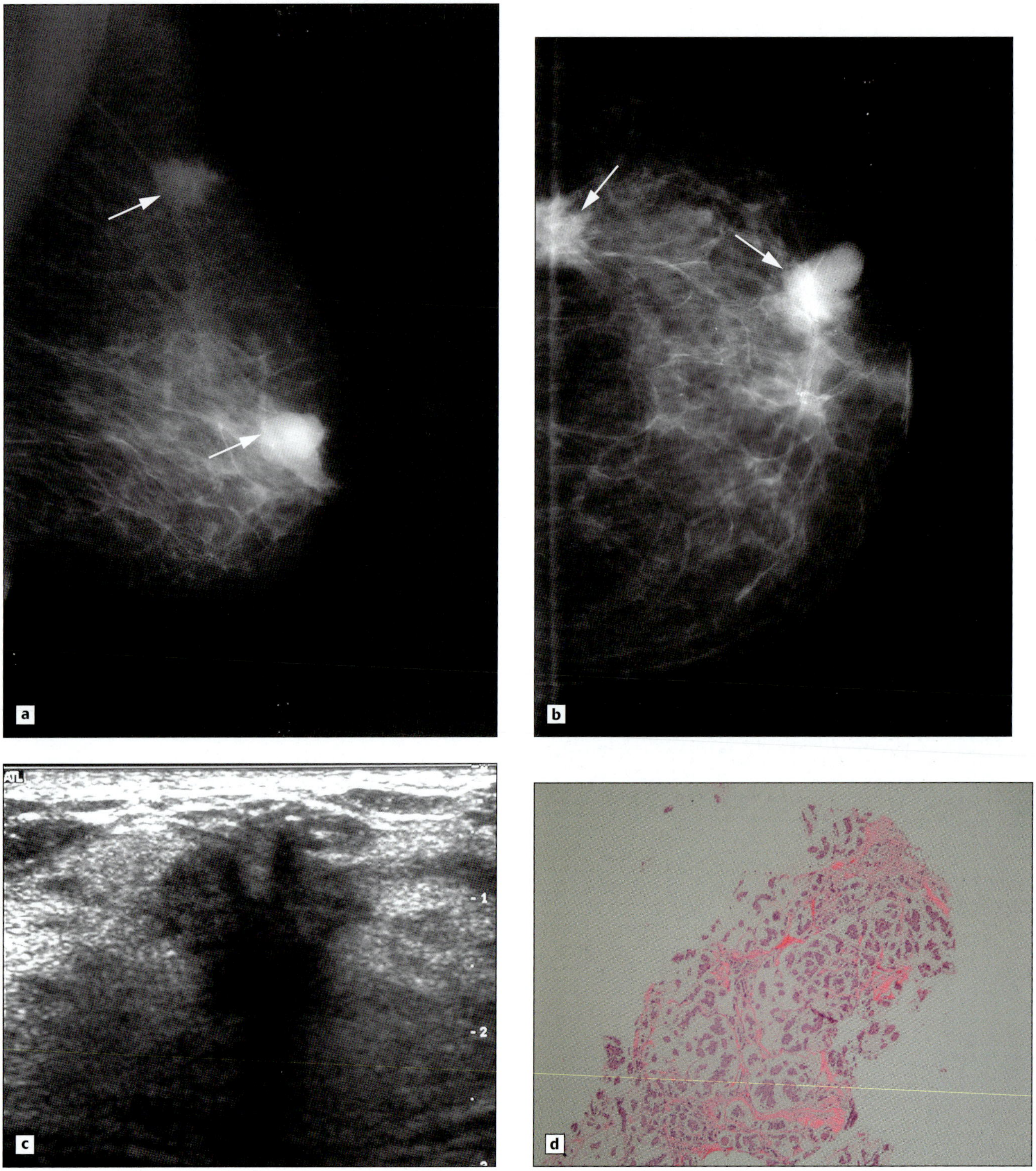

FIGURE 7.4 Multifocal invasive duct carcinoma, micropapillary type. **(a)** MLO and **(b)** CC views of two typical invasive breast cancers. One lesion shows spiculated margins, while the second nodule is dense with multilobulated margins. **(c)** Sonogram revealed a third lesion which was an irregular, taller than wide, hypoechoic mass with angulated margins. **(d)** Core biopsy of all three lesions reveals invasive duct carcinoma composed of groups of tumor cells in mucinous areas as well as in artefactual retraction spaces. The mucinous areas were particularly prevalent in the cores taken from the mammographically dense, microlobulated lesion.

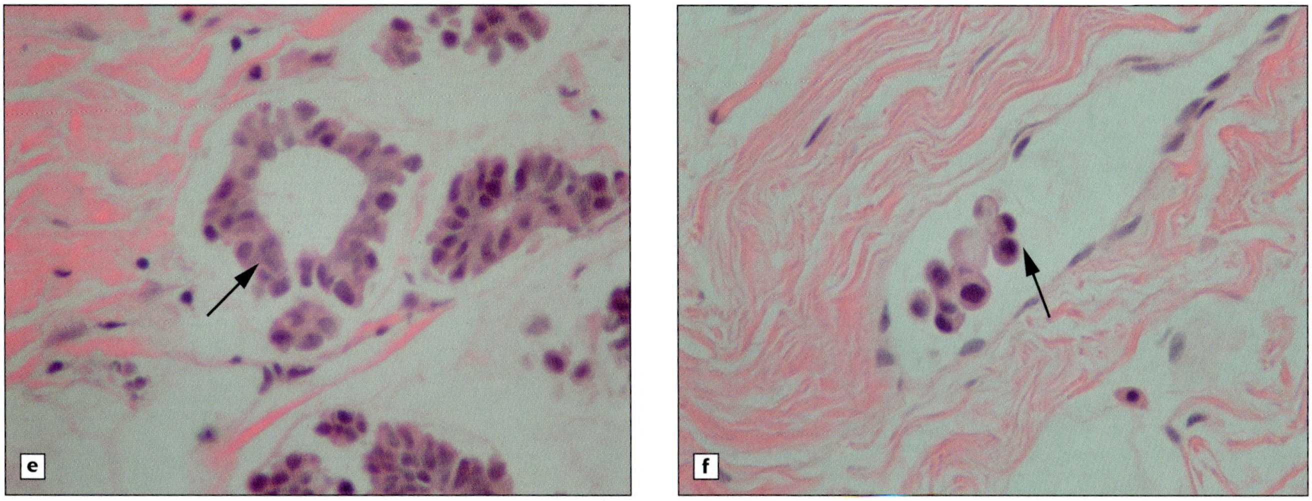

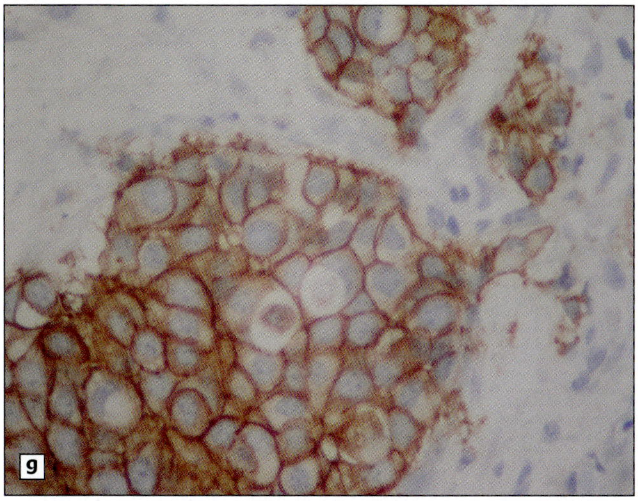

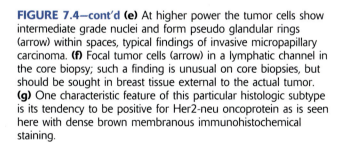

FIGURE 7.4—cont'd **(e)** At higher power the tumor cells show intermediate grade nuclei and form pseudo glandular rings (arrow) within spaces, typical findings of invasive micropapillary carcinoma. **(f)** Focal tumor cells (arrow) in a lymphatic channel in the core biopsy; such a finding is unusual on core biopsies, but should be sought in breast tissue external to the actual tumor. **(g)** One characteristic feature of this particular histologic subtype is its tendency to be positive for Her2-neu oncoprotein as is seen here with dense brown membranous immunohistochemical staining.

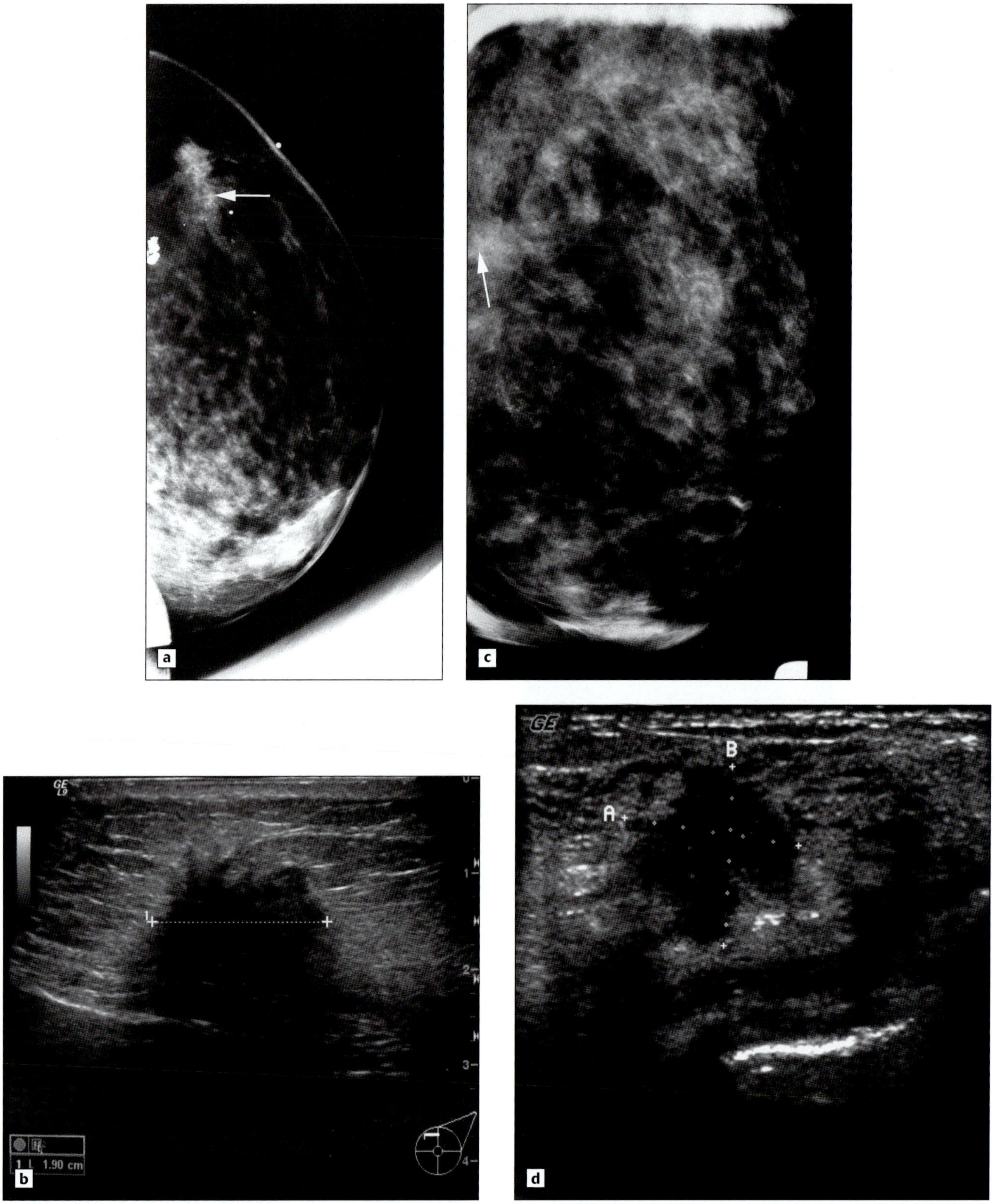

FIGURE 7.5 Two examples of invasive duct carcinoma with calcifications. **(a)** Mammography shows a spiculated density which is associated with a few calcifications (arrow). This mammographic appearance would be suspicious for invasive carcinoma without an extensive intraductal component. **(b)** On sonogram the solid irregular mass measures up to 1.9 cm. **(c)** Mammography of a second case shows a spiculated density (arrow) associated with pleomorphic calcifications which extend outside the mass to widely involve the same quadrant of the breast. This mammographic appearance would be suspicious for invasive carcinoma with extensive intraductal component (EIC). **(d)** Sonography of the second case reveals the hypoechoic irregular mass, measuring up to 1.45 cm.

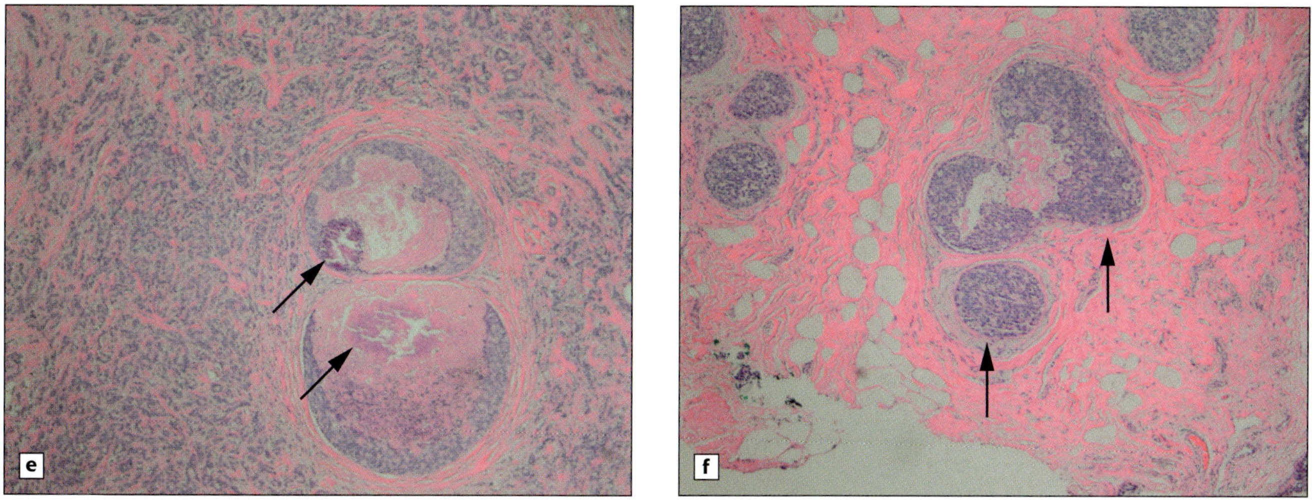

FIGURE 7.5—cont'd **(e)** Core biopsy of both cases revealed identical histology, namely invasive duct carcinoma surrounding intraductal carcinoma of solid type with necrosis and calcification (arrows). Both the intraductal and invasive carcinoma have an intermediate degree of nuclear pleomorphism. **(f)** In both cases, on excision intraductal carcinoma fills ducts (arrows) in breast tissue clearly external to the tumor mass.

with that assessed on excision;[8,9] histologic grade, however, does show a greater rate of discordance in most series.[10–13] Similarly, routine markers such as estrogen receptor protein (ER), progesterone receptor protein (PR), and Her2-neu oncoprotein have correlated well when studied on both types of specimen.[14–18] We routinely assess invasive tumor type and grade since they can be clinically useful parameters when reported on core biopsies. Armed with the knowledge that an invasive duct carcinoma is tubular or well differentiated, a surgeon might perform only a sentinel lymph node biopsy rather than remove any additional lymph nodes because of the low likelihood of nodal metastasis in these tumors. Conversely, a diagnosis of invasive micropapillary carcinoma with lymphatic invasion would tell the surgeon that he or she should perform a sentinel node procedure and at least minimal additional axillary dissection since lymphatic invasion is one of the factors associated with increased risk of non-sentinel lymph node metastasis;[19] therefore, sentinel node sampling alone may not be adequate axillary surgery in such patients. Occasionally histologic problems in classification of malignancy can be aided by knowledge of imaging findings. For example, colloid carcinoma can be seen in combination with invasive micropapillary carcinoma; however, a true mucinous carcinoma with its attendant excellent prognosis is a well-circumscribed tumor as opposed to invasive micropapillary carcinoma which is usually irregular.[20] Simple excision (lumpectomy) and sentinel node excision are nearly always sufficient for the former but often not for the latter.

We do not as a rule report invasive tumor size or perform marker studies on core biopsies unless the entire infiltrating tumor has been removed by the biopsy or the patient will be receiving preoperative chemotherapy (in which case we will perform ER/PR and Her2-neu testing). Reporting the size of invasive tumor on a core biopsy may be inaccurate and potentially misleading. We believe size is more accurately assessed by a combination of gross and microscopic measurement performed on surgical excision and that its measurement is not significantly altered by core biopsy.[21] By judiciously withholding this information on core, we avoid the possible situation whereby a clinician may unwittingly overestimate the invasive tumor size by adding together the tumor size reported on core biopsy and that on excision. The potential clinical applications are profound since most patients with invasive tumors measuring greater than 1.0 cm are treated with some form of chemotherapy. We prefer to perform ER/PR and Her2-neu on excision specimens since these specimens simply contain more tumor tissue to evaluate. Since the tests' interpretation depends in part on the percentage of tumor cells that are positive, the results are more representative of the entire tumor when a block of the excision specimen is selected for study. More importantly perhaps, no clinical decisions are generally made on the basis of this information at the time of core biopsy.

Of course, not all image-detected irregular densities of the breast prove to be invasive carcinomas. The differential diagnosis includes fat necrosis, post-surgical scarring, duct ectasia, and radial scar. Fat necrosis (essentially an inflammatory reaction with damage to adipocytes) can be traumatic or idiopathic in origin but can be accompanied by dense, even hyalinizing, fibrosis which can simulate malignancy.[22] It has a broad spectrum of presentation ranging from a palpable mass, spiculated mass on mammography (Fig 7.6), to oil cysts, or eggshell, lacy, coarse, and fine calcifications (see Chap. 12). Sometimes the patient relates a history of trauma; however the most common external etiology is prior biopsy, lumpectomy, or reduction mammoplasty. Core biopsies will reveal variably sized fat-containing histiocytes, chronic inflammation, and fibrosis. Such lesions should, however, be examined carefully for malignancy since fat necrosis can accompany carcinoma.

Scarring and a foreign body reaction are usually encountered in core biopsies performed to evaluate mammographic changes in follow-up studies months to years after surgery, lumpectomy, and/or radiation therapy. A spiculated mass may be the result of scarring from prior surgery (Fig 7.7). This focal distortion is often connected to localized changes in the overlying skin, i.e., retraction. Scars should diminish in density with time, are often seen better in one compression view than another, and tend to change configuration with cone compression or rolled views, while a breast cancer will maintain its shape on two views and often becomes more prominent when the surrounding breast tissue is compressed with a cone view.

Duct ectasia can simulate invasive carcinoma when it occurs at branching points of major ducts.[23] Core biopsy will show fibrosis and histologic findings identical to those described above (Fig. 7.7) except for the changes attributable to the cyst wall and the prominence of foamy histiocytes in the cystic form.

Radial scars are irregular spiculated lesions that can mimic a breast cancer both mammographically and sonographically (see also chapter 8 on architectural distortion), although classically the spicules are thinner and longer in a radial scar, and there is often central lucency on mammography. The histologic distinction of radial scar from invasive carcinoma on core biopsy can be difficult but often depends on the lack of glands directly invading adipose tissue (see Chap. 8 for a full discussion).

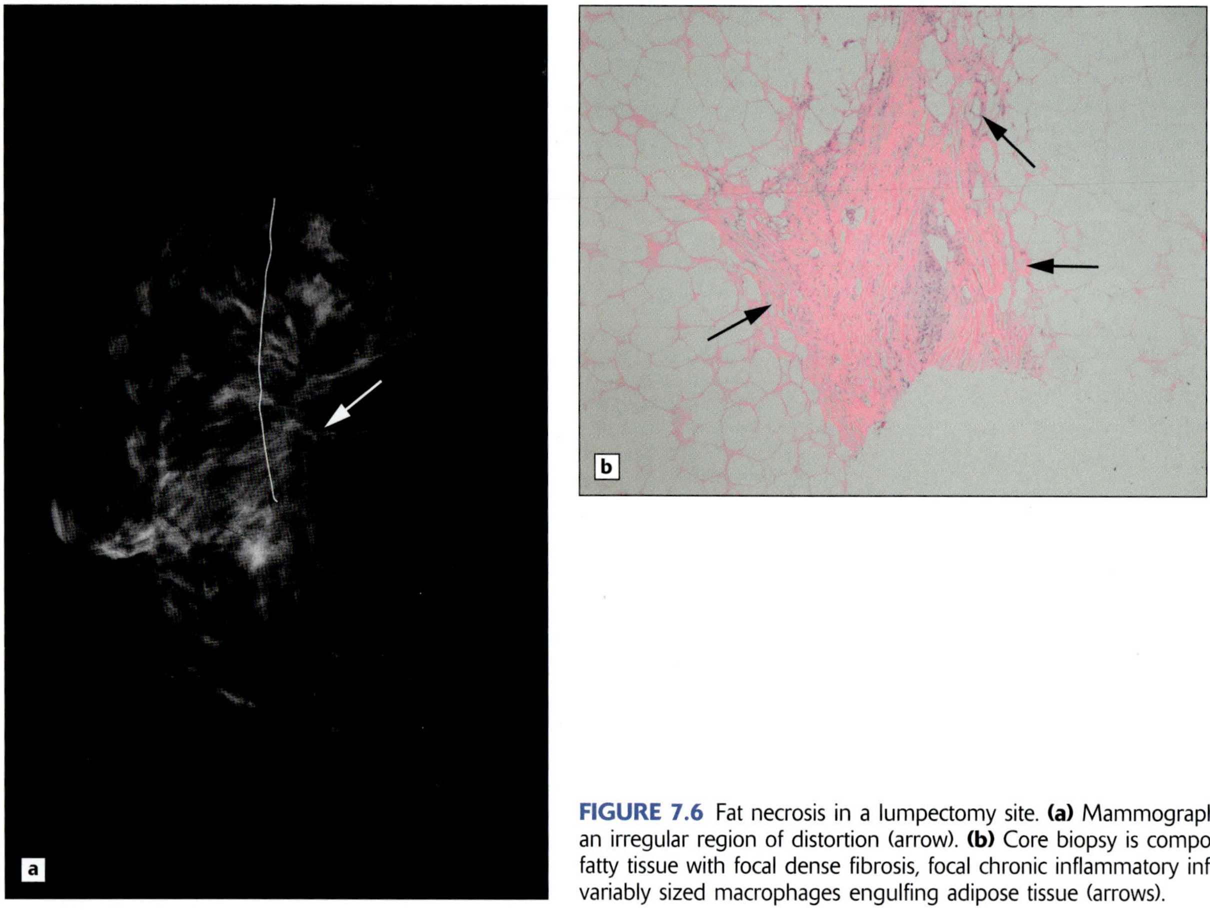

FIGURE 7.6 Fat necrosis in a lumpectomy site. **(a)** Mammography shows an irregular region of distortion (arrow). **(b)** Core biopsy is composed of fatty tissue with focal dense fibrosis, focal chronic inflammatory infiltrate, and variably sized macrophages engulfing adipose tissue (arrows).

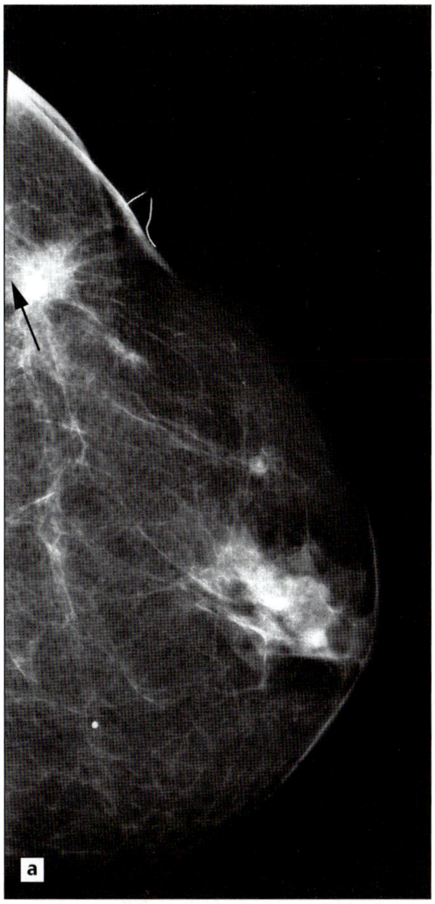

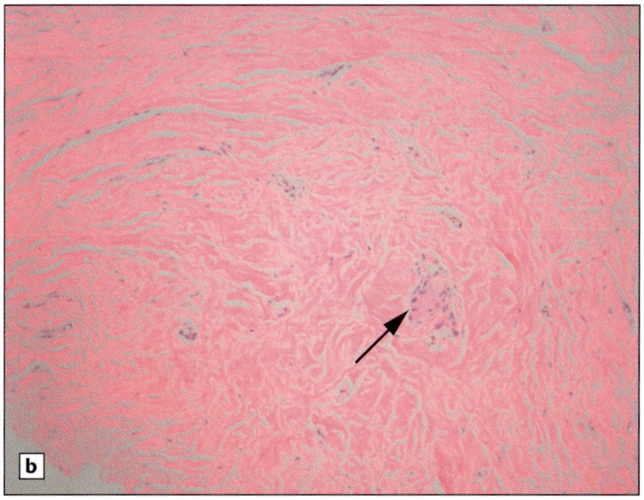

FIGURE 7.7 Scar in a lumpectomy site. **(a)** Mammography reveals an irregular radiodensity (arrow) with retraction of the overlying skin. **(b)** Histologically scarring is composed of dense fibrosis and clustered foreign body type giant cells (a granulomatous reaction – arrow) indicating prior manipulation.

Differential diagnoses of irregular densities

- Infiltrating duct carcinoma
- Fat necrosis
- Scar
- Duct ectasia

POINTS TO REMEMBER

1. The grade and type of invasive carcinoma on core biopsy may influence the choice of subsequent surgical procedure.
2. Reporting size of invasive tumor on core biopsy can be inaccurate and misleading.
3. ER/PR/Her2-neu testing is usually unnecessary on core biopsy and is more representative on excision specimens.

REFERENCES

1. Luna-More S, Gonzalez B, Acedo C, et al. Invasive micropapillary carcinoma of the breast. A new special type of invasive mammary carcinoma. Pathol Res Pract 190:668–674,1994.
2. Walsh MM, and Bleiweiss IJ. Invasive micropapillary carcinoma of the breast: Eighty cases of an under recognized entity. Hum Pathol 32:583–589,2001.
3. Paterakos M, Watkin WG, Edgerton SM, et al. Invasive micropapillary carcinoma of the breast: a prognostic study. Hum Pathol 30:1459–1463,1999.
4. Connolly JL, Schnitt SJ. Evaluation of breast biopsy specimens in patients considered for treatment by conservative surgery and radiation therapy for early breast cancer. Pathol Annu 23:1–23,1988.
5. Jimenez RE, Bongers S, Bouwman D, et al. Clinicopathologic significance of ductal carcinoma in situ in breast core needle biopsies with invasive cancer. Am J Surg Pathol 24:123–128,2000.
6. Dzierzanowski M, Melville KA, Barnes PJ, et al. Ductal carcinoma in situ in core biopsies containing invasive breast cancer: correlation with extensive intraductal component and lumpectomy margins. J Surg Oncol 80:71–76,2005.

*7. Hoda SA, Rosen PP. Practical considerations in the pathologic diagnosis of needle core biopsies of breast. Am J Clin Pathol 118:101–108,2002.

8. Deshpande A, Garud T, Holt SD. Core biopsy as a tool in planning the management of invasive breast cancer. World J Surg Oncol 3:1;2005.
9. Harris GC, Denley HE, Pinder SE, et al. Correlation of histologic prognostic factors in core biopsies and therapeutic excisions of invasive breast carcinoma. Am J Surg Pathol 27:11–15;2003.
10. Connor CS, Tawfik OW, Joyce AJ, et al. A comparison of prognostic tumor markers obtained on image-guided breast biopsies and final surgical specimens. Am J Surg 184:322–324,2002.
11. Badoual C, Maruani A, Ghorrra C, et al. Pathological prognostic factors of invasive breast carcinoma in ultrasound-guided large core biopsies-correlation with subsequent surgical excisions. Breast 14:22–27;2005.
12. Monticciolo DL. Histologic grading at breast core needle biopsy: comparison with results from the excised breast specimen. Breast J 11:9–14;2005.
13. Andrade VP, Gobbi H. Accuracy of typing and grading invasive mammary carcinoma on core needle biopsy compared with the excisional specimen. Virchows Arch 445:597–602;2004.
14. Jacobs T, Siziopikou KP, Prioleau JE, et al. Do prognostic marker studies on core needle biopsy specimens of breast carcinoma accurately reflect the marker status of the tumor? Mod Pathol 11: 259–264,1998.
15. Hodi Z, Chakrabarti J, Lee AH, et al. The reliability of oestrogen receptor expression on needle core biopsies of invasive carcinoma of the breast. J Clin Pathol 60:299–302,2007.
16. Cahill RA, Walsh D, Landers RJ, Watson RG. Preoperative profiling of symptomatic breast cancer by diagnostic core biopsy. Ann Surg Oncol 13:45–51,2006.
17. Al Sarakbi W, Salhab M, Thomas V, Mokbel K. Is preoperative core biopsy accurate in determining the hormone receptor status in women with invasive breast cancer? In press Int Semin Surg Oncol 2:15,2005.

18. Burge CN, Chang HR, Apple SK. Do the histologic features and results of breast cancer biomarker studies differ between core biopsy and surgical excision specimens. Breast 15:167–172,2006.
19. Sachdev U, Murphy K, Derzie A, et al. Predictors of nonsentinel lymph node metastasis in breast cancer patients. Am J Surg 183:213–217,2002.
20. Gunhan-Bilgen I, Zekioglu O, Ustun EE, et al. Invasive micropapillary carcinoma of the breast: clinical, mammographic, and sonographic findings with histopathologic correlation. AJR Am J Roentgenol 179:927–931,2002.
21. Charles M, Edge SB, Winston JS, et al. Effects of stereotactic core needle biopsy on pathologic measurement of tumor size of T1 breast carcinomas presenting as mammographic masses. Cancer 97:2137–2141,2003.
22. Bilgen IG, Ustun EE, Memis A. Fat necrosis of the breast: clinical, mammographic and sonographic features. Eur J Radiol 2001 39:92–99,2001.
23. Sweeney DJ, Wylie EJ. Mammographic appearances of mammary duct ectasia that mimic carcinoma in a screening programme. Australas Radiol 39:18–23,1995.

CHAPTER

8

Spiculated architectural distortion

A radial scar may present as a spiculated mass or region of architectural distortion on mammography.[1] The spicules are often longer with less central density than those seen in a carcinoma (Fig. 8.1). This appearance corresponds to the pathologic condition in which ductal elements are surrounded by bands of fibrous connective tissue radiating from a central sclerotic focus. Radial scars may also contain microcalcifications. Despite the name, radial scars are not related to scarring. Their etiology is a matter of some controversy with some authors hypothesizing that they result from local inflammation and or chronic ischemia,[2] while others believe they are related to intraductal papilloma.[3] Most radial scars are microscopic in size (<4.0 mm) and thus are often incidental findings.[4] The small proportion that are detected clinically are identified mammographically or sonographically since they are too small to be palpable.

Radial scar is most confidently diagnosed by evaluating the entire lesion as a continuous whole. Characteristically it consists of a relatively fibrotic center and a more cellular periphery. The peripheral zones show florid duct hyperplasia often forming papillae with fibrous cores. Small tubular glands composed of two cell layers are present in both zones but are more frequent peripherally. The glands are round or elongated and, importantly, do not directly invade the fat. Varying amounts of elastosis are characteristic but by no means pathognomonic of radial scar (Fig. 8.2). Given the importance of examining the overall architecture of the entire lesion, it may be difficult to definitively diagnose radial scar on the basis of core biopsy alone. Partly for this reason, we generally recommend surgical excision unless the radial scar is tiny and incidental to the density or calcifications being targeted, in which case it has probably already been totally excised. As is the case with atypical duct hyperplasia (see Chap. 13), with the advent of vacuum-assisted stereotactic core biopsies the rate of underestimation for radial scars has also decreased and is directly related to retrieval of multiple larger tissue specimens. In one study, the false negative rate was non-existent for vacuum assisted mammotome core biopsies in contrast to 9% using a spring-loaded device.[5] Core biopsy based diagnosis of radial scar is more reliable when the lesion presents as a mammographic mass rather than architectural distortion and when >12 samples are obtained.

The most obvious differential diagnosis for a radial scar is tubular carcinoma, both from pathologic and imaging points of view. While the two cannot be distinguished based on imaging studies, histologically tubular carcinoma is composed of small, well-formed, focally angulated glands lined by a single cell layer and occasional calcifications (Fig. 8.3). The glands should be evenly dispersed across both the center and periphery of the lesion and directly invade into adipose tissue. Thus, as with radial scar, the ideal situation would include evaluation of the entire geography of the lesion, yet, in our experience, a definitive core biopsy-based diagnosis of tubular carcinoma is possible. We require the direct invasion of fat at the periphery of the lesion to make the diagnosis on core biopsy and reserve immunohistochemistry (to demonstrate lack of myoepithelial cells) for difficult lesions (Fig. 8.4).

One of the more frequent diagnostic dilemmas which we see in our consultation practice is the distinction between DCIS involving a radial scar and invasive duct carcinoma. When DCIS (of any grade) is present in an area otherwise showing the typical configuration of radial scar (Fig. 8.5), we are averse to diagnosing invasive carcinoma unless the tumor cells directly invade adipose tissue. In a similar vein, one will occasionally find DCIS involving foci of sclerosing adenosis (Fig. 8.6a). In such areas microinvasion is considered when the tumor cells no longer reside in rounded, well-defined structures and/or directly infiltrate fat (Fig. 8.6b). We believe it is impossible to rule out microinvasive carcinoma in some such situations, even with the use of immunohistochemistry, and therefore we feel that excision with or without sentinel lymph node sampling is an acceptable next step in management regardless of whether or not invasion is definitively diagnosed in such lesions.

The above situations bring up the question of the premalignant potential of radial scars. In the literature radial scars have been associated with atypia[6] or malignancy (up to 50% of cases), specifically tubular carcinoma[7] (Fig. 8.7). Some authors[4,7] have noted not only the differential diagnosis of tubular carcinoma but also the association

Text continued on p. 90

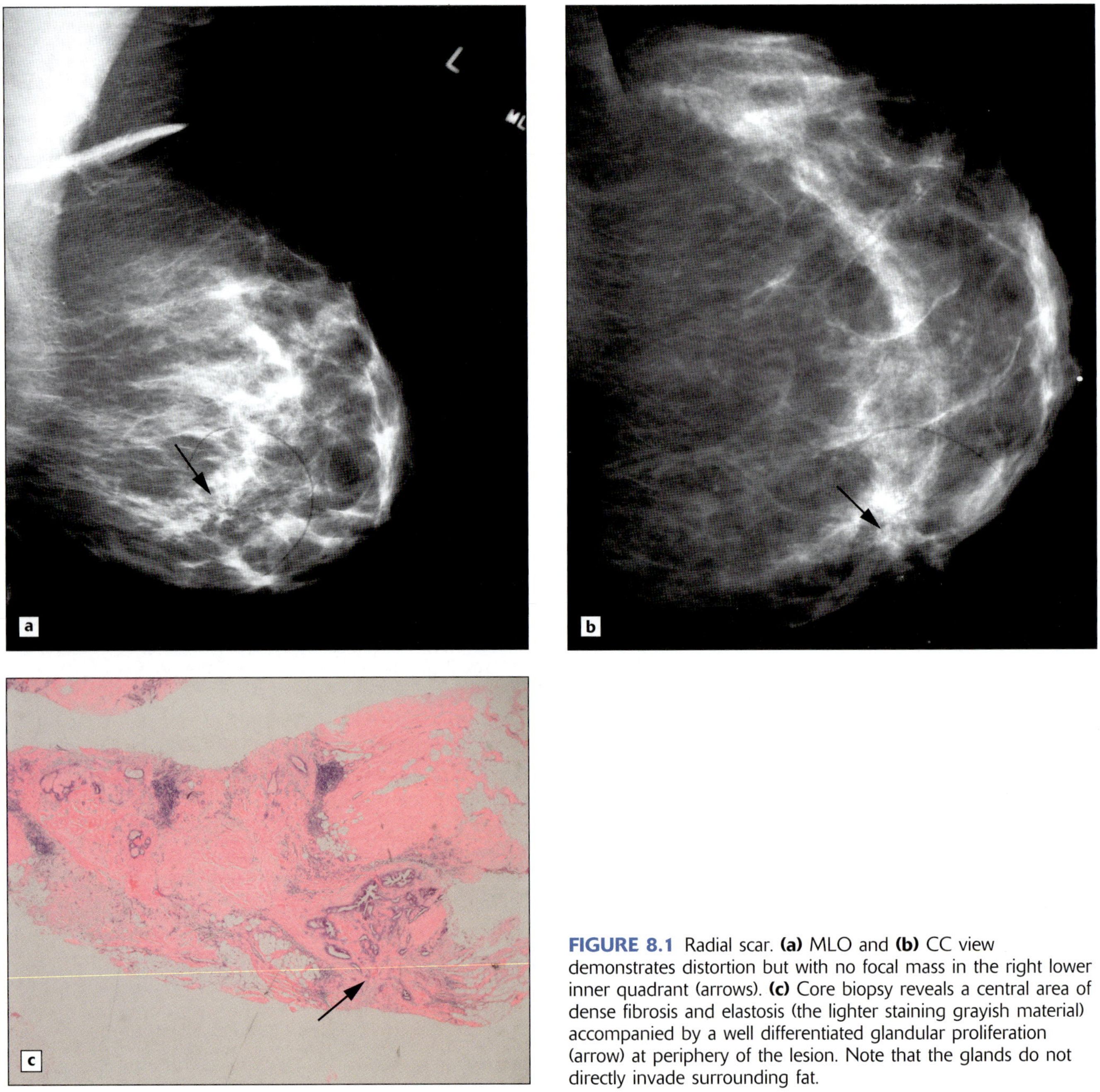

FIGURE 8.1 Radial scar. **(a)** MLO and **(b)** CC view demonstrates distortion but with no focal mass in the right lower inner quadrant (arrows). **(c)** Core biopsy reveals a central area of dense fibrosis and elastosis (the lighter staining grayish material) accompanied by a well differentiated glandular proliferation (arrow) at periphery of the lesion. Note that the glands do not directly invade surrounding fat.

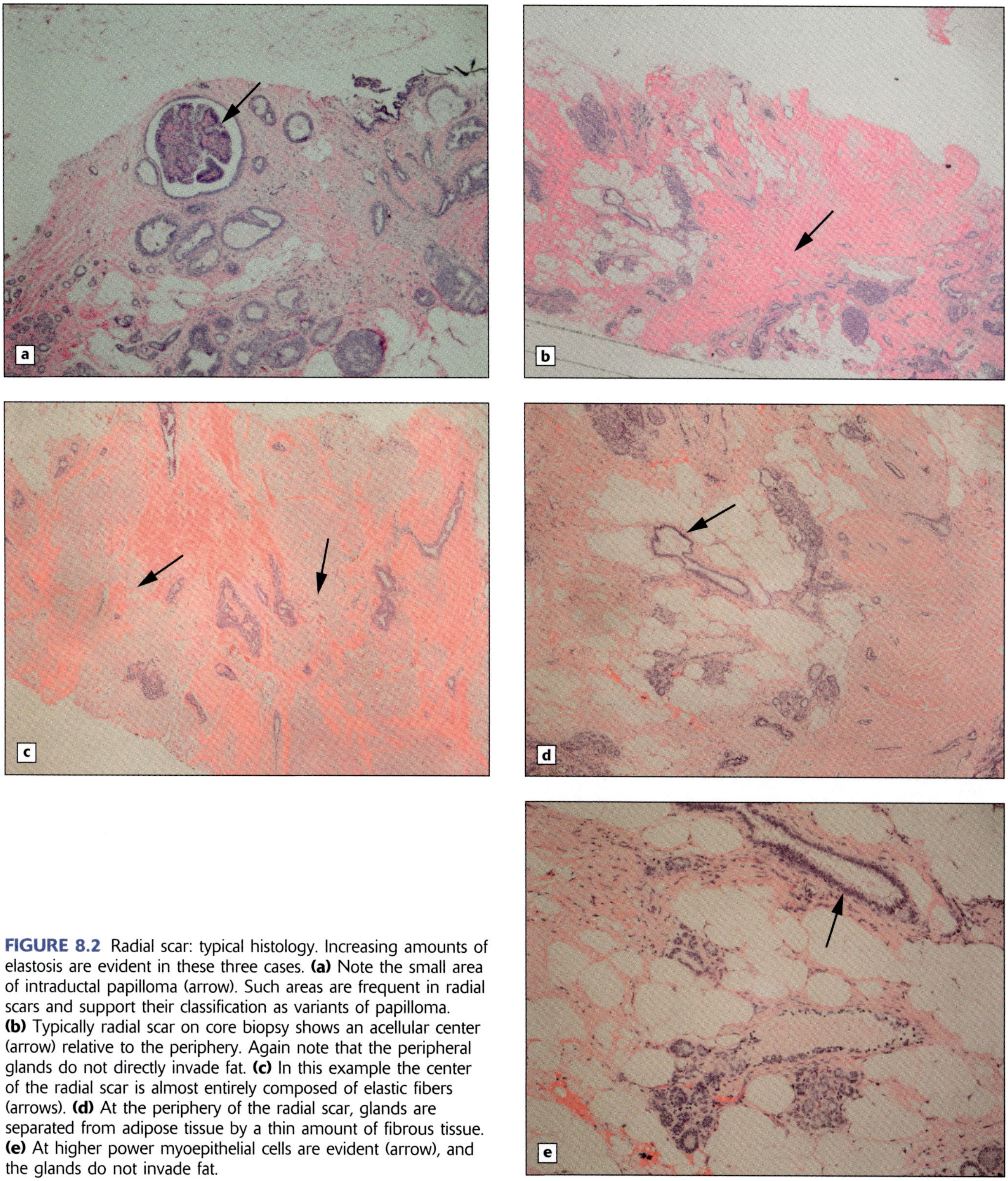

FIGURE 8.2 Radial scar: typical histology. Increasing amounts of elastosis are evident in these three cases. **(a)** Note the small area of intraductal papilloma (arrow). Such areas are frequent in radial scars and support their classification as variants of papilloma. **(b)** Typically radial scar on core biopsy shows an acellular center (arrow) relative to the periphery. Again note that the peripheral glands do not directly invade fat. **(c)** In this example the center of the radial scar is almost entirely composed of elastic fibers (arrows). **(d)** At the periphery of the radial scar, glands are separated from adipose tissue by a thin amount of fibrous tissue. **(e)** At higher power myoepithelial cells are evident (arrow), and the glands do not invade fat.

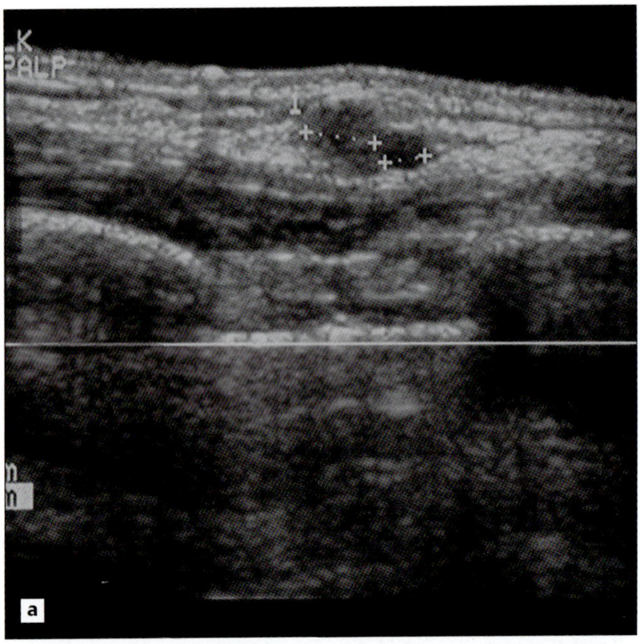

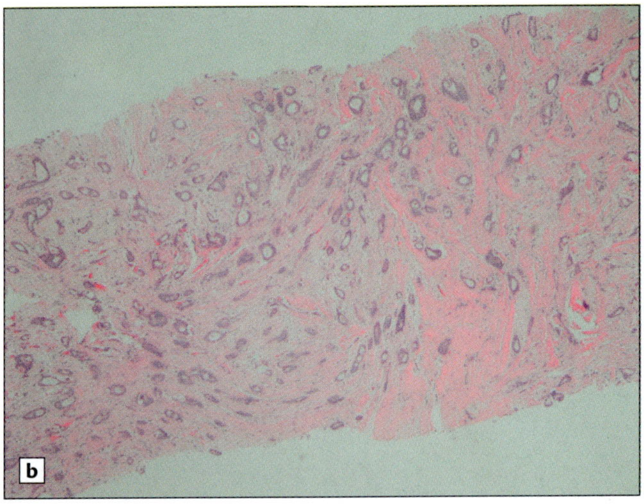

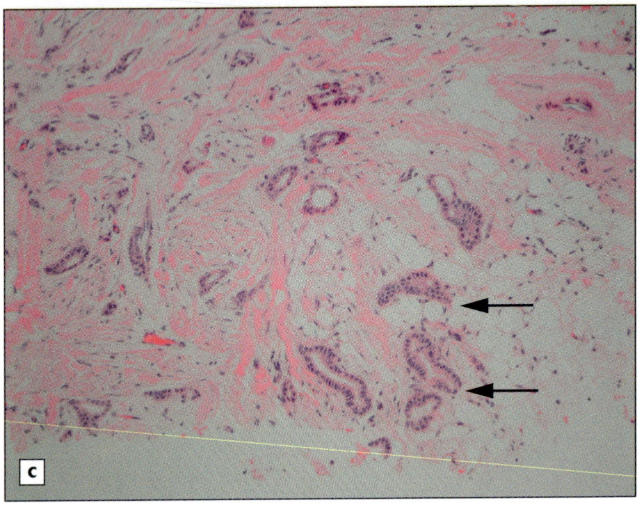

FIGURE 8.3 Tubular carcinoma. **(a)** Sonography demonstrates a hypoechoic slightly taller than wide microlobulated solid mass. This is superficial and palpable in nature. **(b)** Core biopsy reveals a uniform glandular proliferation which is dispersed evenly across the core. **(c)** At higher power the well-formed glands are composed of a single cell population, devoid of myoepithelial cells, directly invading adipose tissue (arrows) at the periphery of the core.

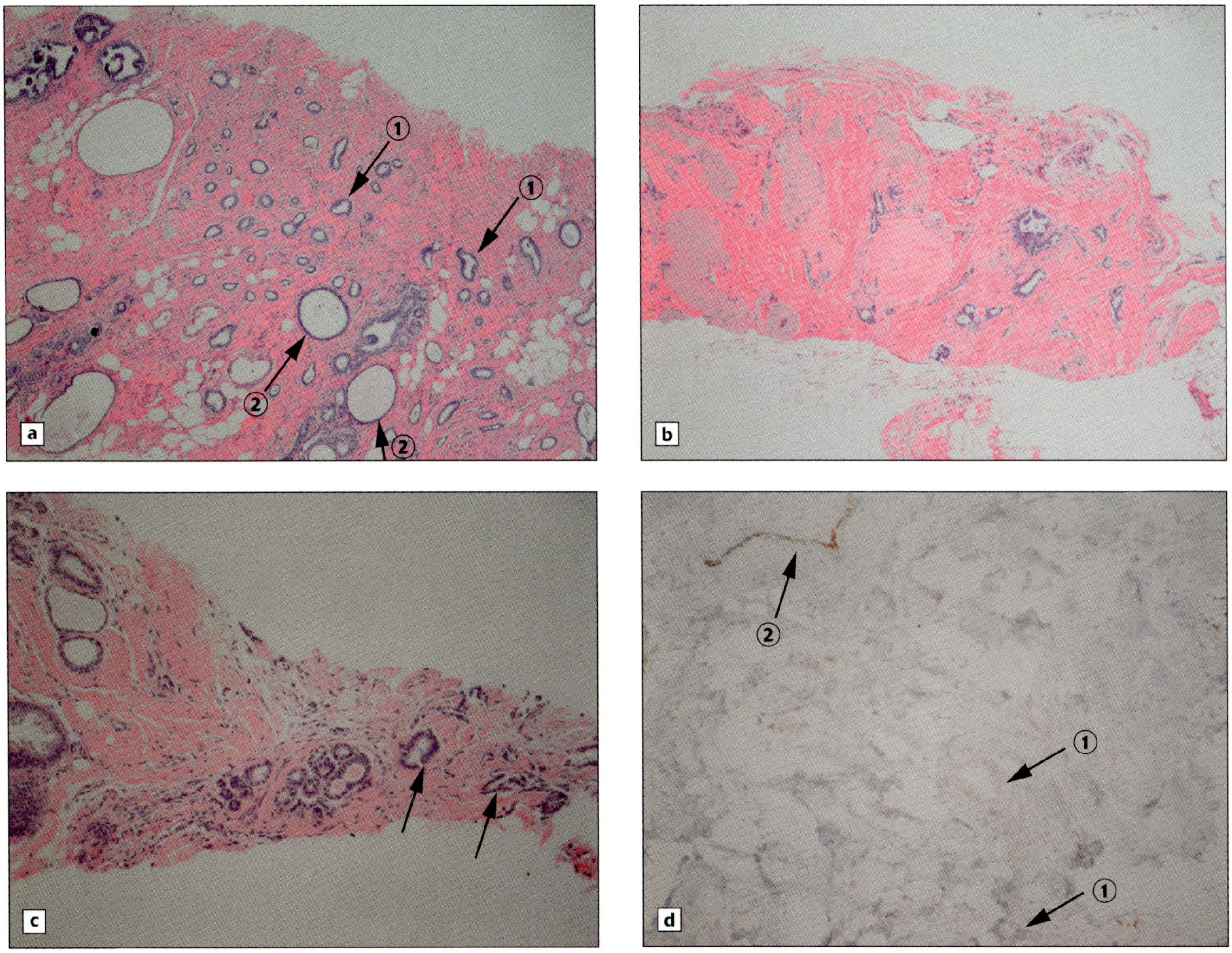

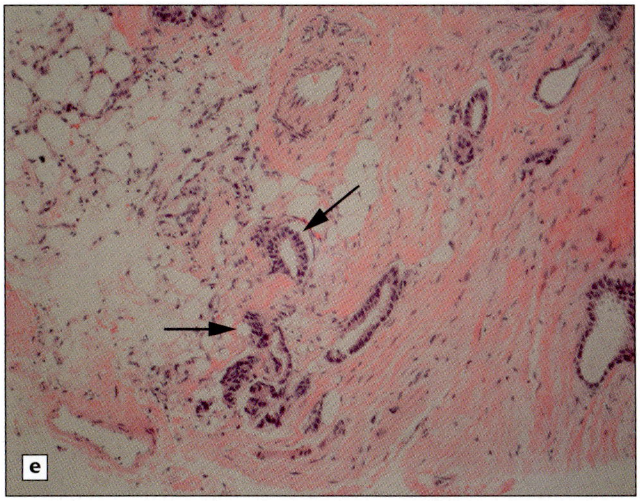

FIGURE 8.4 Tubular carcinoma. **(a)** Occasional cases may present difficulty either in separating the neoplastic glands (arrow 1) from the surrounding normal breast tissue (arrow 2) or **(b)** because the glandular proliferation is central amidst elastosis, blurring the distinction from radial scar. **(c)** In this example several glands are suspicious (arrows), and, in difficult cases such as this, immunohistochemistry **(d)** is valuable in order to demonstrate lack of myoepithelial cells (p-63 negativity for example – arrow) 1 in tubular carcinoma. The benign glands at the top left (arrow 2) serve as a built-in positive control. **(e)** We have found direct invasion of adipose tissue (arrows) to be a reliable criterion for the diagnosis of tubular carcinoma.

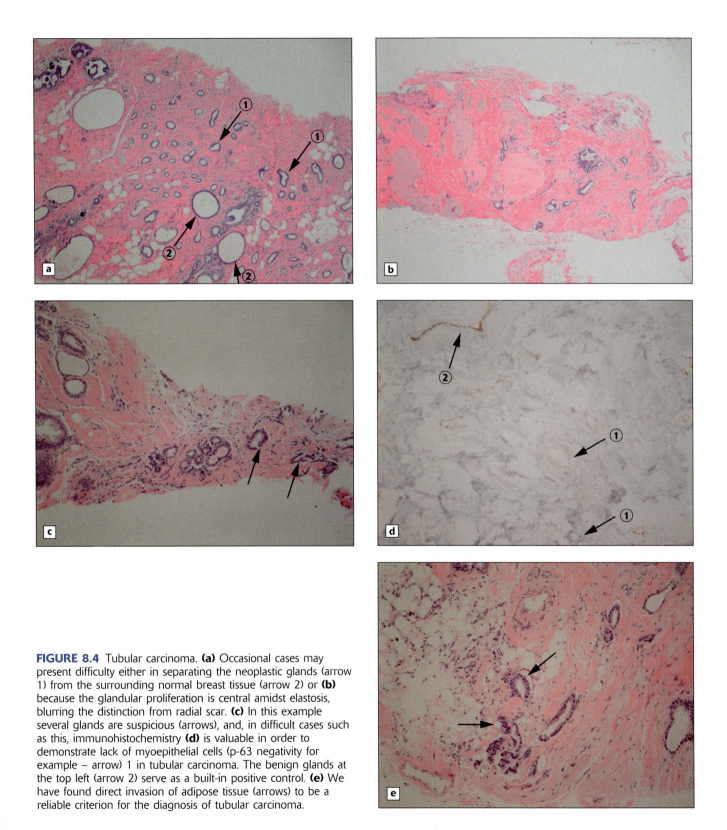

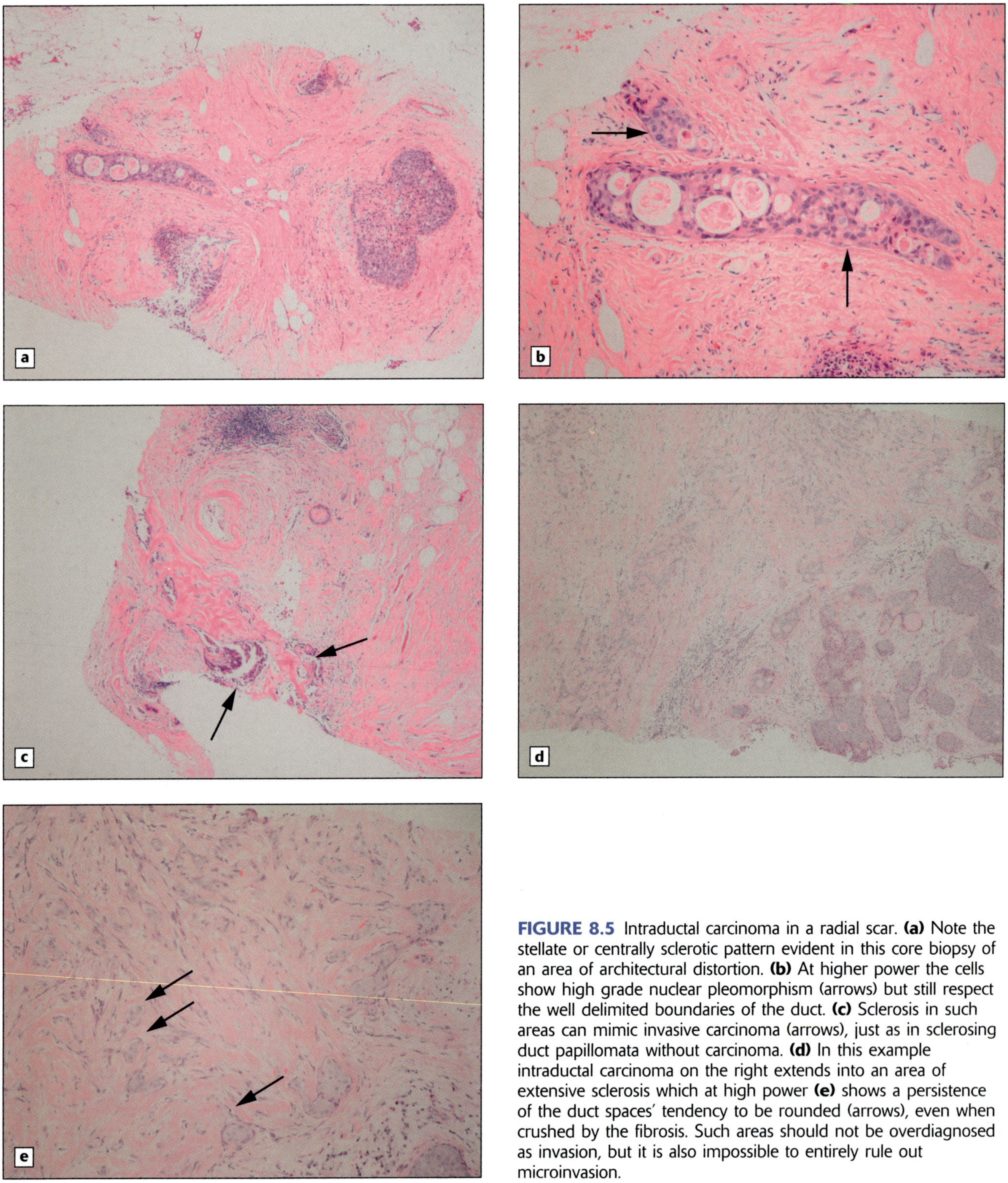

FIGURE 8.5 Intraductal carcinoma in a radial scar. **(a)** Note the stellate or centrally sclerotic pattern evident in this core biopsy of an area of architectural distortion. **(b)** At higher power the cells show high grade nuclear pleomorphism (arrows) but still respect the well delimited boundaries of the duct. **(c)** Sclerosis in such areas can mimic invasive carcinoma (arrows), just as in sclerosing duct papillomata without carcinoma. **(d)** In this example intraductal carcinoma on the right extends into an area of extensive sclerosis which at high power **(e)** shows a persistence of the duct spaces' tendency to be rounded (arrows), even when crushed by the fibrosis. Such areas should not be overdiagnosed as invasion, but it is also impossible to entirely rule out microinvasion.

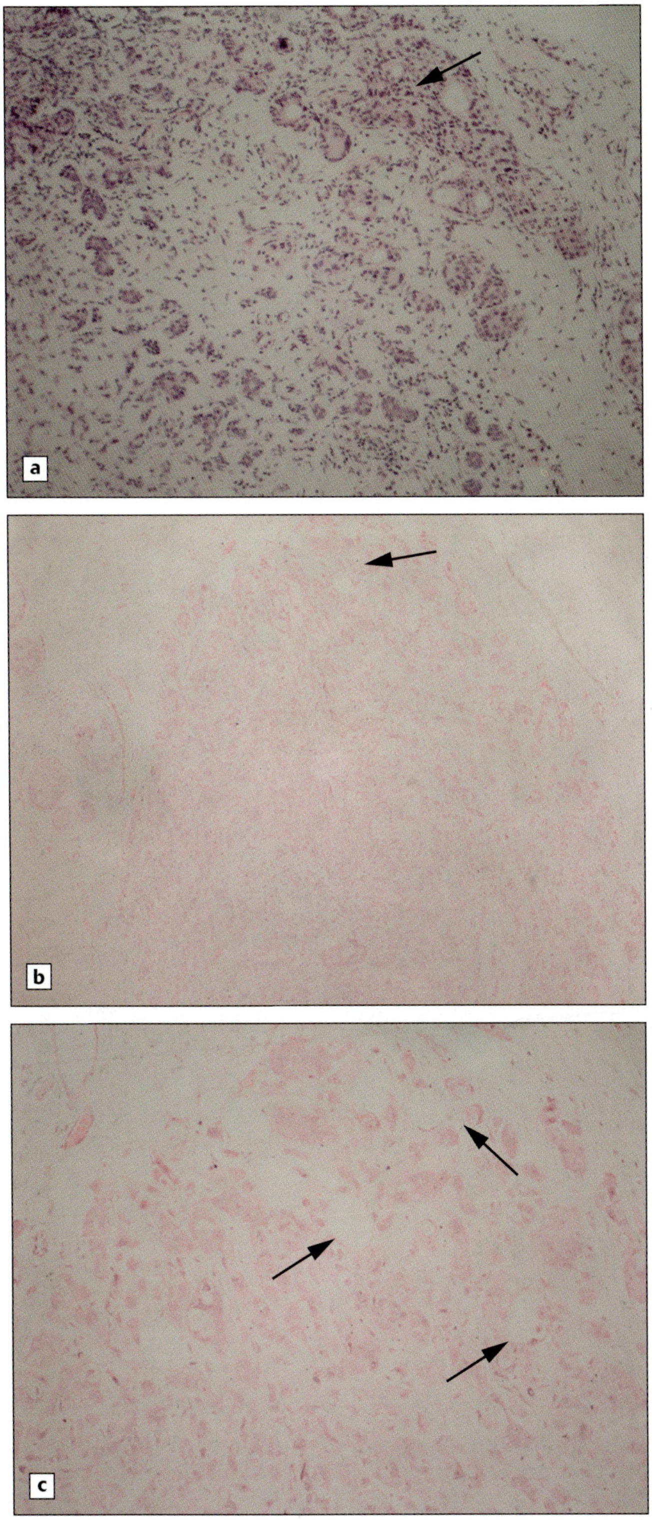

FIGURE 8.6 Intraductal carcinoma involving sclerosing adenosis. **(a)** High nuclear grade intraductal carcinoma (arrow) extending into areas of sclerosing adenosis by expanding the acini, but maintaining the underlying benign pattern. **(b)** In contrast invasive carcinoma can sometimes mimic this pattern, causing diagnostic difficulties; however, the distinction can be made by recognizing direct invasion of fat (arrow) in the latter. **(c)** Note the remaining adipocytes enveloped by the tumor at its leading edge (arrows).

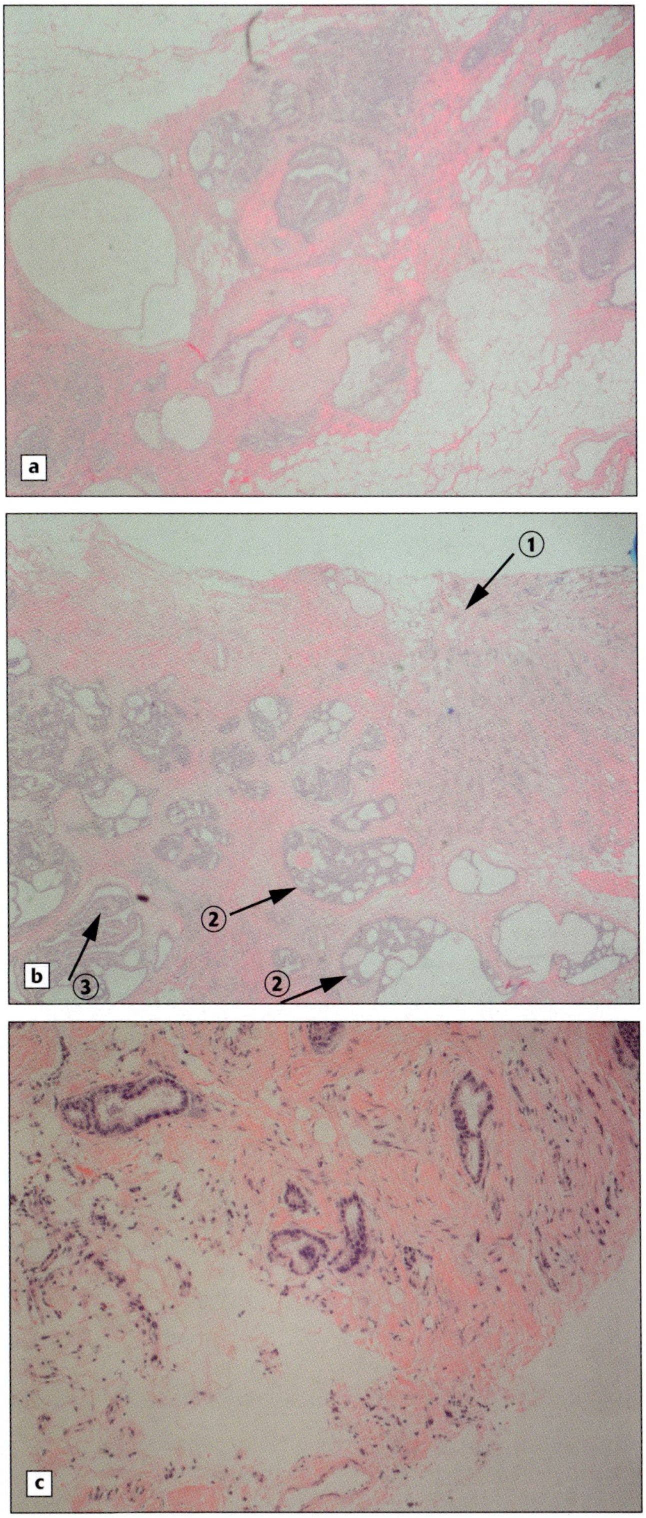

FIGURE 8.7 Tubular carcinoma and intraductal carcinoma in radial scar. **(a)** This core biopsy of architectural distortion shows typical radial scar histology with peripheral glands, central elastosis, and tiny foci of intraductal papilloma, yet a second core biopsy of the same lesion **(b)** reveals tubular carcinoma (arrow 1) adjacent to intraductal carcinoma (arrow 2) involving the radial scar. Note the small area of intraductal papilloma (arrow 3) and the fact that the tubular carcinoma invades fat, seen best at high power of a different focus **(c)**.

of radial scar with tubular and other forms of invasive carcinoma elsewhere in the breast, i.e., that radial scar is at least a twofold risk factor for the development of infiltrating carcinoma in either breast (somewhat akin to a diagnosis of atypical duct hyperplasia or lobular neoplasia), especially with increasing size (>4.0–6.0 mm) and increasing age of the patient (>50 years).[8] Some authors (ourselves included) consider radial scar to be a variant of sclerosing duct papilloma.[3] Thus, if one considers sclerosing duct papilloma a premalignant lesion, one's opinion should carry forward to radial scar as well. For this and all the other reasons outlined above, we feel that all radial scars diagnosed on core biopsy should be surgically excised if they constitute the lesion of radiographic interest.[9] Logically, it is the larger radial scars that are detected mammographically, and these are more likely to be associated with carcinoma. Finally while tubular carcinomas are indolent, extremely slow growing tumors with excellent prognoses, they can occasionally progress in grade (Fig. 8.8) and thus warrant complete excision.

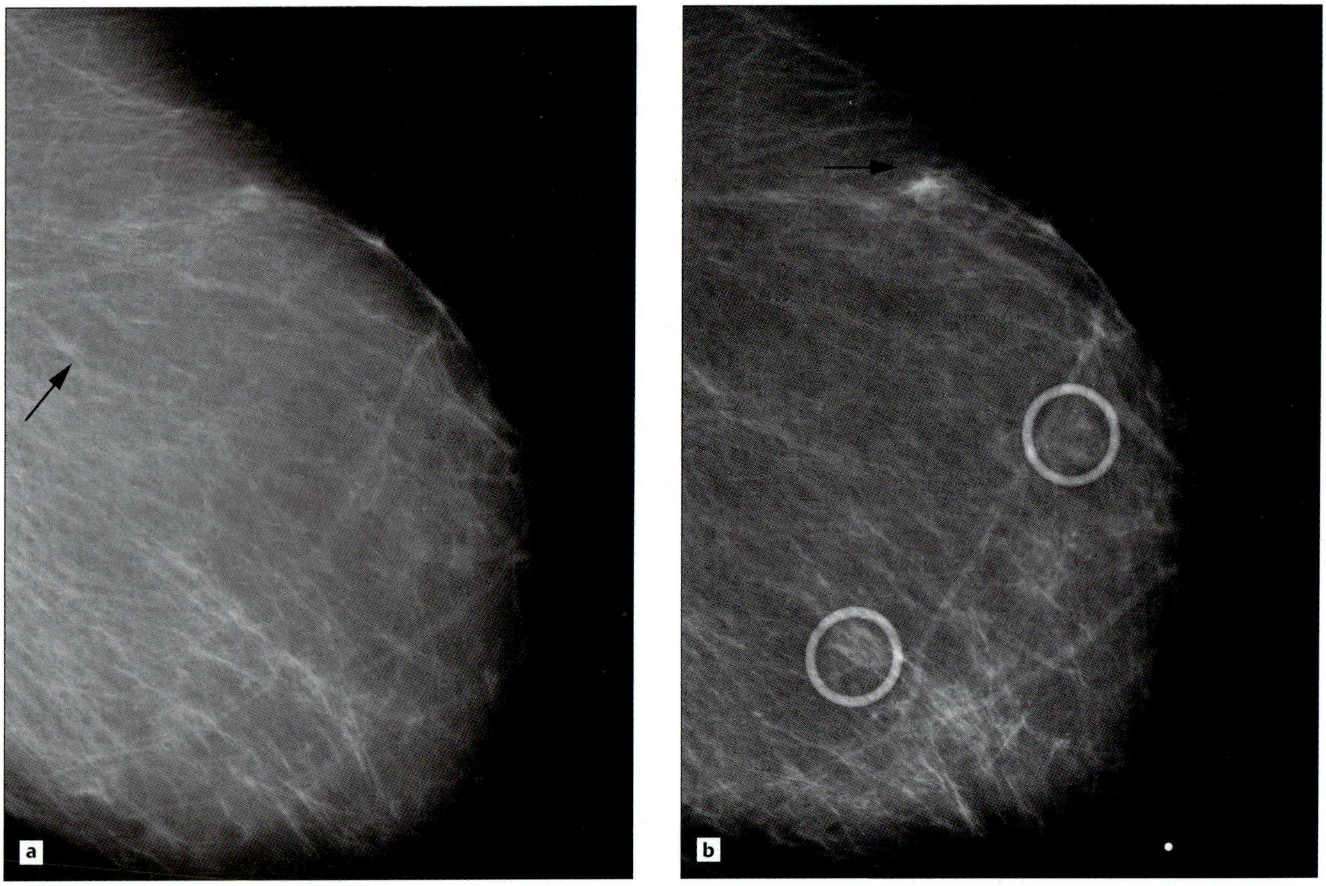

FIGURE 8.8 Tubular carcinoma and invasive well differentiated duct carcinoma. **(a)** Screening mammography in a 61-year-old woman demonstrated an irregular nodular density that measured 4 mm (arrow) in diameter at the upper outer quadrant of her right breast. **(b)** Two years later the nodule appeared denser and larger (arrow), measuring approximately 5 mm in diameter.

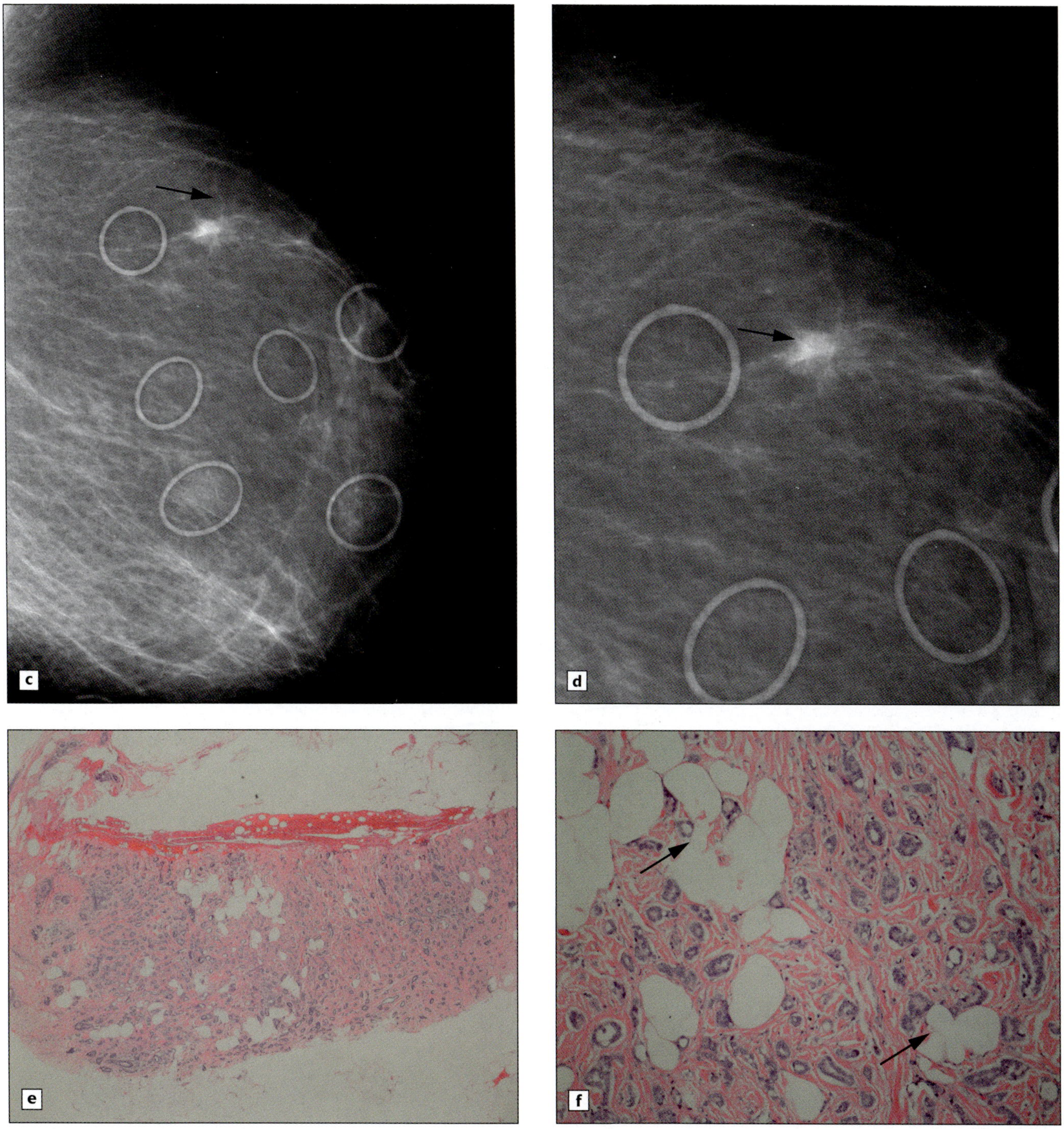

FIGURE 8.8—cont'd One year later, follow-up mammogram **(c)** and magnified view **(d)** showed that the nodule had became larger, indistinct and denser (arrow). There was no calcification present. The rings represent markers of skin lesions. Ultrasound failed to detect the abnormality. **(e)** Core biopsy shows tubular carcinoma composed of a uniform evenly dispersed proliferation of well formed glands which **(f)** directly invade adipose tissue (arrows). Note the low grade nuclei typical of tubular carcinoma.

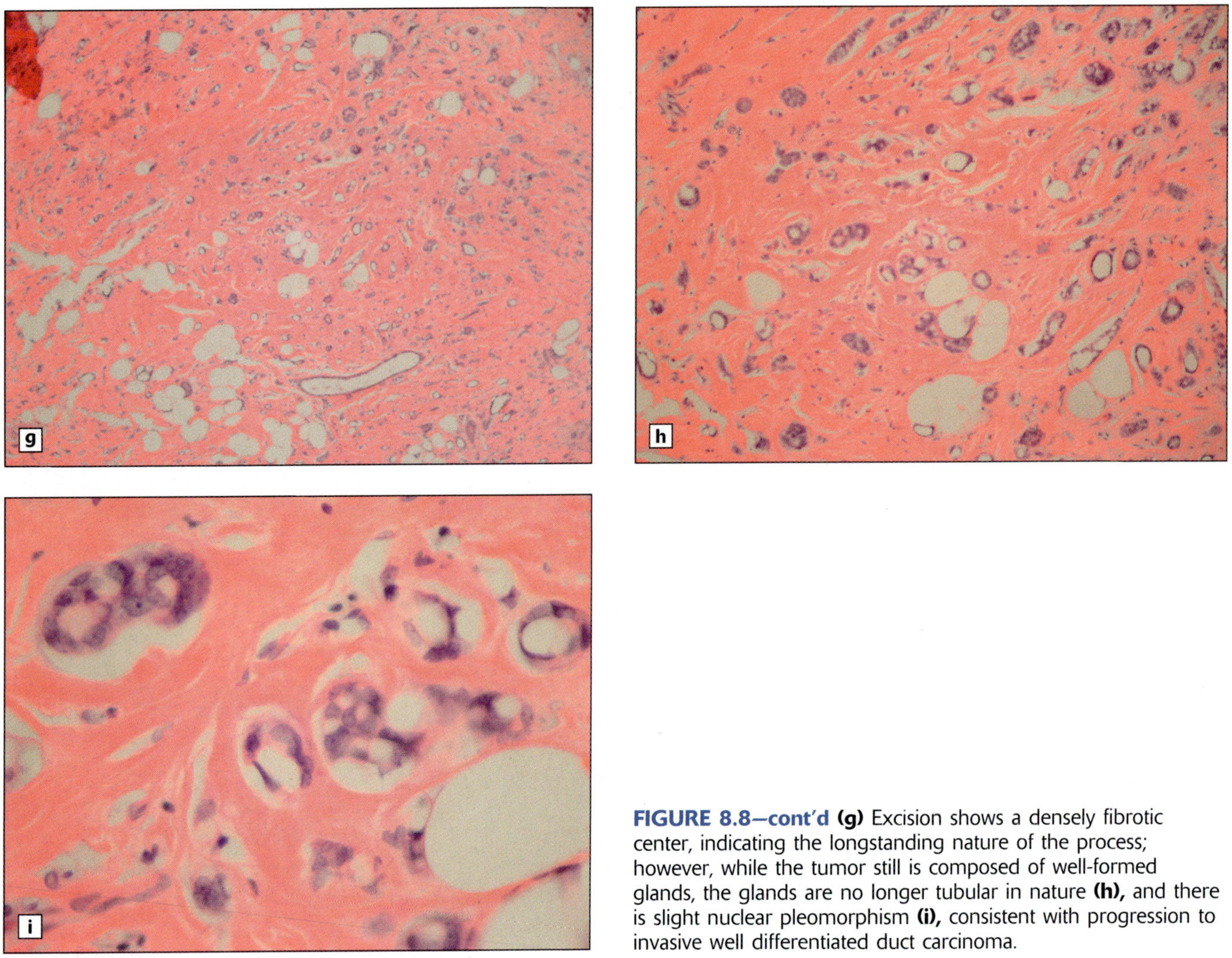

FIGURE 8.8—cont'd (g) Excision shows a densely fibrotic center, indicating the longstanding nature of the process; however, while the tumor still is composed of well-formed glands, the glands are no longer tubular in nature **(h),** and there is slight nuclear pleomorphism **(i),** consistent with progression to invasive well differentiated duct carcinoma.

Differential diagnoses of stellate architectural distortion

- Radial scar
- Radial scar containing DCIS
- Tubular carcinoma

POINTS TO REMEMBER

1. Radial scar is best definitively diagnosed on excisional biopsy.
2. DCIS can involve radial scar.
3. Invasive carcinoma in areas of DCIS involving radial scar or sclerosing adenosis should be diagnosed cautiously and be based on invasion of fat.
4. Radial scar may be premalignant and/or a risk factor for invasive breast cancer.
5. Core biopsy diagnosis of tubular carcinoma should be based on invasion of fat.

REFERENCES

1. Alleva DQ, Smetherman DH, Farr GH, Cederbom GJ. Radial scar of the breast: radiologic-pathologic correlation in 22 cases. RadioGraphics 19: S27–S35,1999.
2. Wellings SR, Alpers CE. Subgross pathologic features and incidence of radial scars in the breast. Hum Pathol 15:475–479,1984.
3. Fenoglio C, Lattes R. Sclerosing papillary proliferations in the female breast. A benign lesion often mistaken for carcinoma. Cancer 33:691–700,1974
4. Jacobs TW, Byrne C, Colditz G, et al. Radial scars in benign breast-biopsy specimens and the risk of breast cancer. N Engl J Med 340:430–436,1999.
5. Brenner RJ, Jackson RJ, Parker SH, et al. Percutaneous core needle biopsy of radial scars of the breast: when is excision necessary? AJR Am J Roentgenol 179:1179–1184,2002.

*6. Philpotts LE, Shaheen NA, Jain KS, et al. Uncommon high-risk lesions of the breast diagnosed at stereotactic core-needle biopsy: Clinical importance. Radiology 216:831–837,2000

7. Frouge C, Tristant H, Guinebretiere JM, et al. Mammographic lesions suggestive of radial scars: microscopic findings in 40 cases. Radiology 195:623–625,1995.
8. Sloane JP, Mayers MM. Carcinoma and atypical hyperplasia in radial scars and complex sclerosing lesions: importance of lesion size and patient age. Histopathology 23:225–231,1993.
9. Douglas-Jones AG, Denson JL, Cox AC, et al. Radial scar lesions of the breast diagnosed by needle core biopsy – analysis of cases containing occult malignancy. J Clin Pathol 60:295–298,2007.

CHAPTER 9

Architectural distortion

The classic malignancy presenting as radiographic architectural distortion is invasive lobular carcinoma. The majority of infiltrating lobular carcinomas are indistinguishable mammographically and sonographically from infiltrating duct carcinomas; however, the imaging features of infiltrating lobular carcinomas may be more subtle because of their growth pattern. Single rows of infiltrating carcinoma cells can diffusely invade surrounding breast parenchyma without creating a central mass, generating little in the way of a host connective tissue reaction. The mass like features of infiltrating lobular carcinoma can be more impressive on one mammographic view, as the lesion is often better seen on the craniocaudal image as opposed to the mediolateral oblique projection (Fig. 9.1). Physical examination may demonstrate only a vaguely palpable region even with large tumors. The tumor size is also often underestimated by imaging because of the relative lack of a peripheral desmoplastic reaction. Sonography is a helpful adjunct in the workup of occult palpable abnormalities or mammographically subtle lesions, many of which represent early infiltrating lobular carcinomas. The most common sonographic feature of invasive lobular carcinoma is that of a hypoechoic, heterogeneous mass with irregular or indistinct margins and posterior acoustic shadowing (Fig. 9.1c). In addition, the finding of focal acoustic shadowing without a discrete mass is more often seen in infiltrating lobular carcinoma than in infiltrating duct carcinoma. The differential diagnosis of invasive lobular carcinoma in a core biopsy is no different from that in a surgical specimen; however, in difficult cases the distinction is aided by knowledge of the radiologic appearance (Fig. 9.2). Invasive lobular carcinoma does not typically present as a well- circumscribed lesion, and thus the diagnosis should be questioned in such an instance (see above discussion of myoid hamartoma, Chapter 3). Extreme examples of sclerosing adenosis are often difficult to differentiate from infiltrating lobular carcinoma and should be distinguished by the maintenance of the lobulocentric, organized growth pattern in the former and the direct invasion of adipose tissue in the latter (see Fig. 8.6b). Nodules of sclerosing adenosis (so-called adenosis tumor) are also fairly well-circumscribed lesions and knowledge of the lesion as such should throw caution on a diagnosis of invasion. Finally intraductal carcinoma may extend into sclerosing adenosis or adenosis tumor, mimicking invasive lobular carcinoma, but the radiologic characteristics would be those of the nodule, not those of invasive lobular carcinoma (see Fig. 8.6a). We are loath to diagnose invasion in this context; however, we also feel it is impossible to absolutely rule out invasion in such lesions. Therefore, we typically advise excision with possible sentinel lymph node sampling in these rare instances in order to create a compromise in which the patient might be spared the additional surgical procedure which would be performed if invasion were definitively diagnosed upon lumpectomy alone.

In large series of patients the distinction between invasive duct carcinoma and invasive lobular carcinoma has never been prognostically significant after the size of the tumor is taken into account.[1] However, this does not mean that proper classification of these lesions is irrelevant. The distinction assumes greater importance with respect to considerations of multifocality, multicentricity, local treatment, and prevention of local recurrence. Invasive lobular carcinomas are more frequently present in multiple, isolated foci in the same quadrant, different quadrants of the same breast (Fig. 9.3), and the opposite breast.[2] Despite this tendency, a higher local recurrence rate for lumpectomy patients with invasive lobular or lobular "features" has never been shown in large series.[3] Whether or not this may be ascribed to theoretical considerations of small residual tumor volume being successfully treated by radiation and tamoxifen and/or cytotoxic chemotherapy must remain a matter for further study; however, it is accepted that all malignancy that is radiologically and/or pathologically evident at initial diagnosis should be surgically treated with the goal of at least histologically clear margins. Thus, "lobular" may matter.

In our view the primary responsibility of the pathologist in evaluating a malignancy on core biopsies is to determine the presence or absence of invasive carcinoma. Subtyping and grading the invasive component is somewhat secondary, but it should still be performed to the best of one's ability since it can contribute to decisions in the next treatment steps. The appellation "lobular" has traditionally been applied to an invasive carcinoma based

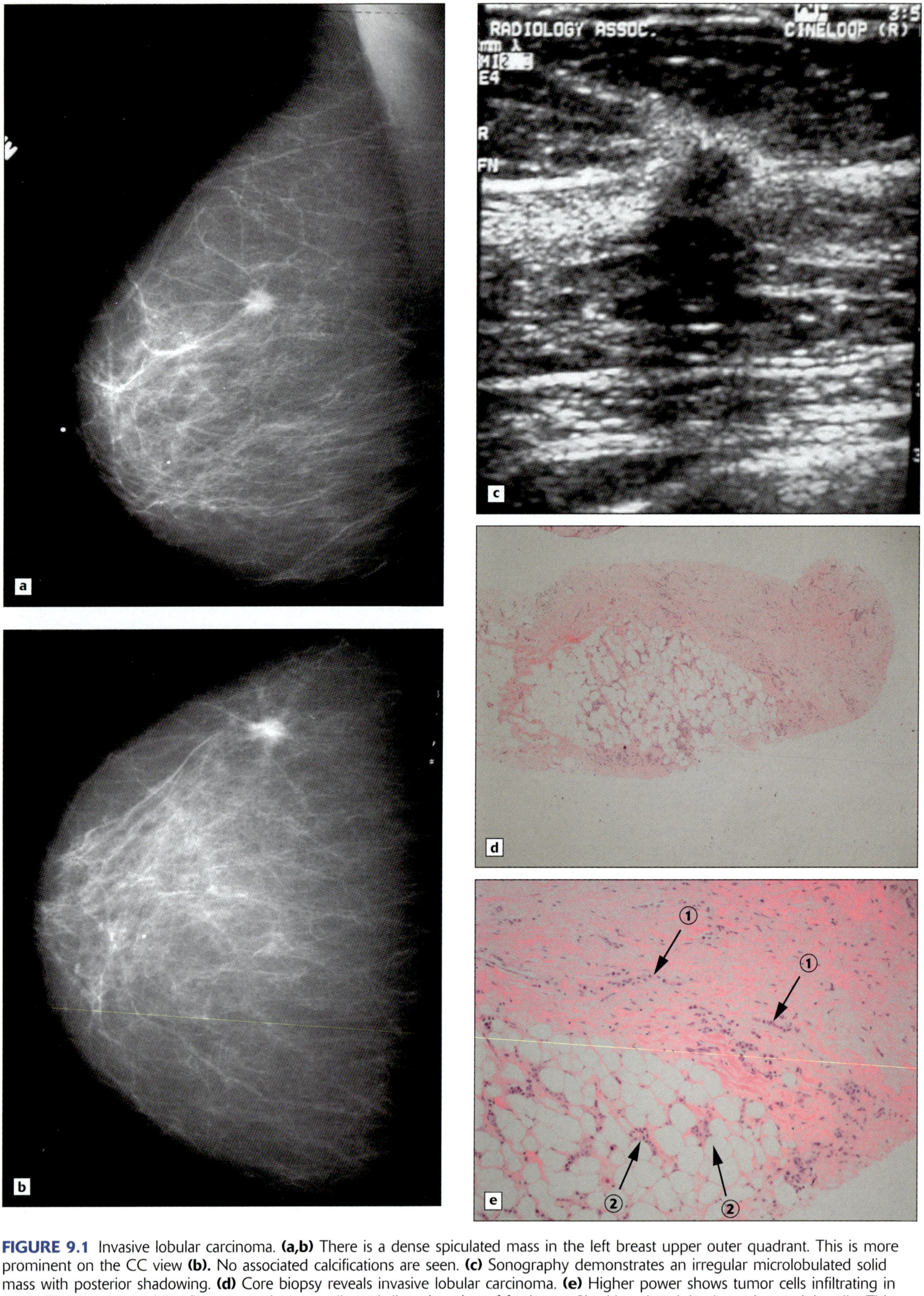

FIGURE 9.1 Invasive lobular carcinoma. **(a,b)** There is a dense spiculated mass in the left breast upper outer quadrant. This is more prominent on the CC view **(b).** No associated calcifications are seen. **(c)** Sonography demonstrates an irregular microlobulated solid mass with posterior shadowing. **(d)** Core biopsy reveals invasive lobular carcinoma. **(e)** Higher power shows tumor cells infiltrating in single files (arrow 1) with a fibrous reaction centrally and direct invasion of fat (arrow 2) with only minimal reaction peripherally. This accounts for the fact that invasive lobular carcinoma is often larger than is apparent clinically or radiographically.

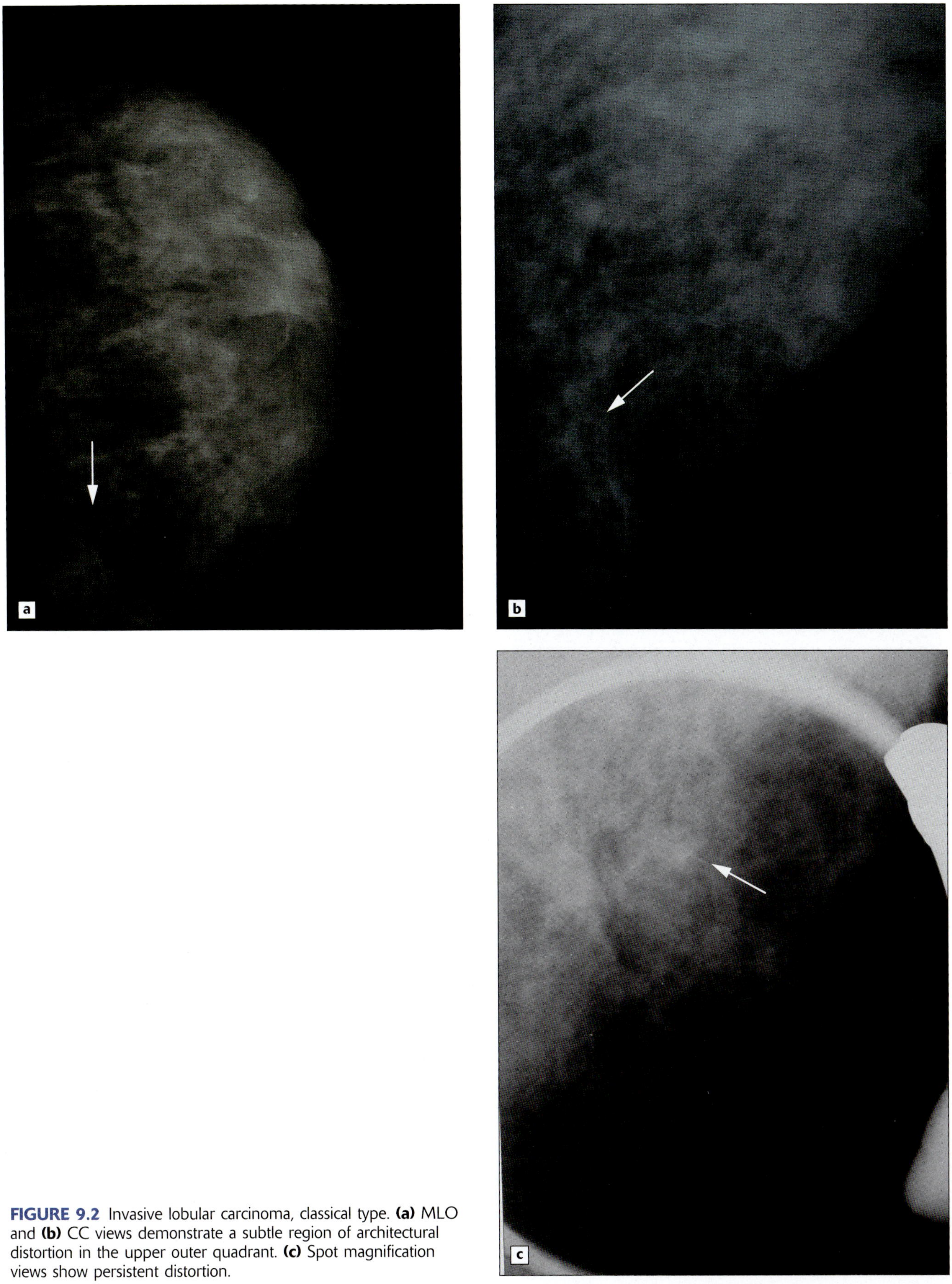

FIGURE 9.2 Invasive lobular carcinoma, classical type. **(a)** MLO and **(b)** CC views demonstrate a subtle region of architectural distortion in the upper outer quadrant. **(c)** Spot magnification views show persistent distortion.

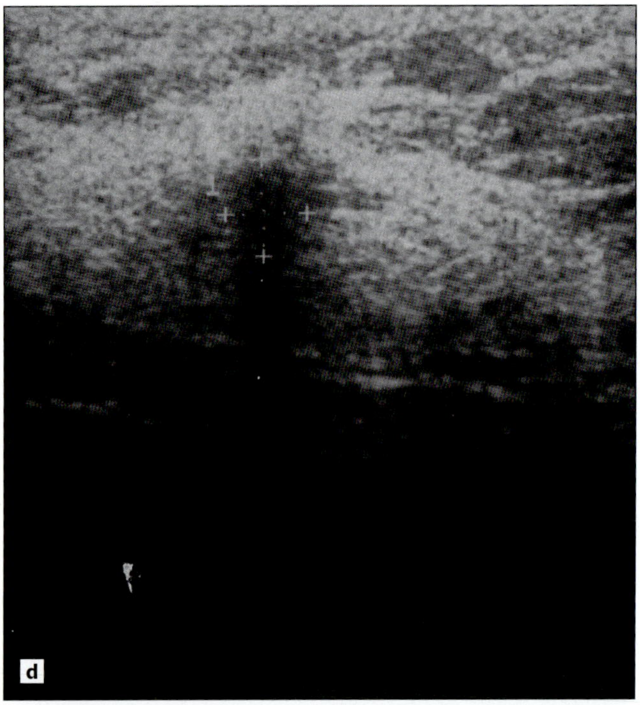

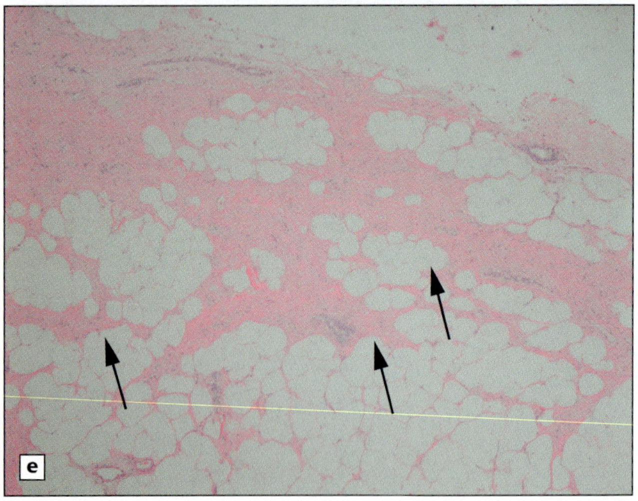

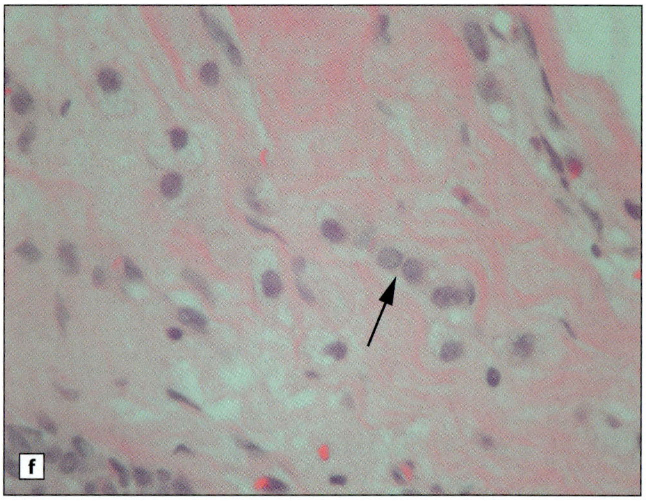

FIGURE 9.2—cont'd (d) Sonography demonstrates a markedly hypoechoic microlobulated solid mass with dense posterior shadowing. **(e)** At low power the histology of this core biopsy may appear innocuous except for the odd interconnecting bands of fibrous tissue in fat (arrows); however, **(f)** higher power examination of these fibrous bands reveals classical invasive lobular carcinoma with uniform low grade nuclei and lack of mitoses (arrow). Note the cytologic resemblance of these tumor cells to those of epithelioid cells in myoid hamartoma (see Fig. 3.6).

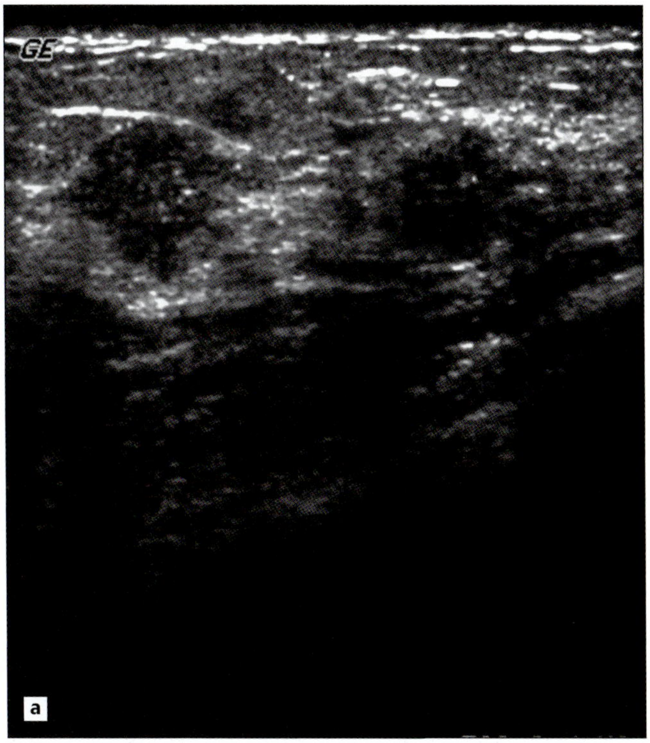

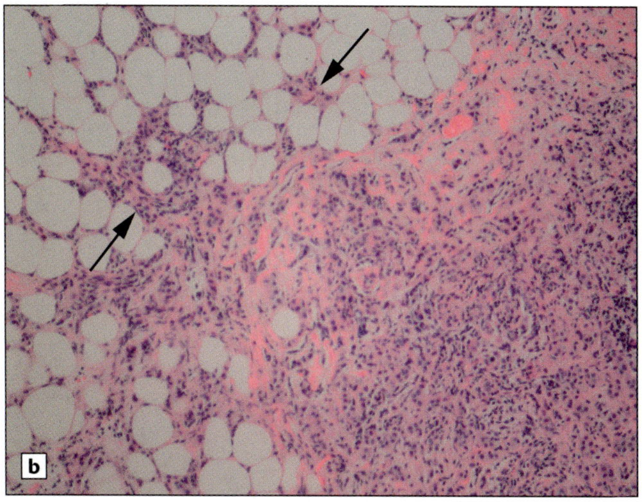

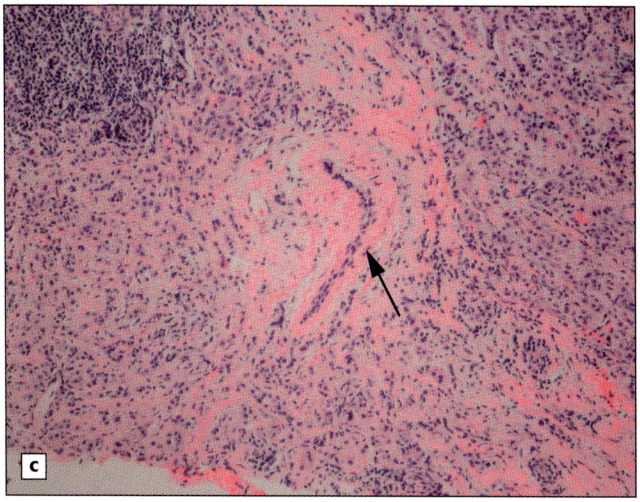

FIGURE 9.3 Multifocal invasive lobular carcinoma. **(a)** Sonography shows multiple solid irregular masses. Only one lesion was apparent mammographically as architectural distortion. Core biopsies of each mass showed identical histology with **(b)** single file invasion of tumor cells. Radiologic images typically underestimate the actual size of invasive lobular carcinoma because of the relative lack of desmoplastic reaction, histologically corresponding to tumor cells investing themselves between adipocytes (arrows) without fibrosis. **(c)** Invasive lobular carcinoma typically surrounds normal breast structures (arrow), the so called targetoid pattern of invasion.

on the combined evaluation of: pattern of infiltration (single files of uniform, small, dyscohesive, plasmacytoid cells surrounding normal structures, culminating in a targetoid appearance), gland formation (a relative paucity for lobular), and cytologic characteristics (smaller cells with less cytoplasm, relatively small and uniform nuclei, and lack of mitoses). Such lesions typically evoke far less of a desmoplastic reaction than do their ductal cousins. Variants of invasive lobular carcinoma (Fig. 9.4) have been described (pleomorphic,[4] signet ring cell,[5] histiocytoid,[6] alveolar,[7] and tubulolobular[8]) to account for lesions which have a mixed histologic character and correspond at least in part to tumors often diagnosed as "invasive mammary carcinoma with mixed ductal and lobular features. Pleomorphic lobular applies to lesions such as that above with severe nuclear atypia and mitotic activity but maintenance of the lobular growth pattern. Signet ring cell and histiocytoid variants are dominated by their corresponding cytologic features, alveolar carcinoma is composed of cells with lobular cytology invading in nests usually accompanying the more typical invasive pattern, and tubulolobular combines the classical invasive lobular carcinoma with areas of well differentiated gland formation by the same cells.

It is especially important to recognize the pattern of invasive tubulolobular carcinoma on core biopsy and to not simply diagnose it as invasive well or moderately differentiated duct carcinoma (Fig. 9.5). In general, tubulolobular carcinoma has the same predilection for multiple lesions as does invasive lobular carcinoma and shows the same infiltration pattern, surrounding normal structures;[9] thus, the diagnosis should initiate the search for other imaging-detected lesions, and often, in our experience, multiple lesions have already been found and biopsied. Prognostically tubulolobular carcinoma is similar to invasive moderately differentiated duct carci-

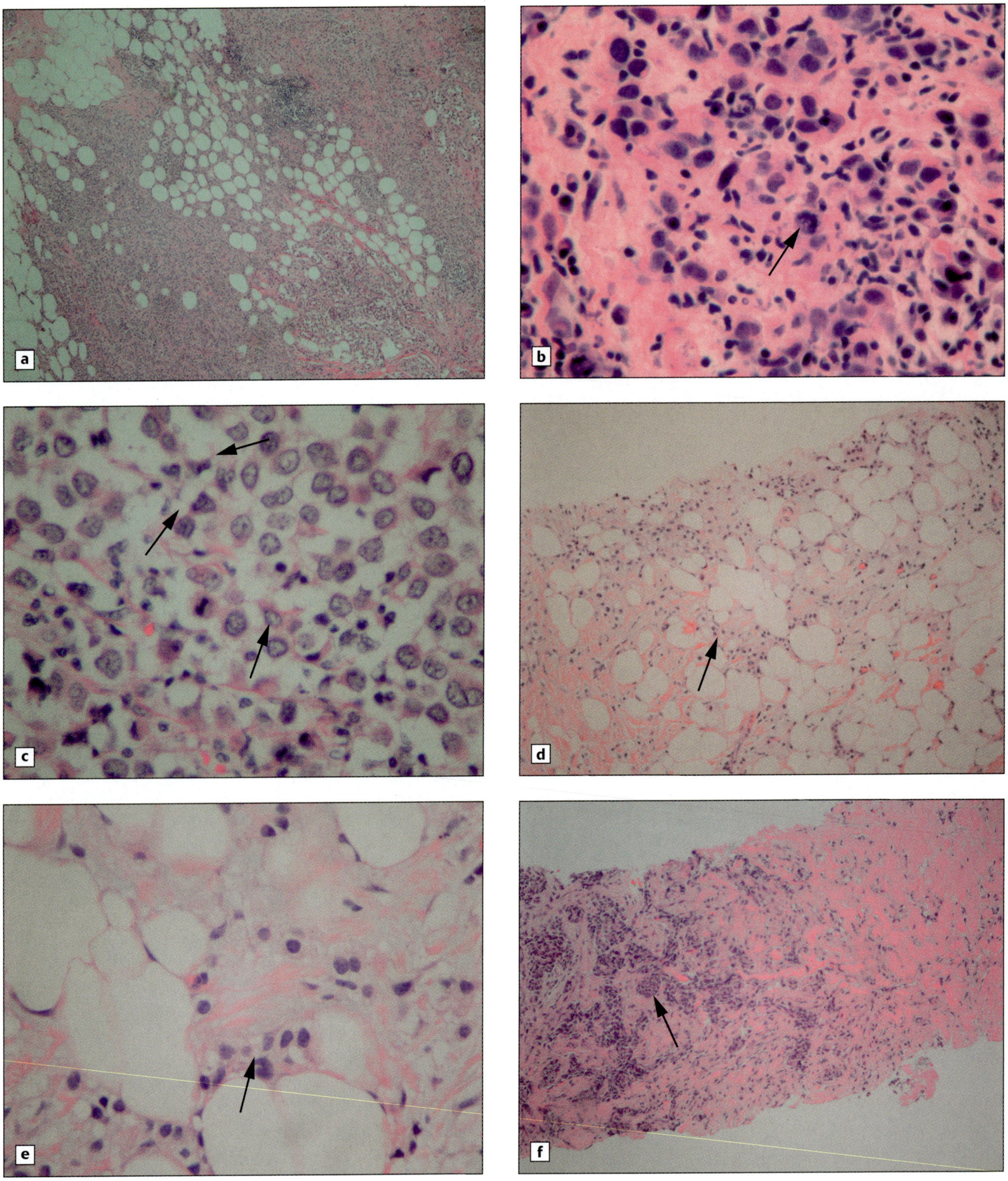

FIGURE 9.4 Variants of invasive lobular carcinoma. All histologic variants of invasive lobular carcinoma share the same relative lack of fibrous reaction **(a).** Pleomorphic lobular carcinoma **(b)** consists of high grade nuclear pleomorphism and mitotic activity (arrow); signet ring cell carcinoma cells **(c)** show nuclei pushed aside by cytoplasmic mucin (arrows); **(d,e)** histiocytoid lobular carcinoma cells (arrows) resemble histiocytes and thus can be very deceptive, occasionally requiring immunohistochemical stains for keratins to prove their epithelial nature; and **(f)** alveolar lobular carcinoma cells form invasive nests (arrow).

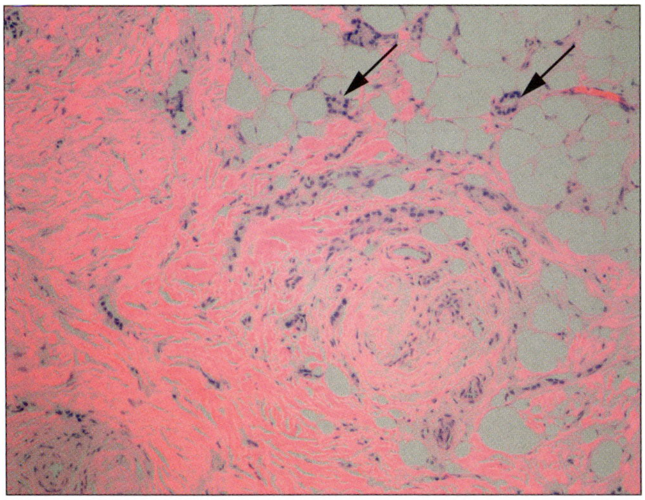

FIGURE 9.5 Invasive tubulolobular carcinoma. In this variant tumor cells merge the pattern of ordinary invasive lobular carcinoma with small well-formed glands (arrows).

noma in terms of its likelihood of being associated with positive lymph nodes, but it is more akin to invasive lobular carcinoma with respect to its local disease characteristics and treatment implications.

While the above lesions have slightly different histologies, they all share the tendency for formation of multiple separate lesions. They also typically share the same radiologic and clinical features. Their relative lack of desmoplastic reaction results in the fact that these tumors are often quite subtle on mammography. In general, in our experience, sonographically determined size of invasive tumor is quite accurate; however, it is less precise in cases of invasive lobular carcinoma and its variants. While any patient diagnosed with a breast malignancy deserves a preoperative imaging workup of both breasts, we believe this is especially important in cases of invasive lobular carcinoma. Despite the inherent imaging difficulties, accurate core biopsy designation of an invasive carcinoma as lobular or a variant thereof may alert the radiologist to evaluate other subtle areas in the breast(s) which might otherwise be overlooked. Finally it eventually serves as a warning to the pathologist to be wary of the oft-times subtle lobular metastases when evaluating the sentinel and non-sentinel lymph nodes.

Differential Diagnoses of architectural distortion

- Invasive lobular carcinoma
- Invasive lobular carcinoma (pleomorphic, signet ring, histiocytoid, alveolar variants)
- Invasive tubulolobular carcinoma
- Radial scar
- Tubular carcinoma

POINTS TO REMEMBER

1. Variants of invasive lobular carcinoma share classical lobular's propensity to form multiple lesions.
2. Invasive lobular carcinoma should not be definitively diagnosed in the context of a well-circumscribed lesion on imaging.
3. Extreme examples of sclerosing adenosis or adenosis tumor can closely mimic invasive lobular carcinoma.

REFERENCES

1. Rosen PP. Rosen's Breast Pathology, 1st ed. New York: Lippincott-Raven, pp. 557–562,1997.
2. Rosen PP. Rosen's Breast Pathology, 1st ed. New York: Lippincott-Raven, pp. 546,1997.
3. Peiro G, Bornstein BA, Connolly JL, et al. The influence of infiltrating lobular carcinoma on the outcome of patients treated with breast-conserving surgery and radiation therapy. Breast Cancer Res Treat 59:49–54,2000.
4. Weidner N, Semple JP. Pleomorphic variant of invasive lobular carcinoma of the breast. Hum Pathol 23:1167–1171,1992.
5. Frost AR, Terahata S, Yeh IT, et al. The significance of signet ring cells in infiltrating lobular carcinoma of the breast. Arch Pathol Lab Med 119:64–68,1995.
6. Walford N, ten Velden J. Histiocytoid breast carcinoma: an apocrine variant of lobular carcinoma. Histopathology 14:515–522,1989.
7. Shousha S, Backhous CM, Alaghband-Zadeh J, Burn I. Alveolar variant of invasive lobular carcinoma of the breast. A tumor rich in estrogen receptors. Am J Clin Pathol 85:1–5,1986.
8. Fisher ER, Gregorio RM, Redmond C, Fisher B. Tubulolobular invasive breast cancer: a variant of lobular invasive cancer. Hum Pathol 8:679–83,1977.
9. Green I, McCormick B, Cranor M, Rosen PP. A comparative study of pure tubular and tubulolobular carcinoma of the breast. Am J Surg Pathol 21:653–657,1997.

CHAPTER 10

Introduction to stereotactic core biopsies for calcifications

Calcium deposits are extremely common in the breast and are known to be more numerous microscopically than they are radiologically apparent. Calcification may be the result of active cell secretion, a response to inflammation, trauma, radiation or foreign body, the end result of necrosis (usually in intraductal carcinoma), or of unknown pathogenesis. Calcifications can be found within the ducts, alongside or around the ducts, in the lobular acini, in vascular structures, in the interlobular stroma, in fat, or in the skin. The majority of calcifications form in benign processes. The recognition that certain clustered patterns of calcifications can be found in early stage breast cancer forms the basis for mammographic screening and early detection.

Mammography is the only reliable examination able to depict calcifications within the breast. Thus, specimen radiography is the most precise method of verifying the inclusion of the targeted calcifications in the core biopsy or excisional biopsy specimen. For approximately 50% of nonpalpable mammographically detected breast cancers, calcifications are the only radiographic sign that leads to a diagnosis. Duct carcinoma in situ comprises an enlarging subset of breast malignancies because of the advent of mammographic screening. Spot compression magnification, in lateral and or tangential views, are essential in characterizing the mammographic morphology of calcifications. When assessing calcifications, radiologists evaluate the particle size, shape, number, and distribution, as well as association with any soft tissue density (see Figure 1.13). We can first attempt to categorize calcifications as benign or malignant and then to define the remainder as indeterminate. "Malignant" calcifications may occur with or without the presence of a mass. Benign calcifications tend to be fewer in number and less tightly clustered with dot-like or punctate forms which are round and often coarser than "malignant" calcifications (Fig. 10.1). The size, shape and distribution, and/or other characteristic appearances of some types of calcifications enable them to be classified as definitively benign:

- secretory calcifications-thick linear and coarse rounded;
- vascular calcifications-double linear tracks ("railroad tracks");
- radiolucent centered, eggshell, secretory-fat necrosis, silicone granulomata;
- small cysts-milk of calcium, teacups-layering of calcifications within cysts on special views;
- macrocysts;
- fibroadenomas;
- fat necrosis-post-surgical or post-traumatic;
- suture calcifications; and
- metabolic-renal failure, hyperparathyroidism, dermatomyositis

Fibroadenomas are the most common benign solid tumors of the female breast. As mentioned previously only rarely do they arise or enlarge in postmenopausal women; however, they may present as calcifications in older women as part of a degenerative hyalinizing process. Coarse or popcorn-like calcifications are typical of fibroadenomas undergoing such involution (Fig. 10.2). The calcifications usually begin inside the mass and increase centripetally; some residual mass may be visible, or the lesion may be entirely calcified. Early calcifications within a fibroadenoma may be indistinguishable from carcinoma, thus requiring biopsy. These early calcifications may be fine and irregular, with forms varying in size and shape. Masses with peripheral type calcifications in a rim-like pattern are almost always benign (see Chaps 4 and 12). Fibroadenomas, cysts with calcified walls, and calcified fat necrosis commonly have these rim-like deposits. Large solitary calcifications often develop in calcified fibroadenomas, but may also arise in the irradiated breast (see Chap. 12, Figs 12.1–12.3). Fibroadenomas when seen on ultrasound present as a smooth, oval, well-defined solid mass with homogeneous internal echoes and often a small amount of posterior through transmission (see Chapter 2). The coarse calcifications within the mass may be brightly reflective and, even when very dense, demonstrate posterior shadowing.

When a mass is associated with the calcifications, the lesions' borders as well as the morphology of the calcifications can help determine its etiology. As mentioned above fibroadenomas have large confluent calcifications associated with smoothly circumscribed, or lobulated borders. When the calcifications are pleomorphic and

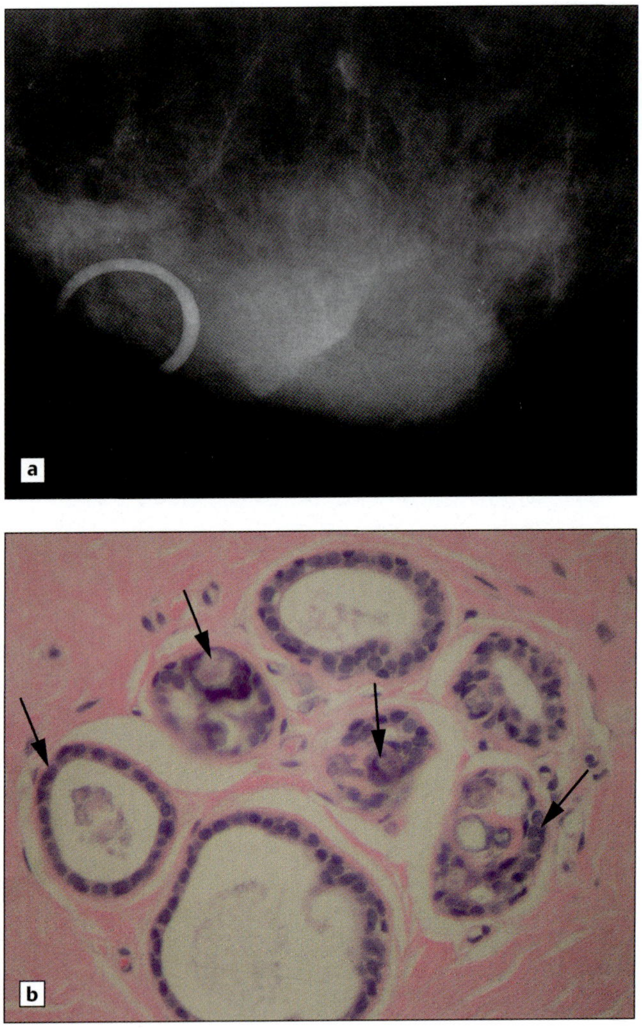

FIGURE 10.1 Magnified view of a mammogram **(a)** showing calcifications which appear as round, loosely clustered, dot-like or punctate forms. These correlated with fibrocystic changes with calcifications **(b)** (arrows).

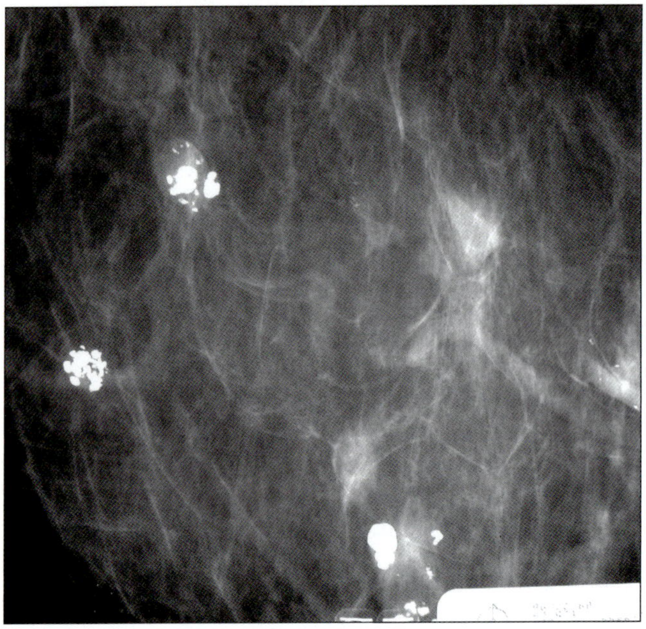

FIGURE 10.2 Mammogram showing multiple fibroadenomas with typical popcorn-like calcifications

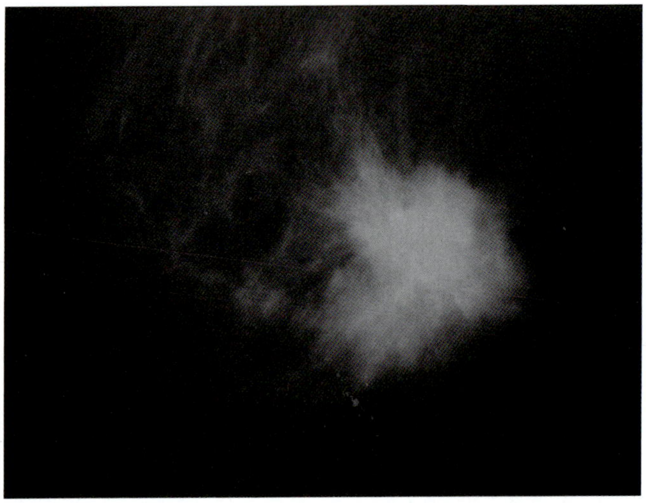

FIGURE 10.3 Mammogram showing irregular linear branching clustered calcifications associated with a spiculated dense mass.

irregular it is the analysis of the calcifications that takes precedence, even if the margins of the mass are circumscribed, biopsy is indicated. The calcifications are defining the intraductal component and the solid mass is likely the invasive component. Irregular linear branching or pointed punctate clustered calcifications associated with a spiculated dense mass are characteristic of a breast cancer (Fig. 10.3).

"Malignant" calcifications tend to be more tightly clustered; these forms are heterogeneous or pleomorphic, may be linear or irregular, and their individual particle size is small (Fig. 10.4). The morphology and distribution of breast calcifications can often indicate their etiology. Some calcifications form in the extralobular stroma, but most occur within the lobules and ducts. The risk of malignancy increases when there are five or more isolated calcifications visible in a 1 ml volume. The morphology of the calcification is the most important feature in mammographic analysis.

Malignant calcifications

- particle morphology-particles vary in size and shape with granular or linear branching forms of calcifying necrotic intraductal material (casting calcifications);
- particle size-generally small, often <0.5 mm;
- distance between particles is often less in a malignant process than benign one, i.e., they are tightly clustered;
- distribution-cluster, ductal distribution;

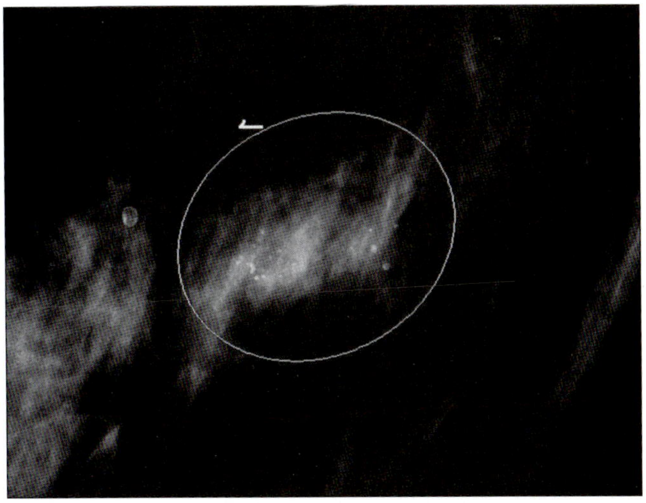

FIGURE 10.4 Mammogram showing malignant calcifications which appear more numerous, finer and tightly clustered compared to benign calcifications. Note the pleomorphic, linear and irregular nature of the calcifications.

- cluster-linear, irregular, disorganized, pleomorphic; and
- associated ill-defined soft tissue mass.

In the diagnosis and treatment of duct carcinoma in situ (DCIS) it is important to be aware of the subtypes of DCIS and their differences in mammographic presentation. High grade comedo carcinoma often manifests as casting pleomorphic calcifications which appear as linear, branching, heterogeneous forms which represent calcification of intraductal necrotic material (Fig. 10.5). Although prognosis is worse with comedocarcinoma than with noncomedo lesions, the extent of disease may often be more accurately mammographically estimated in the comedo type. In the low to intermediate grade cribriform and micropapillary subtypes of DCIS, the calcifications form as stagnation of secretions within cystic spaces and cleft like openings or within the interstices of the intraluminal papillary projections. These calcifications are thus punctate, granular and sand-like, but do

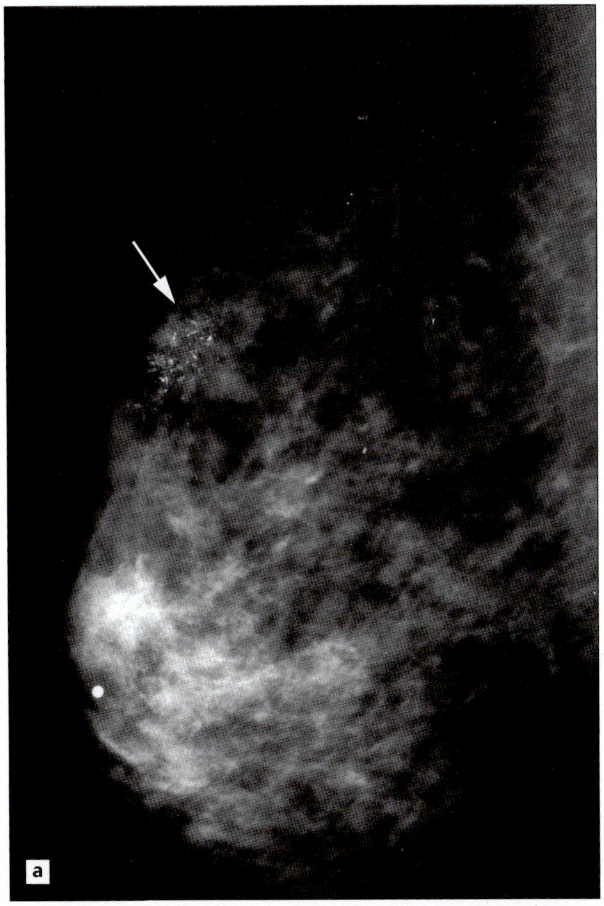

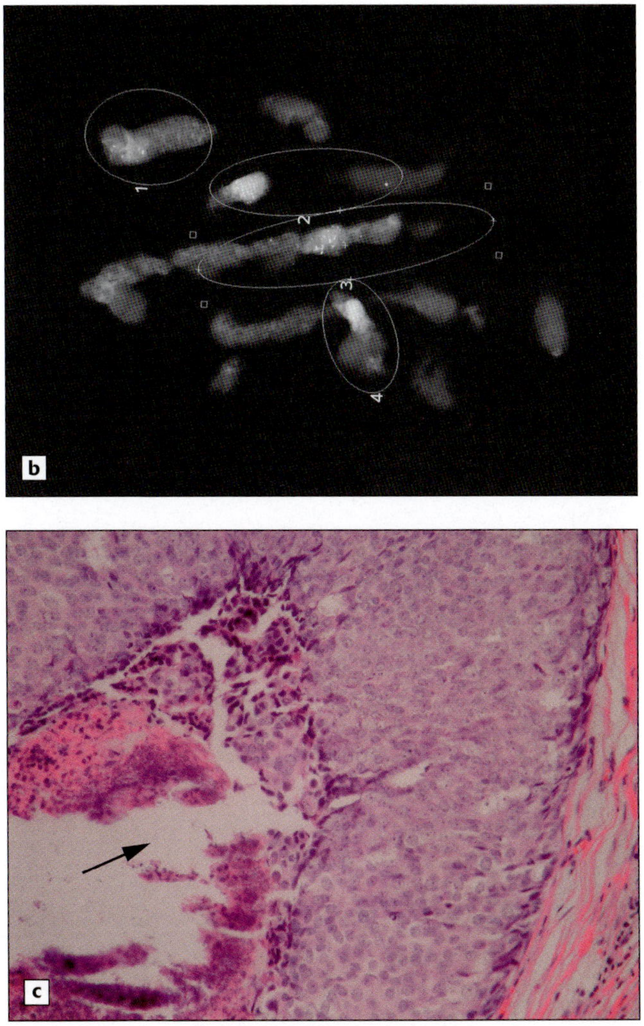

FIGURE 10.5 **(a)** Mammogram showing linear and branching calcifications (arrow). **(b)** These were also seen on the specimen radiograph. **(c)** H&E sections show comedo DCIS with determinant calcifications (arrow).

vary in size and shape (Fig. 10.6). Such noncomedo patterns of DCIS, especially the cribriform and micropapillary types are less consistently identified mammographically, and their extent of disease is more often underestimated. It is our experience, however, that the occurrence of a one-to-one correlation between the calcifications and DCIS (so-called determinant calcifications) is extremely unusual in any form of DCIS, with the exception of some cases of comedo type (Fig. 10.5). Frequently microscopic calcifications are also found in benign breast tissue accompanying the DCIS, distorting this 1:1 ratio (see Chap. 14, Figs 14.2, 14.5 and 14.6). Occasionally DCIS may not be associated with calcifications i.e. occult, being detected due to benign calcifications (Fig. 10.7). Comedo DCIS with its characteristic calcifications notably enables a precise correlation between the type of calcification and pathology, and also the extent of disease.

When microcalcifications have a high imaging probability of being malignant, the type of sampling used should reflect the size of the cluster, whether or not there is more than one cluster, and the calcifications' location. Stereotactic vacuum assisted biopsy is an accurate and cost effective[1] alternative to surgical excisional biopsy in the evaluation of mammographically detected calcifications.[2,3] The issue of underestimation of the presence of invasive carcinoma persists in lesions percutaneously diagnosed as DCIS and atypical duct hyperplasia (ADH), as is also the case for DCIS if ADH is the core biopsy diagnosis.[4,5] However, the frequency of underestimation has decreased with the 11-gauge biopsy instrument compared to 14 gauge cores obtained with the automated biopsy gun,[6,7] especially when the targeted calcifications have been completely removed.[8] The issue of underestimation has also been addressed more recently by the

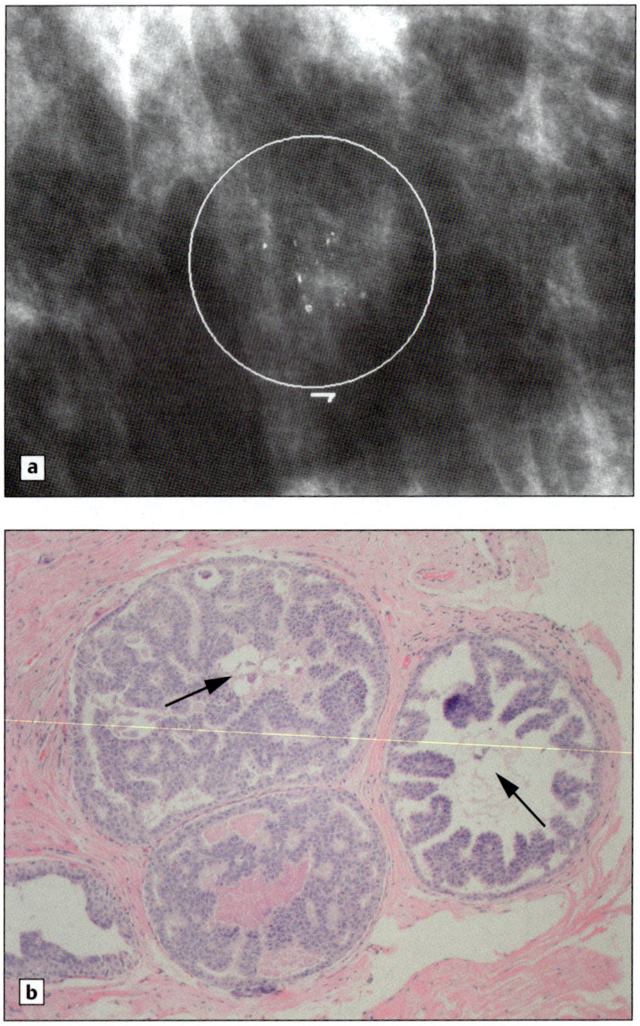

FIGURE 10.6 **(a)** Mammogram showing punctate, granular sand like calcifications that are also pleomorphic correlating with low grade DCIS **(b)** with calcifications (arrows).

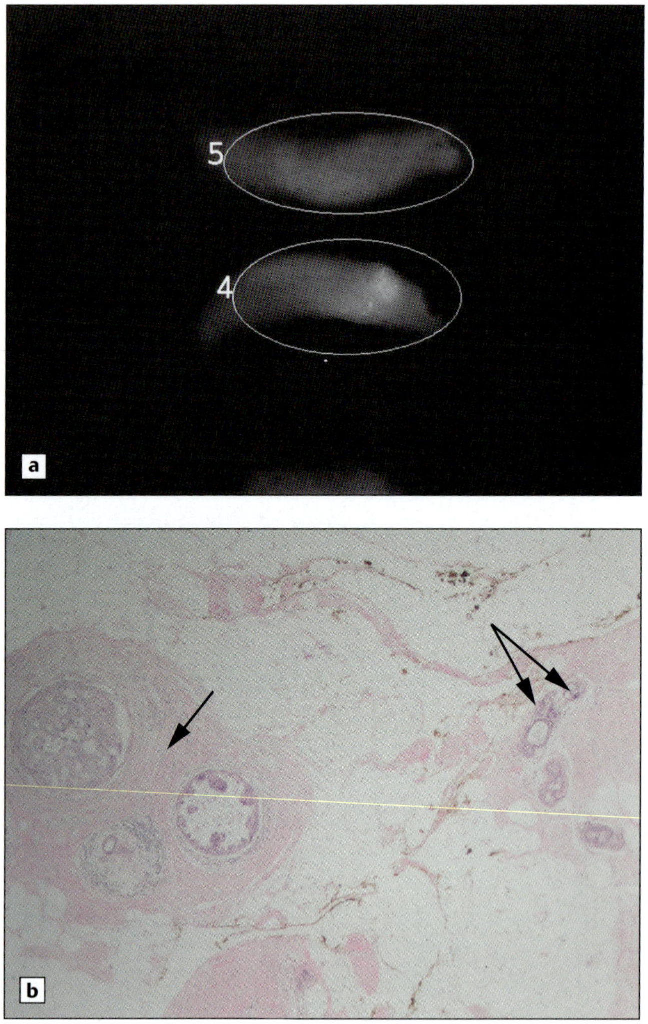

FIGURE 10.7 **(a)** Specimen radiograph shows few punctate calcifications that correlate with calcifications in fibrocystic changes (**b,** right arrows). Notice the occult DCIS not associated with calcifications (left arrow).

more frequent use of an 8-gauge vacuum-assisted biopsy instrument when sampling clustered broad region of calcifications. This is related to the greater volume of tissue obtained with the larger size gauge instrument, and the contiguous nature of sampling with the vacuum-assisted device. As expected, underestimation of the invasive component occurs more frequently in large DCIS lesions than in small lesions wherein most or the entire tumor may be removed by the cores. When a lesion is removed in its entirety, the standard of care is to place a stainless steel or titanium marker or clip through the biopsy probe to mark its location. If the calcifications or mass are malignant or atypical, then the breast surgeon can accurately locate the site of the prior percutaneous biopsy via preoperative wire localization. If the lesion is benign the clip remains in place with no ill effects.

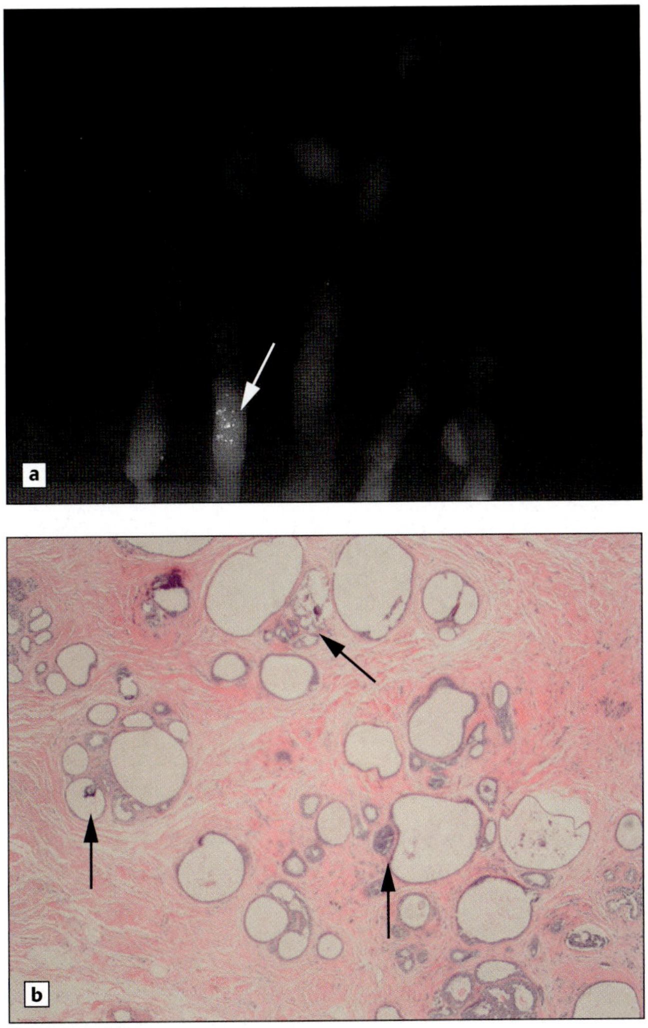

FIGURE 10.8 A 1 : 1 correlation between **(a)** specimen radiograph and **(b)** H&E section. The specimen radiograph shows punctate calcifications (arrow) present on a core which correlates with those found in the fibrocystic changes with calcifications (arrows).

GENERAL ASPECTS OF HISTOLOGIC EVALUATION OF CORE BIOPSIES FOR CALCIFICATIONS

The Pathologist's goal: to identify in the tissue sample the histological correlate of the calcifications present on the specimen radiograph both in terms of number and pattern (Fig. 10.8).

1. Radiologic-pathologic correlation using the specimen radiograph. At our institution, we require utilization of specimen radiographs to sign out mammotome core biopsies performed for calcifications. After completion of the biopsy, the radiologist places the tissue core biopsy fragments on a petri dish or solid media to be x-rayed so as to be able to distinguish tissue cores with calcifications from those without. These cores are then separated in containers designated as such, i.e., "with calcifications" and "without calcifications", enabling the pathologist to perform a focused search for calcifications from the containers labeled as such.
2. Discordance between the slides and specimen radiograph should prompt radiography of the paraffin blocks. At our institution, we utilize the digital faxitron machine using 35 kV for 22 seconds to x-ray blocks, then develop it digitally, such that within minutes we can determine if residual calcifications are present on the block.
3. Residual calcifications on the paraffin blocks (Fig.10.9) necessitate additional sections until the calcifications are found.

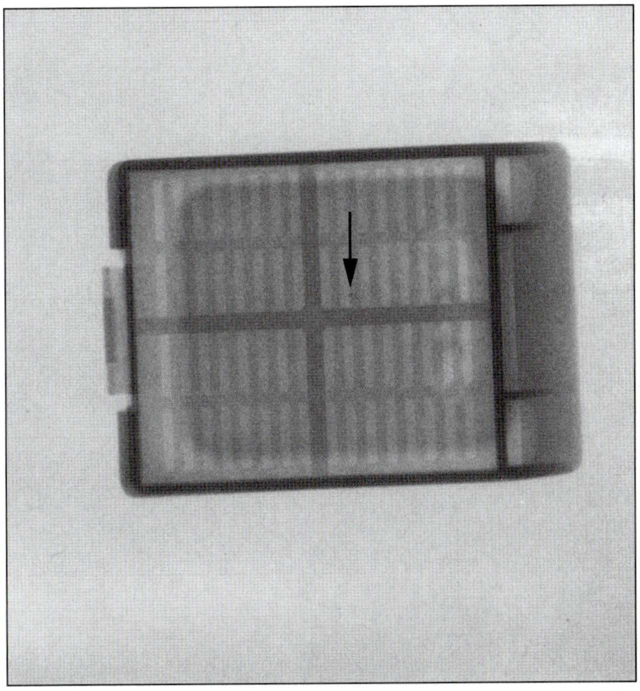

FIGURE 10.9 Paraffin block radiograph showing residual calcifications (arrow), necessitating additional levels.

4. Lack of radiologic–pathologic correlation (points 1–3) should prompt careful re review of the original slides with examination under polarized light and a search for histologic evidence of cysts.

REFERENCES

1. Lee CH, Egglin TK, Philpotts L, et al. Cost-effectiveness of stereotactic core needle biopsy: analysis by means of mammographic findings. Radiology 202:849–854,1997.
2. Meyer JE, Smith DN, Dipiro PJ, et al. Stereotactic breast biopsy of clustered microcalcifications with a directional, vacuum-assisted device. Radiology 204:575–576,1997.
3. Reynolds HE, Poon CM, Goulet RJ, et al. Biopsy of breast microcalcifications using an 11-gauge directional vacuum-assisted device. AJR Am J Roentgenol 171:611–613,1998.
4. Liberman L, Dershaw DD, Glassman JR. Analysis of cancers not diagnosed at stereotactic core breast biopsy. Radiology 203:151–157,1997.
5. Jackman RJ, Nowels KW, Rodriguez-Soto J, et al. Stereotactic, automated, large-core needle biopsy of nonpalpable breast lesions: false-negative and histologic underestimation rates after long-term follow-up. Radiology 210:799–805,1999.
6. Philpotts LE, Shaheen NA, Carter D, et al. Comparison of rebiopsy rates after stereotactic core needle biopsy of the breast with 11-gauge vacuum suction probe versus 14-gauge needle and automatic gun. AJR Am J Roentgenol 172:683–687,1999.
7. Liberman L, Smolkin JH, Dershaw DD, et al. Calcification retrieval at stereotactic, 11-gauge, directional, vacuum-assisted breast biopsy. Radiology 208:251–260,1998.
8. Liberman L, Kaplan JB, Morris EA, et al. To excise or to sample the mammographic target: What is the goal of stereotactic 11-gauge vacuum-assisted breast biopsy? AJR Am J Roentgenol 179:679–683,2002.

CHAPTER 11

Calcium oxalate crystals

Calcifications in the breast which histologically represent calcium oxalate are typically punctate and somewhat amorphous in character (Fig. 11.1). An absolutely specific radiographic appearance for calcium oxalate crystals has not been described. This is unfortunate because these crystals have almost never been associated with histologic malignancy, and thus their removal is unnecessary.

Histologically, calcium oxalate crystals are seen in two situations. Most commonly they are encountered within cysts lined by apocrine metaplasia (Fig. 11.2). Less frequently, they are seen within a foreign body reaction (Fig. 11.3), usually adjacent to or accompanying such cysts (Fig. 11.4). The two situations are not mutually exclusive, as the second likely represents rupture of a cyst with reactive changes due to spillage of its contents, namely, at least in part, the crystals. The etiology of these crystals is uncertain, but one might assume that apocrine cells have the ability to synthesize, concentrate and secrete oxalic acid. Additionally and alternatively, the rich glycolipid secretory product of apocrine cells may act as an organic matrix and thus binds to the calcium oxalate crystals.

Because of a lack of affinity for hematoxylin and eosin (H&E) stains, the crystals are usually not readily identifiable on routine sections, and may therefore be easily overlooked[1,2] (Fig. 11.4a). They are better visualized utilizing the condenser appearing as crystals with a yellow hue (Fig. 11.4b), but are best seen with polarized light which heightens refractility such that they appear as bright birefrigent crystals (Fig. 11.4c). Larger crystals may partially or completely shatter, leaving only small residual fragments. Though they may easily be mistaken for holes on routine H&E sections, they actually have angulated rather than spherical edges, best visualized under polarized light (Fig. 11.5). Other configurations of intact crystals include overlapping plates, rosettes, sheaves, rods and geometric shapes such as diamonds and pyramids (Fig. 11.6).

As mentioned earlier, the identification and recognition of calcium oxalate in the breast is almost pathognomonic of benign breast disease. Calcium oxalate has only rarely been described in association with atypical lobular hyperplasia/lobular carcinoma in situ[3–5] or invasive carcinoma.[6] In our experience, calcium oxalate is rarely present in cases with malignancy; when present it is always within benign apocrine cysts incidental to the malignancy (Fig. 11.7).[1,7] It is theoretically possible for in situ or invasive carcinoma to involve an apocrine cyst containing calcium oxalate. We have very rarely encountered this scenario (Fig. 11.8).

The deceptive appearance of calcium oxalate can lead to a discrepancy between the calcifications on the specimen radiograph and H&E that may sometimes be resolved with polarized light. However, in some cases even with the use of polarized light, fewer calcium oxalate crystais are seen compared to those on the specimen radiograph (Fig. 11.9). In yet other cases, no calcium oxalate crystal is seen (Fig. 11.10). In both scenarios, paraffin block radiography is indicated, which may reveal similar results i.e. either fewer calcifications than those present on the specimen radiograph or maybe none (Figs 11.9c and 11.10c). In real life, the situation arises in which a number of calcifications are removed by the radiologist, seen on the specimen radiograph, yet far fewer to none are seen histologically (Figs 11.9 and 11.10). Diligent search for calcifications in each of the cores, on additional levels and on the paraffin block radiograph to equate those present on the specimen radiograph proves futile in these cases. In our experience, this discrepancy between the calcifications on the specimen radiograph, the slides, and paraffin block radiograph is actually the norm when dealing with apocrine metaplasia-lined cysts containing calcium oxalate crystals. This phenomenon may occasionally also be encountered with cysts containing calcium phosphate (Fig. 11.11).

Discrepancies between the specimen and paraffin block x-ray have been attributed to various reasons such as loss of calcium during processing or sectioning of the tissue, and destruction or dissolution of calcifications by fixatives.[1,8–11] In cases with calcium oxalate, most attribute the discrepancy to under recognition or microtome knife dislodgement.[1,12] We disagree with the latter, because any calcifications be they calcium oxalate or phosphate, are vulnerable to this procedure. However, we believe there is an alternative simpler explanation to clarify the discrepancy between the specimen radiograph and H&E, particularly in cases with calcium oxalate. To understand this phenomenon, one should review the characteristics of core biopsies of larger cysts (see Chap. 4).

Text continued on p. 112

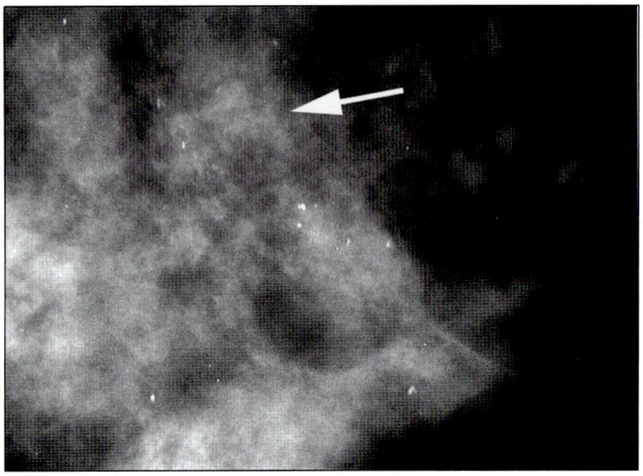

FIGURE 11.1 The typical radiologic appearance of calcium oxalate (arrow) characterized as punctate and somewhat amorphous on mammogram.

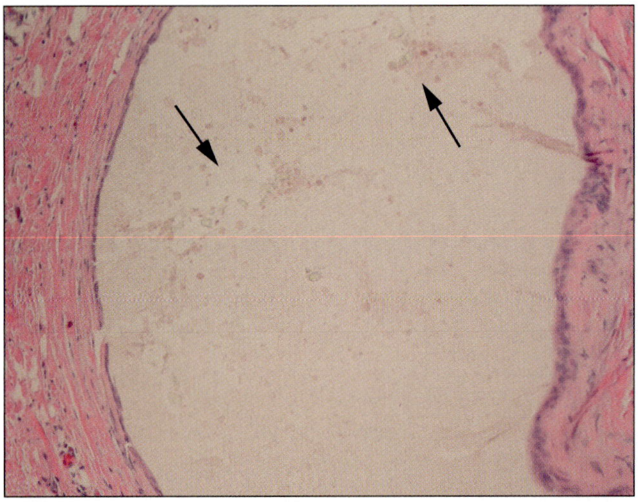

FIGURE 11.2 Calcium oxalate crystals (arrows) in apocrine lined cysts.

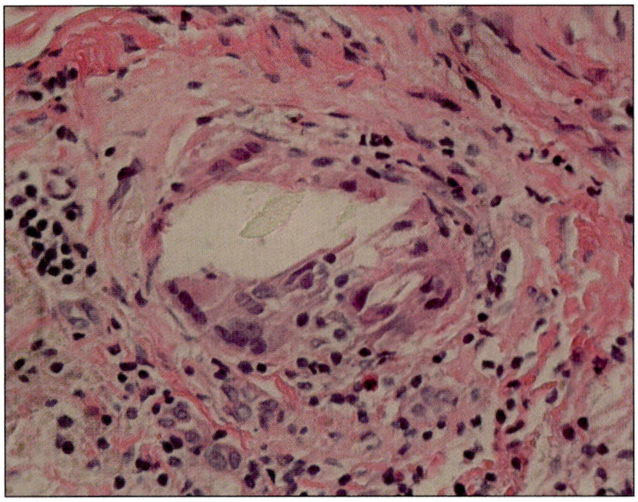

FIGURE 11.3 Calcium oxalate crystals in foreign body giant cell reaction.

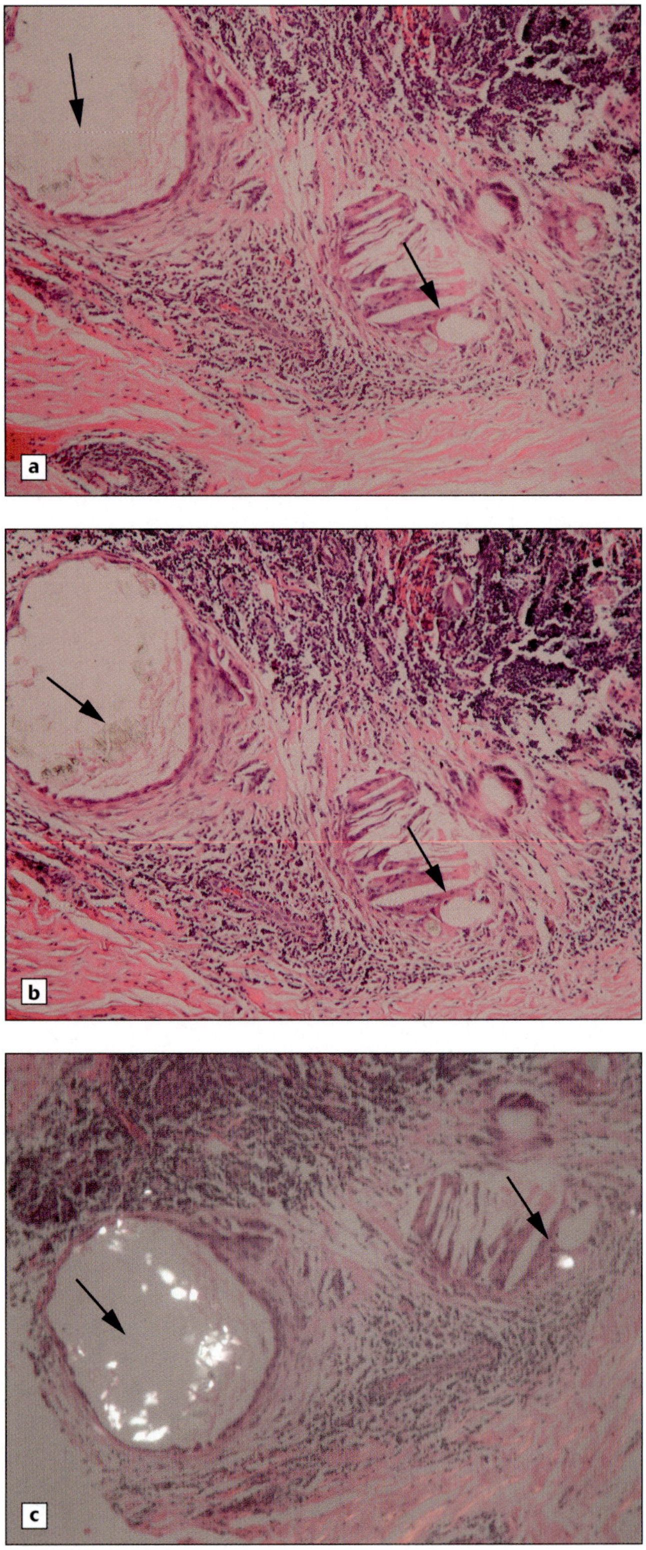

FIGURE 11.4 Comparison of the appearance of calcium oxalate (arrows) on **(a)** H&E, **(b)** with the condenser and **(c)** under polarized light.

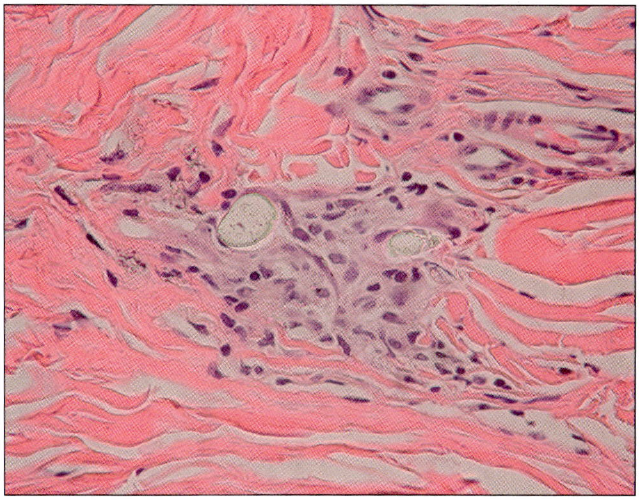

FIGURE 11.5 Deceptive appearance of calcium oxalate crystals as seen with the condenser, such that they may be overlooked on H&E and be mistaken for holes.

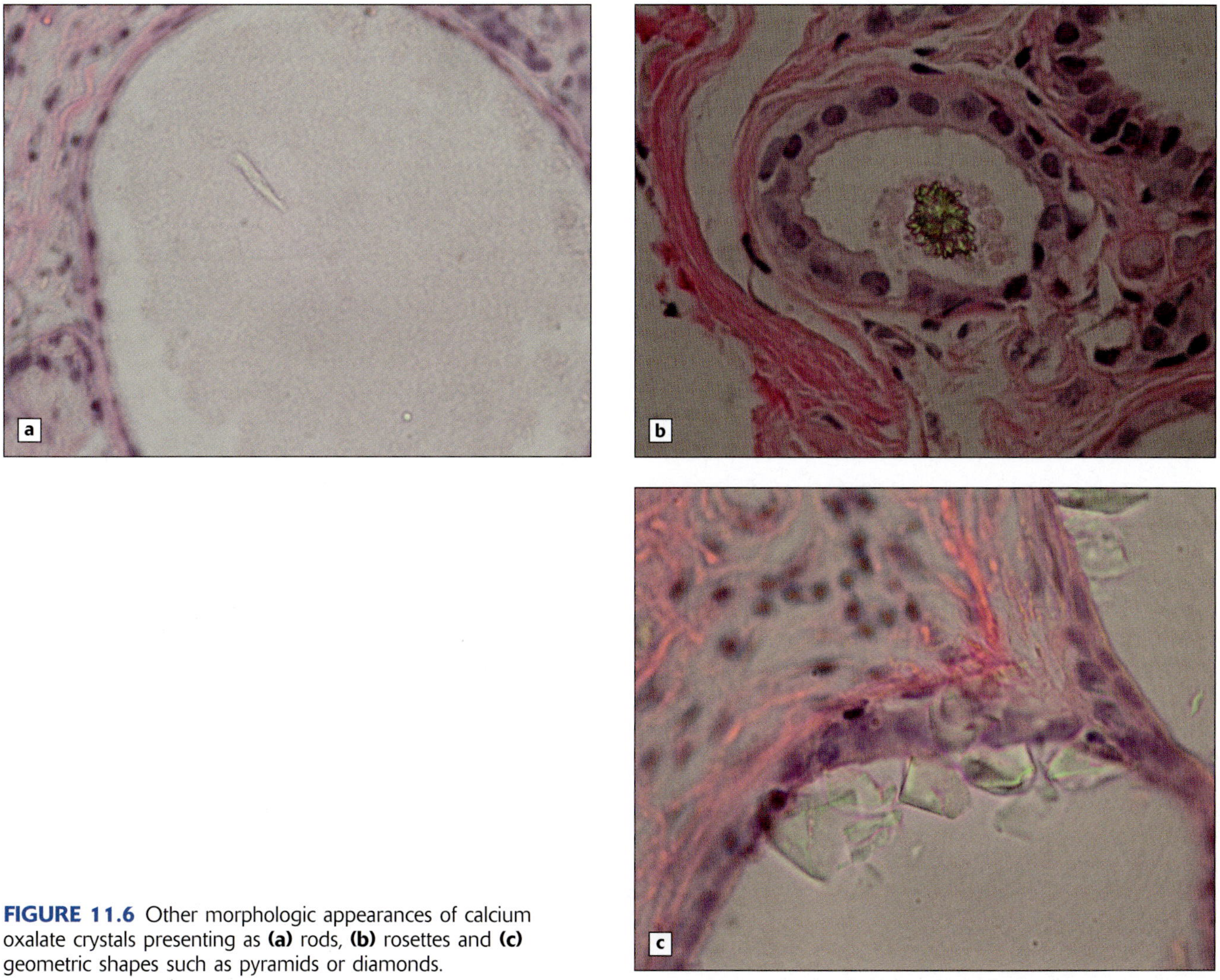

FIGURE 11.6 Other morphologic appearances of calcium oxalate crystals presenting as **(a)** rods, **(b)** rosettes and **(c)** geometric shapes such as pyramids or diamonds.

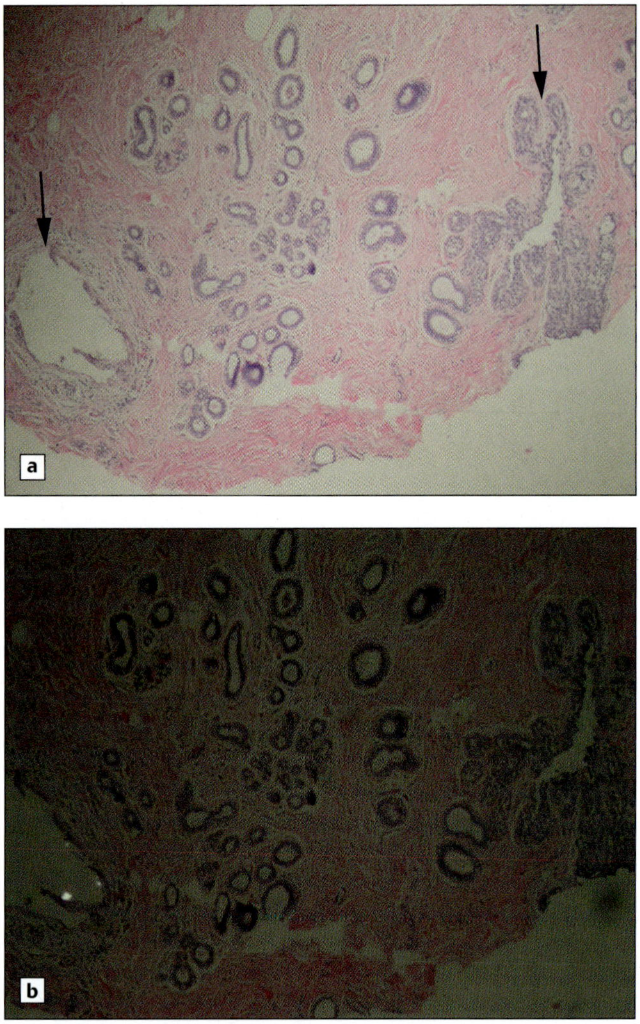

FIGURE 11.7 **(a)** H&E showing calcium oxalate crystals (left arrow) incidental to pagetoid spread of LCIS (right arrow), better appreciated under polarized light **(b).**

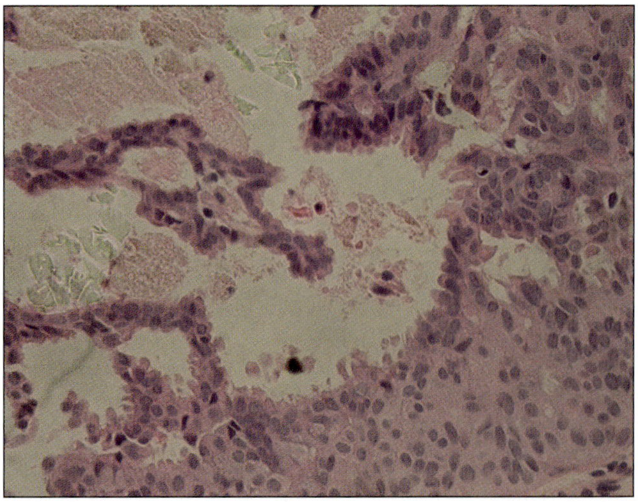

FIGURE 11.8 Calcium oxalate crystals incidental to the pagetoid spread of DCIS along a cyst wall.

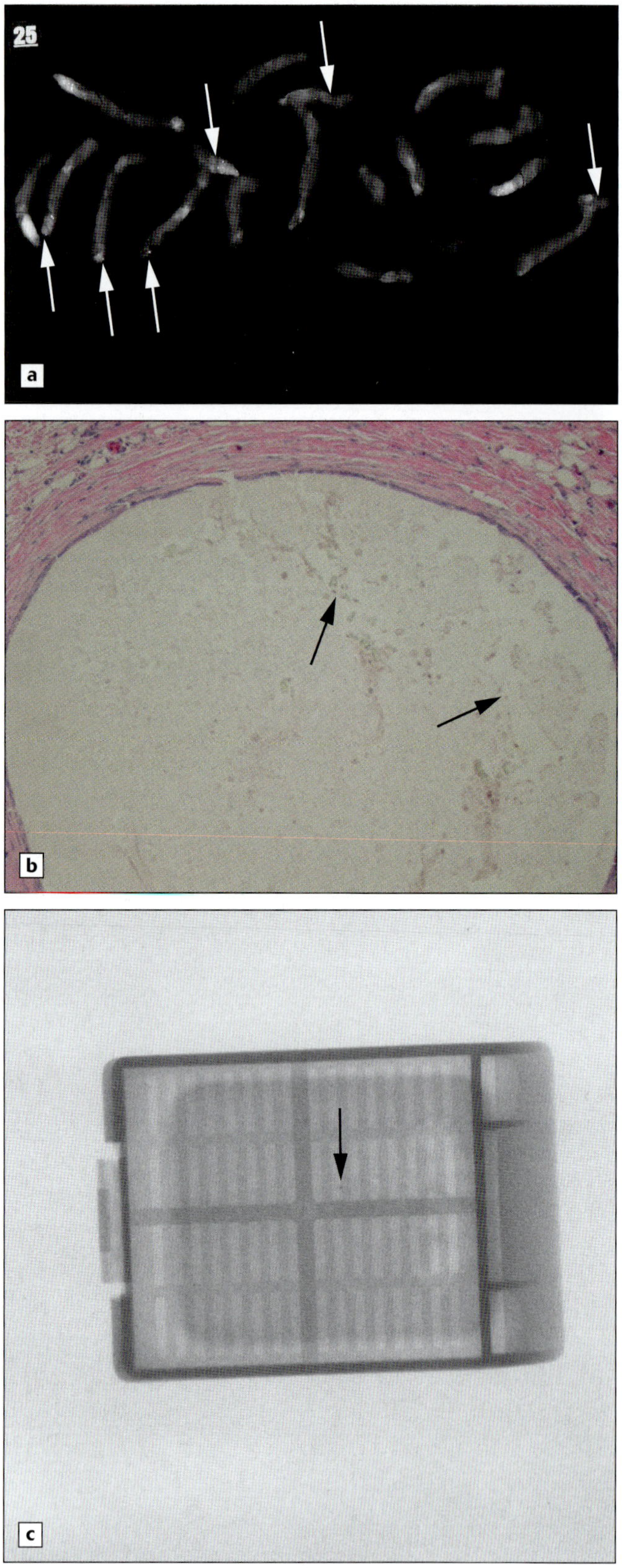

FIGURE 11.9 Specimen radiograph **(a)** shows several cores with numerous calcifications in each (arrows), but only few (calcium oxalate) are found on the H&E **(b)** (arrows) and paraffin block radiograph **(c)** (arrow).

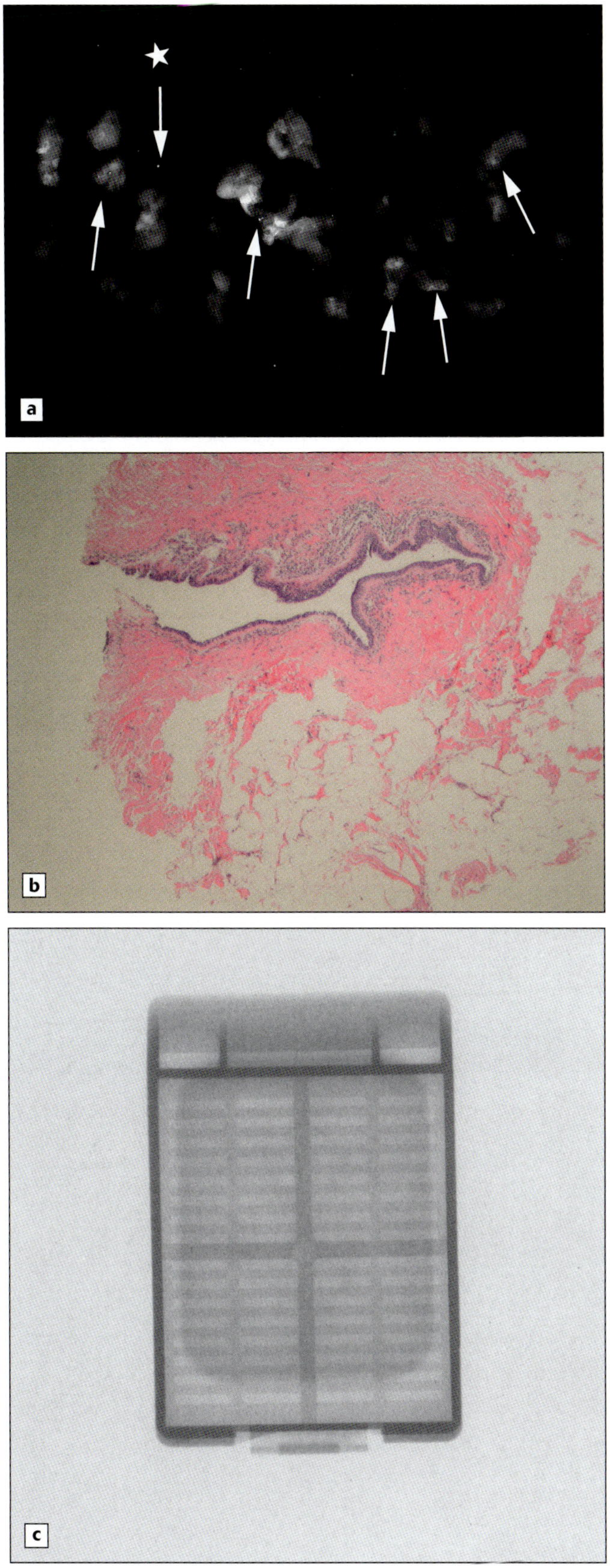

FIGURE 11.10 Specimen radiograph **(a)** shows several cores with numerous calcifications (arrows) in each, few that are dislodged (asterisk). None are found on the H&E **(b)** and paraffin block radiograph **(c).** The H&E shows a ruptured cyst which provides a perfect evacuation route for the calcium oxalate to escape into the formalin bottle.

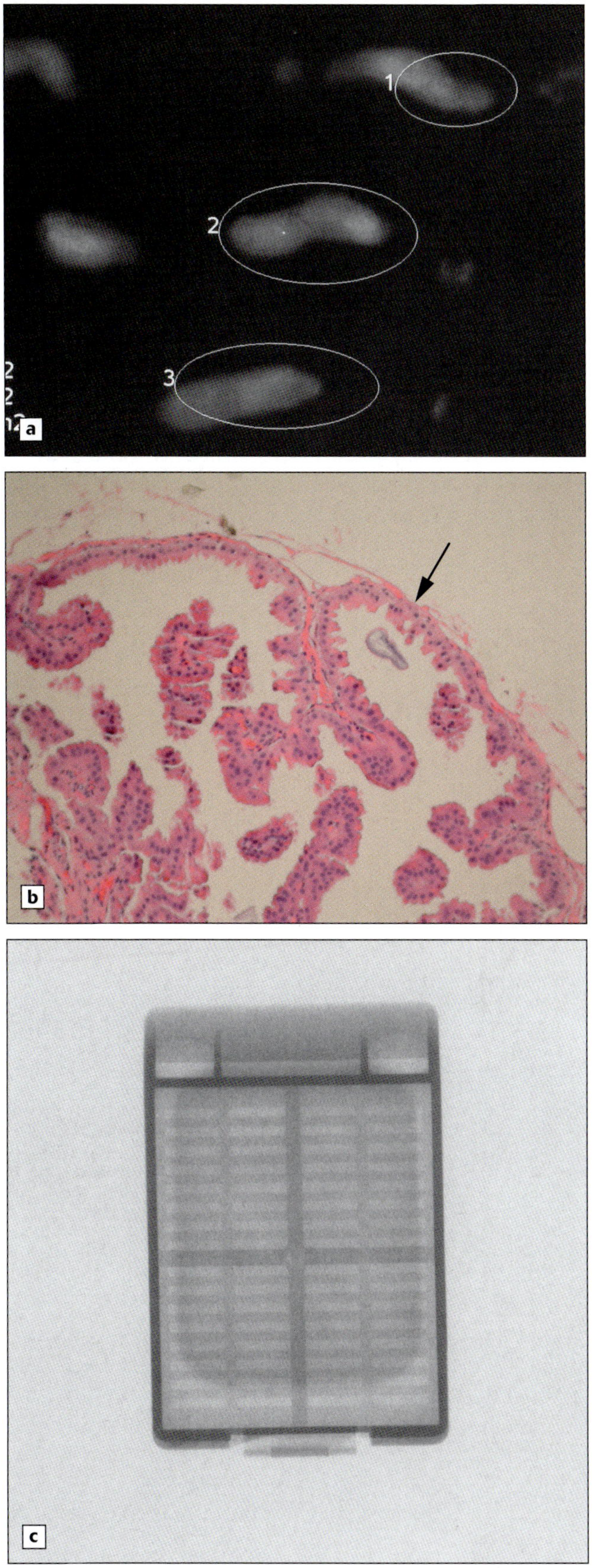

FIGURE 11.11 Specimen radiograph **(a)** shows few cores with dot like calcifications, but only few are found on the H&E (calcium phosphate) **(b)** (arrow) in an apocrine lined cyst. Paraffin block radiograph **(c)** revealed no residual calcifications.

When a cyst is biopsied, regardless of its size, the resultant tissue cores will show the inner lining of the cyst wall either along the peripheral edge (Fig. 11.12a) of the core biopsy or at the tip of the core (Fig. 11.12b). Such microscopic cysts may be removed as a whole and will then be contained intact (with its contents including calcium oxalate) within a single core of tissue (Fig. 11.12b). Alternatively, the cyst maybe ruptured as a result of the biopsy. Consider the fate of any solid contents of a cyst, i.e., calcifications. If the calcifications are removed with the tissue, they will be seen on the specimen radiograph and frequently, in our experience, are present at the periphery (Fig. 11.13) of the individual core, probably loosely adherent, if at all, to the inner lining of the cyst wall. When taken off the Petri dish or other solid base on which they are radiographed, and then placed into a liquid medium, namely formalin, the calcifications will fall out of the tissue cores into the liquid, never to be seen again. Thus, the calcifications that are left to be identified histologically are those which either are more strongly adherent to the cyst wall (Fig. 11.13), those that are present in cysts removed intact within individual cores (Figs 11.2, 11.4, and 11.12) and or adjacent foreign body reaction. As mentioned previously, calcium oxalate is more commonly associated with apocrine lined cysts than calcium phosphate and thus more vulnerable to this phenomenon.

As described above it is not that the missing calcium oxalate crystals are under recognized on the H&E, but rather that they are in the formalin bottle and not on the slides. In fact, when a wet mount of the remaining centrifuged fixative is visualized with polarized light, refrac-

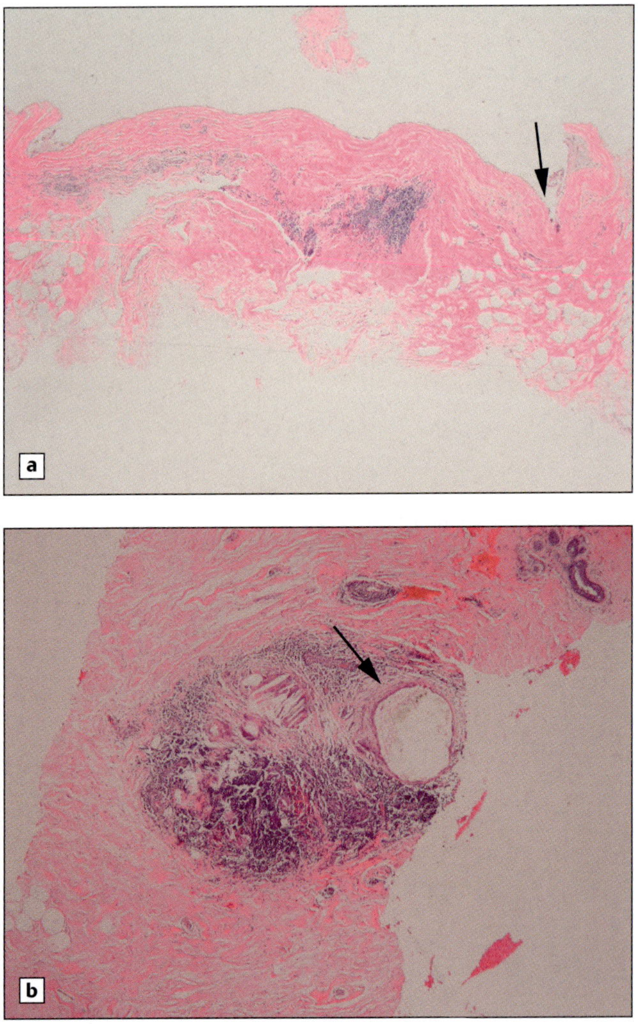

FIGURE 11.12 The fate of a cyst after core biopsy. **(a)** The cyst may rupture such that the inner lining (arrow) is present on the peripheral edge of the biopsy or **(b)** the cyst may be removed en toto within a single core of tissue (arrow) with its contents (calcium oxalate).

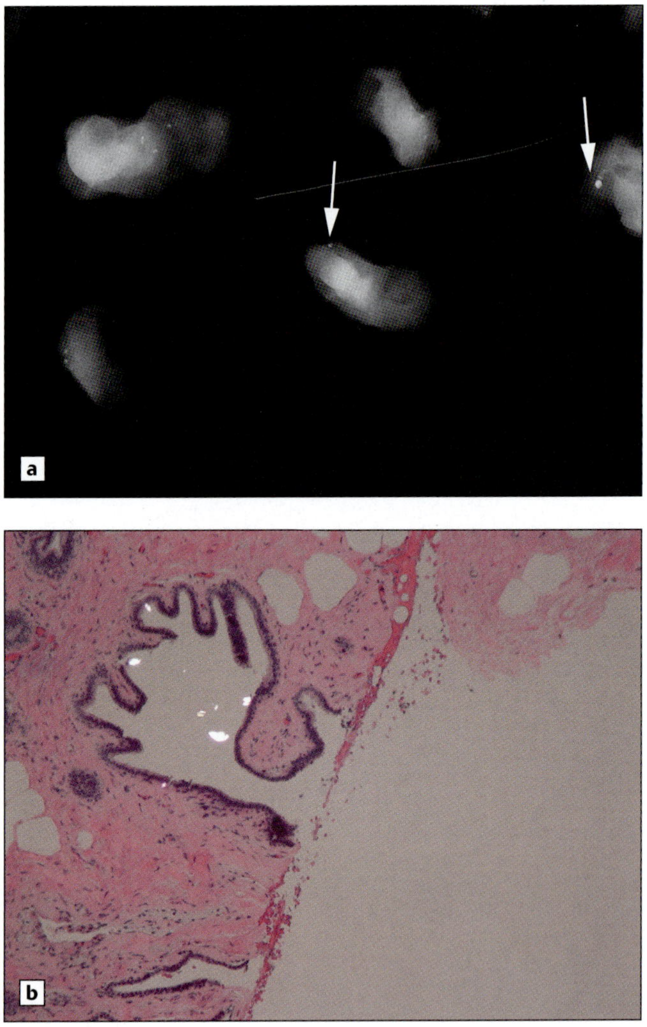

FIGURE 11.13 Specimen radiograph **(a)** showing calcifications at the periphery of tissue core biopsy fragments (arrows). Histologic sections under polarized light **(b)** show a ruptured cyst along the periphery of the core biopsy showing calcium oxalate crystals that are strongly adherent to the cyst wall, the remainder lost in the formalin bottle.

tile crystals are appreciated.[13] Logically, the phenomenon of calcium drop out from cysts would be almost exclusive to calcium oxalate, but may occasionally be seen in the case of calcium phosphate residing in cysts (Fig. 11.11). This scenario may be of more than academic interest since we have spoken to numerous frustrated radiologists who receive reports from pathologists stating that "no calcifications are identified" although specimen radiography demonstrated their removal (Figs 11.9 and 11.10). In part this may be due to the fact that the specimen radiograph is not always available to the pathologist so that he is not certain what he is looking for, but it may also be secondary to the above situation of not only difficult to find but "disappearing" calcifications. Many radiologists may feel obligated to recommend surgical excision of the area just to be safe, especially given the current medico-legal climate in mammography. In our view, however, such unnecessary surgeries can be avoided with careful radiologic–pathologic correlation and knowledge of the tendency for cyst-derived calcifications to result in "discrepancies".

POINTS TO REMEMBER

The work up of discrepant calcifications: (more present on specimen radiograph than on H&E slides)

1. Use polarized light to find calcium oxalate
2. X-ray paraffin block
3. Fewer to no calcifications in the paraffin block x-ray compared to the specimen radiography is nearly always due to dropout of calcium oxalate from apocrine metaplasia lined cysts.

REFERENCES

1. Tornos C, Silva E, el-Naggar A, Pritzker KP. Calcium oxalate crystals in breast biopsies. The missing microcalcifications. Am J Surg Pathol 14:961–968,1990.
2. Truong LD, Cartwright J Jr, Alpert L. Calcium oxalate in breast lesions biopsied for calcification detected in screening mammography: incidence and clinical significance. Mod Pathol 5:146–152,1992.
3. Busing CM, Keppler U, Menges V. Differences in microcalcification in breast tumors. Virchows Arch (A) 393:307–313,1981.
4. Frappart L, Boudeulle M, Boumendil J, et al. Structure and composition of microcalcifications in benign and malignant lesions of the breast. Hum Pathol 15:880–889,1984.
5. Frappart L, Remy I, Chi Lin H, et al. Different types of microcalcifications observed in breast pathology. Virchows Arch (A) 410:179–187,1986.
6. Fandos-Morere A, Prats-Esteve M, Tura-Sotera JM, Traveria-Cros A. Breast tumors: composition of microcalcifications. Radiology 169:325–327,1988.
7. Rosen PPR. Pathological examination of breast specimens. In Rosen's Breast Pathology. New York, Lippincott-Raven Publishers, 848–849,2001.
8. Gonzalez JEG, Caldwell RG, Valaitis J. Calcium oxalate crystals in the breast. Am J Surg Pathol 1991;15:586–591,1991.
9. Dahlstrom JE, Jain S. Histologic correlation of mammographically detected microcalcifications in stereotactic core biopsies. Pathology 33:444–448,2001.
10. Mortitz JD, Luftner-Nagel S, Westerhof JP, et al. Microcalcifications in breast core biopsy specimens: Disappearance at radiography after storage in formaldehyde. Radiology 200:361–363,1996.
11. Liberman L, Evans WP, Dershaw DD, et al. Radiography of microcalcifications in stereotaxic mammary core biopsy specimens. Radiology 190:223–225,1994.
12. Dahlstrom JE, Sutton S, Jain S. Histologic-radiologic correlation of mammographically detected microcalcification in stereotactic core biopsies. Am J Surg Pathol 22:256–259,1998.
13. Cook L, Vinding J, Gordon H.W. Polarizing calcifications. Am J Surg Path 21:255–61,1997.

CHAPTER 12

Linear high-density calcifications

The most important differential diagnosis of linear high-density calcifications (Fig. 12.1) in a post lumpectomy patient is recurrent breast carcinoma. In such patients, frequent follow-up mammograms are indicated in order to detect residual and recurrent breast cancer in the treated breast as early as possible (Figs 12.2 and 12.3). Residual calcifications can be detected by performing mammography including magnification views over the lumpectomy bed in patients post lumpectomy, prior to radiation therapy. Additionally, it is important to be aware of the postoperative, post radiation mammographic changes that occur in these patients. For instance, previously benign calcifications elsewhere in the breast can be pulled into the lumpectomy bed by post surgical distortion (Fig. 12.2).

Calcifications can also form within postoperative fat necrosis. Unlike coarse benign scattered calcifications that may be present in up to 25% of irradiated breasts[1] (Fig. 12.2), these calcifications may initially be faint, fine and hard to distinguish from malignant type calcifications (Fig. 12.4). With time these calcifications are more typical of fat necrosis manifesting as bizarre, disorganized dystrophic forms that may become thick and plaque-like (Fig. 12.5) and others with arc like forms defining radiolucent oil cysts characteristic of fat necrosis (see also Chaps 4 and 10). The presence of new linear and clustered calcifications is worrisome and requires biopsy (Fig. 12.2).

Other benign entities that can present with high-density calcifications (Fig. 12.1) include fibroadenoma, fat necrosis, osseous metaplasia and vascular calcifications. The radiologic features of a calcifying fibroadenoma are straightforward, characterized as containing coarse or popcorn like calcifications (Fig. 12.6a; see also Chap. 10, Fig. 10.2), usually not warranting core biopsy. Histologically, the calcifications correlate with basophilic concretions in the hyalinizing stroma (Fig. 12.6c). Sometimes, these large chunky calcifications cause resistance to the microtome during cutting, causing them to fragment such that they nearly disappear from the tissue, leaving the fibroadenoma itself somewhat fragmented (Fig. 12.7). This shatter artifact may sometimes create a discrepancy between the obvious calcifications typical of fibroadenoma on the specimen radiograph and the H&E that shows a fragmented fibroadenoma with fewer and or smaller calcifications (Fig. 12.7b). Occasionally, the calcifications appear as clusters of tiny, blue-gray, round calcium deposits in the densely hyalinized stroma (Fig. 12.8). Still less frequent is the occurrence of stromal calcifications that track along the periphery of compressed slit shaped ducts, so as to appear as linear and rarely branching forms[2] (Fig. 12.9). These are the cases that must be biopsied to exclude carcinoma particularly in a patient with a history of malignancy.

While in the past, trauma was the most common etiology for fat necrosis, especially in elderly women with pendulous breasts, today, it is seen predominantly as a consequence of surgical and/or radiation treatment of the breast. Mammographically, calcifications may accompany a density (Fig. 12.10) or be present alone. Histological changes vary depending on the timing of the biopsy. Early changes include disruption of adipocytes associated with hemorrhage and histiocytes (Fig. 12.11). Next, the recruited histiocytes coalesce to form multinucleated giant cells associated with hemosiderin and other chronic inflammatory cells (Fig. 12.12). Eventually, peripheral fibrosis takes over to surround the area to form a scar (Fig. 12.13). Histologically the calcifications associated with fat necrosis are usually large (Figure 12.13a), variable in size and shape, and found either in areas of disrupted adipocytes (Fig. 12.14), histiocytes (Fig. 12.14) and or in dense fibrosis (Fig. 12.13). In some cases the fat necrosis may cystify and calcify. The calcifications in cystic fat necrosis are usually dense, present in the fibrous walls, corresponding to rim-like mammographic calcifications (Fig. 12.15; see also Chap 4, Fig. 4.9a).

Patients with fat necrosis as a consequence of previous surgery for malignancy may also most likely have received radiation. Consequently, the surrounding cells may show radiation induced cytologic changes which include: epithelial atrophy, fibrosis and atypical cytological features limited to terminal duct lobular units (Fig. 12.16). Care must be taken in such cases not to over diagnose lobular spread of recurrent intraductal carcinoma, as the cytologic atypia can occasionally become quite worrisome. However, in radiation change, the atypia is limited to individual cells[3] rather than the entire population (Fig. 12.17). Often the cells will also show intranuclear holes

Text continued on p. 122

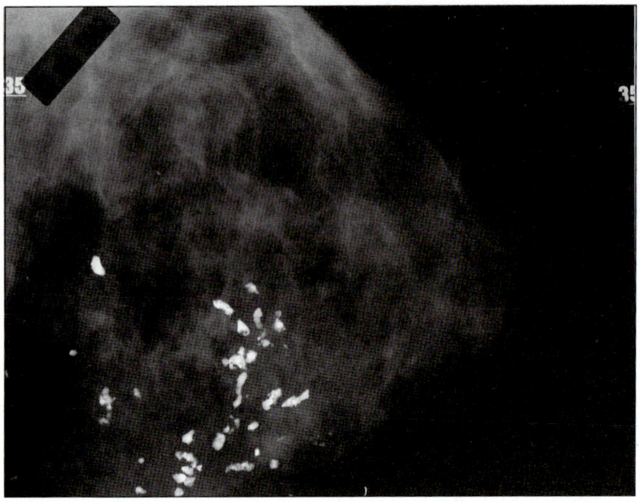

FIGURE 12.1 Mammogram showing high density calcifications.

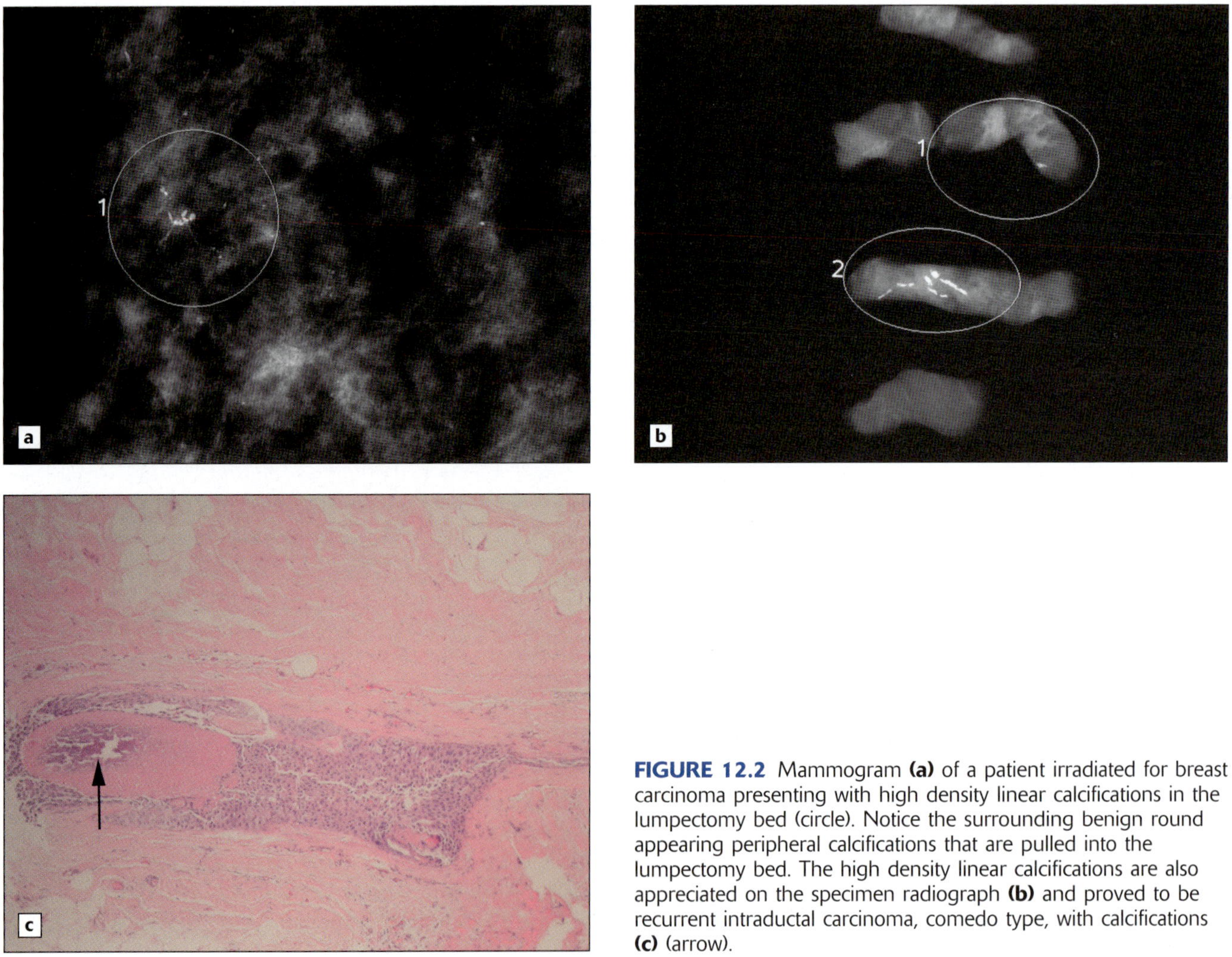

FIGURE 12.2 Mammogram **(a)** of a patient irradiated for breast carcinoma presenting with high density linear calcifications in the lumpectomy bed (circle). Notice the surrounding benign round appearing peripheral calcifications that are pulled into the lumpectomy bed. The high density linear calcifications are also appreciated on the specimen radiograph **(b)** and proved to be recurrent intraductal carcinoma, comedo type, with calcifications **(c)** (arrow).

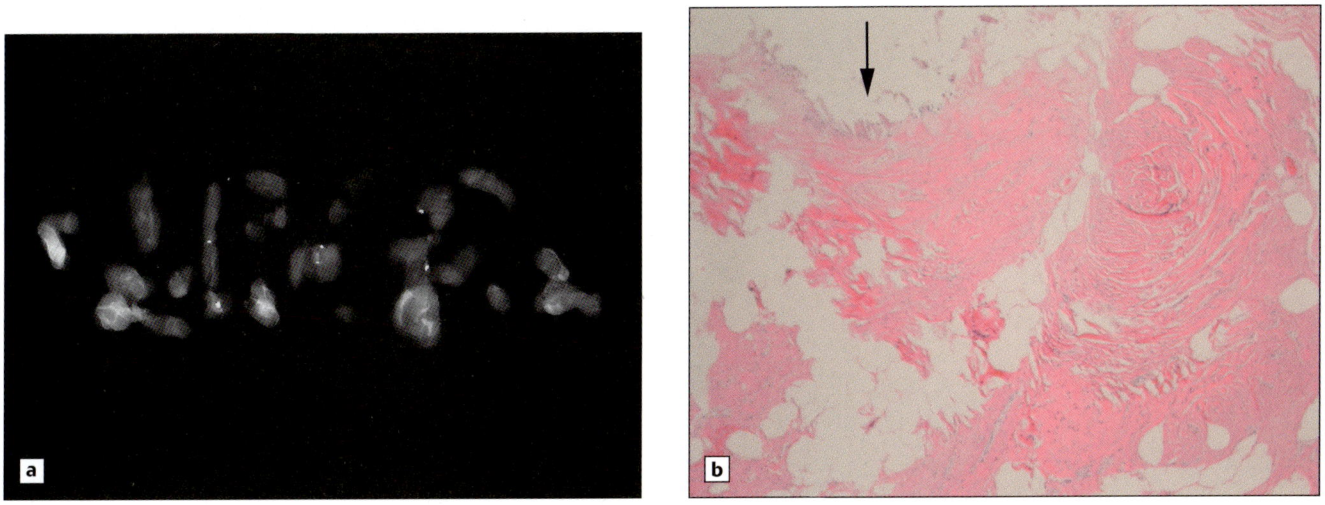

FIGURE 12.3 Specimen radiograph **(a)** showing several cores with coarse calcifications seen after radiation. Core biopsies **(b)** show dense fibrosis consistent with previous surgical scar associated with calcifications (arrow).

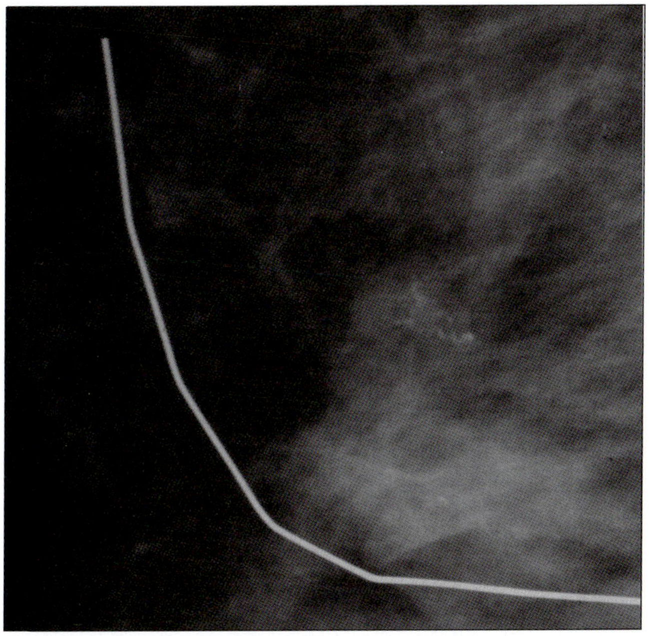

FIGURE 12.4 Calcifications due to early fat necrosis may be faint, fine and hard to distinguish from malignant type calcifications.

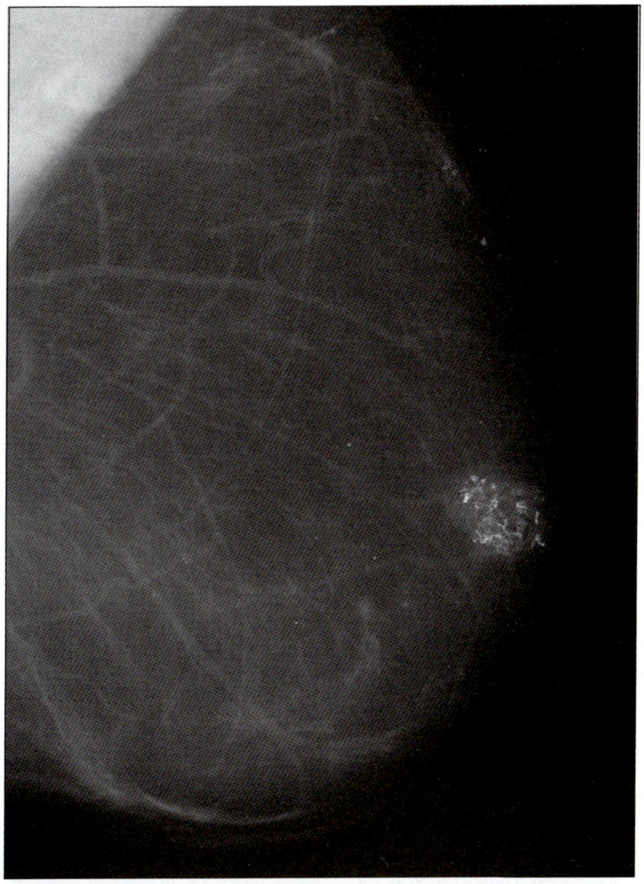

FIGURE 12.5 Mammogram showing high density, bizarre, disorganized dystrophic calcifications that may become thick and plaque-like, typical of fat necrosis.

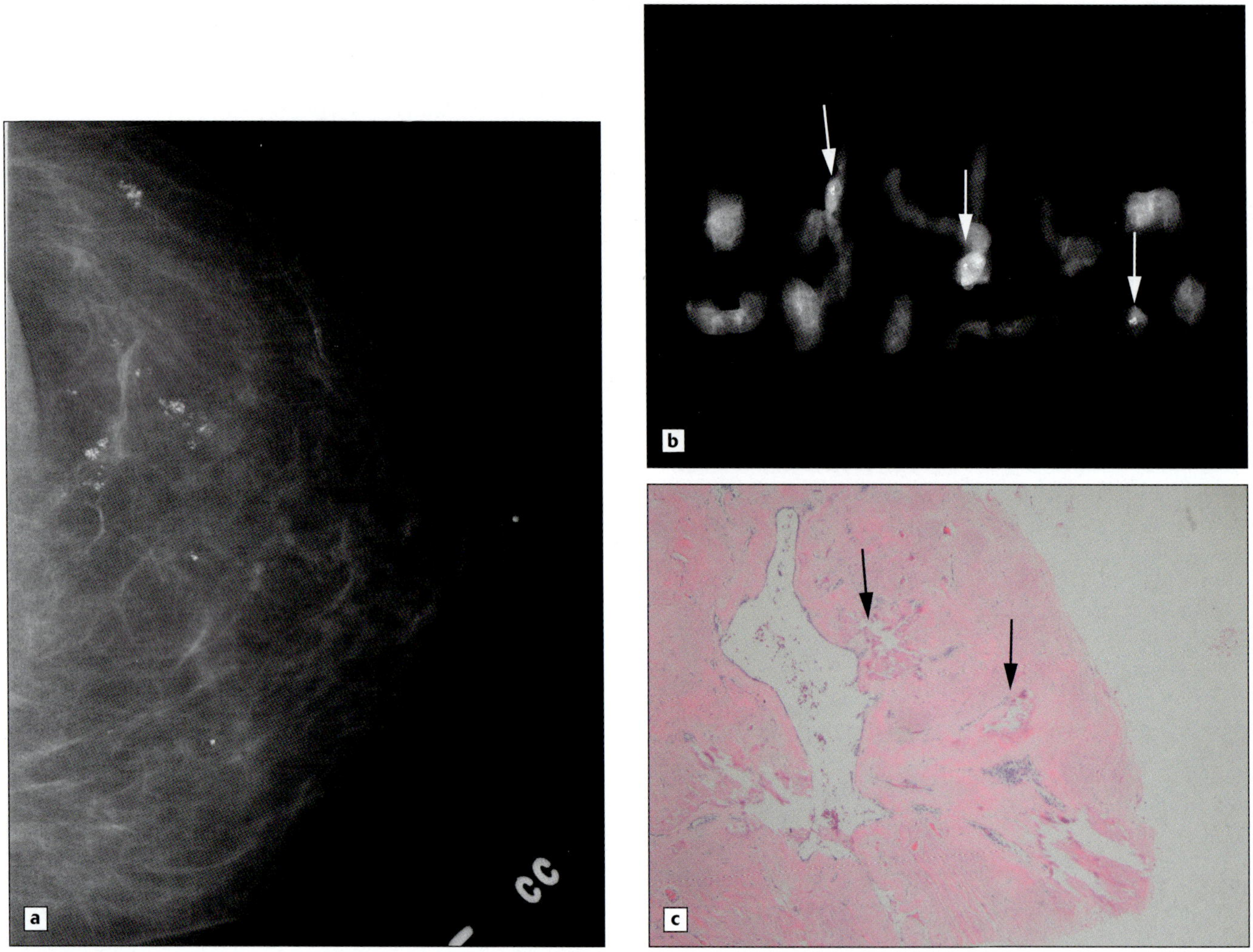

FIGURE 12.6 **(a)** Mammogram, **(b)** specimen radiograph and **(c)** H&E showing chunky popcorn calcifications (arrows) typical of fibroadenoma.

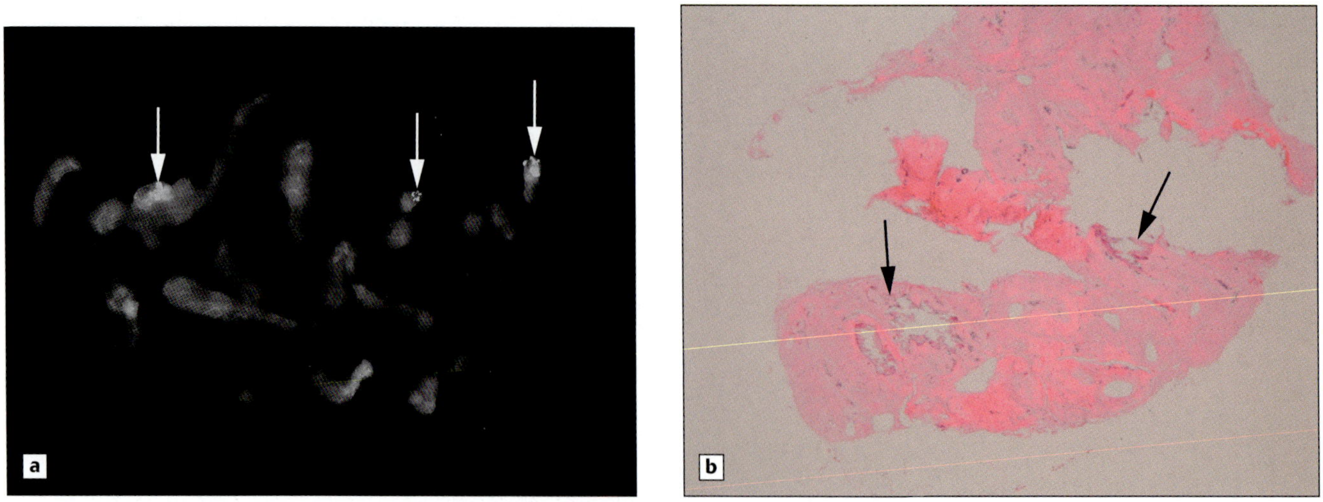

FIGURE 12.7 Although the specimen radiograph **(a)** shows many coarse calcifications (arrows) typical of fibroadenoma, H&E **(b)** shows few shattered calcifications (arrows) within the fibrotic stroma of a disrupted fibroadenoma.

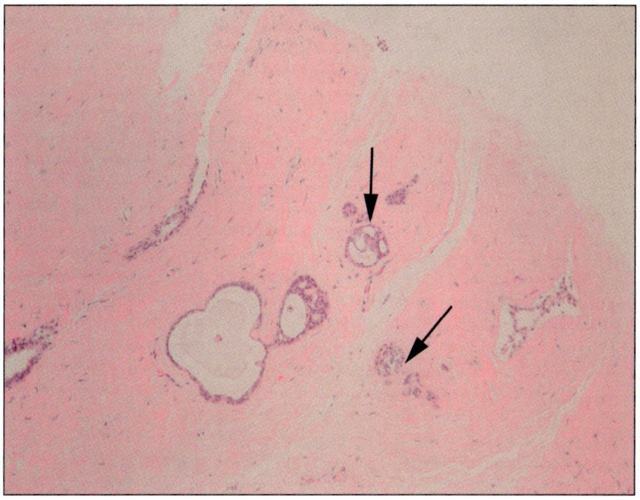

FIGURE 12.8 Clusters of tiny, blue-gray, round calcium deposits (arrows) in the densely hyalinized stroma of a fibroadenoma.

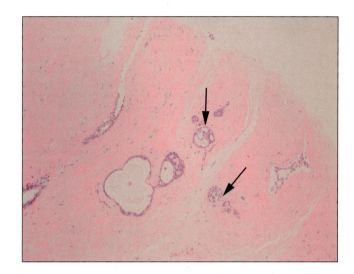

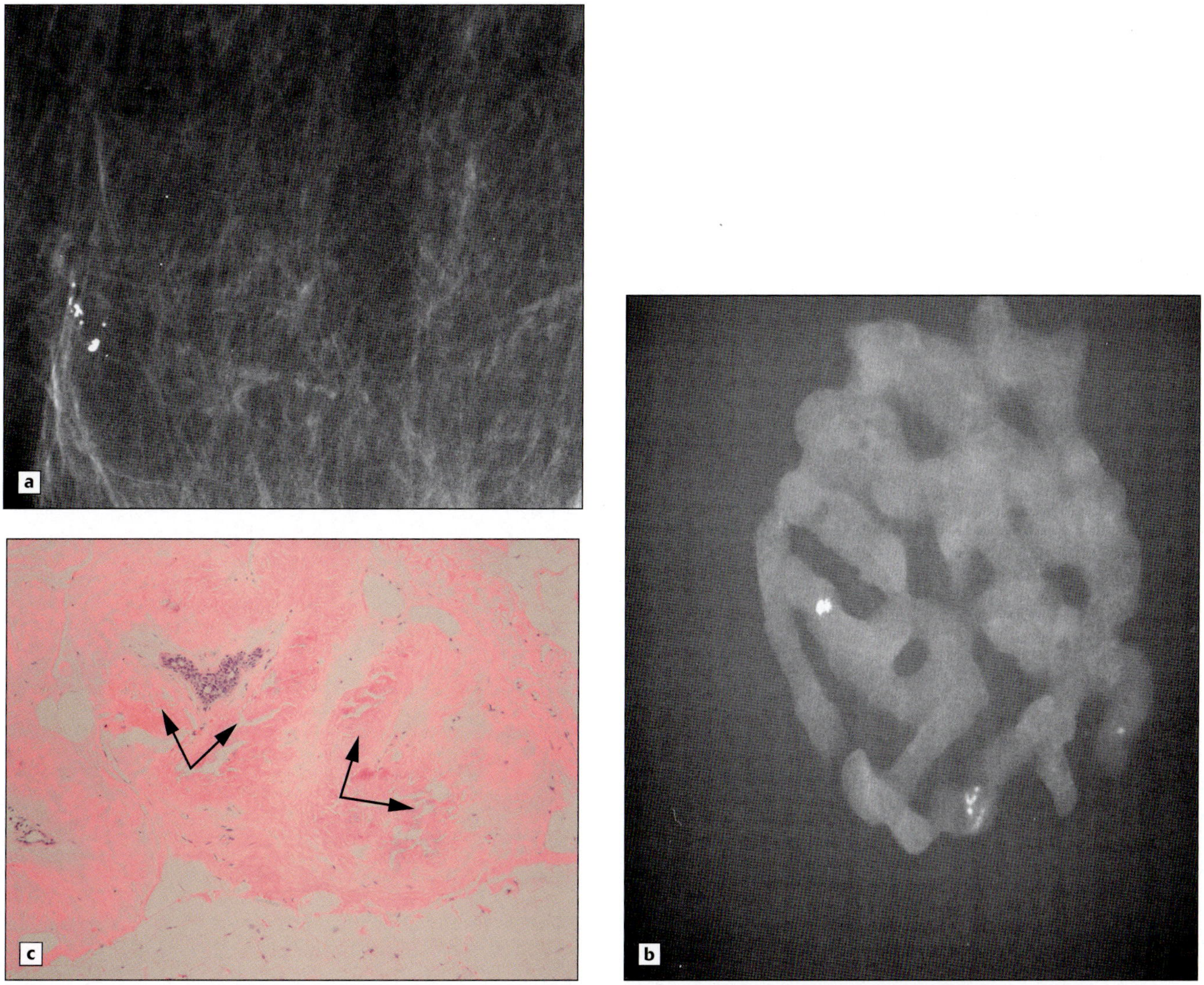

FIGURE 12.9 **(a)** Mammogram and **(b)** specimen radiograph showing high density linear and occasionally branching calcifications which correlate with the periductal stromal branching calcifications **(c)** (arrows) in a fibroadenoma.

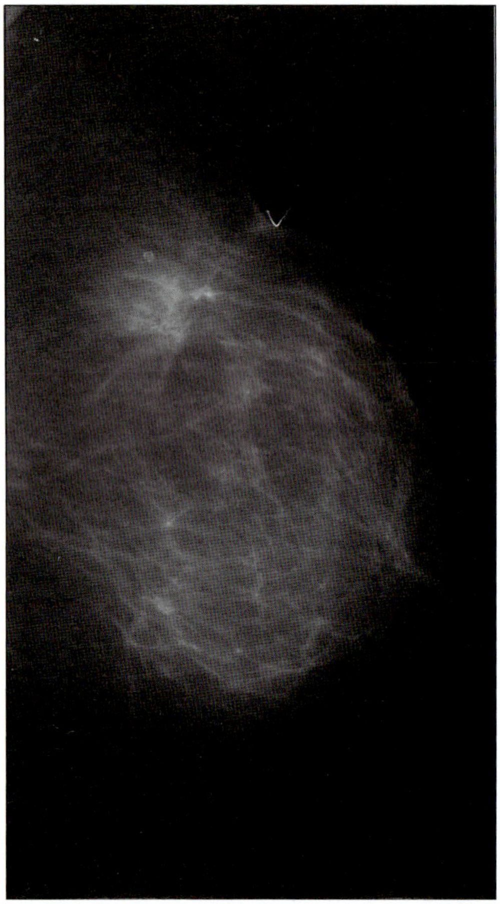

FIGURE 12.10 Mammogram showing fat necrosis presenting as a density and with calcifications.

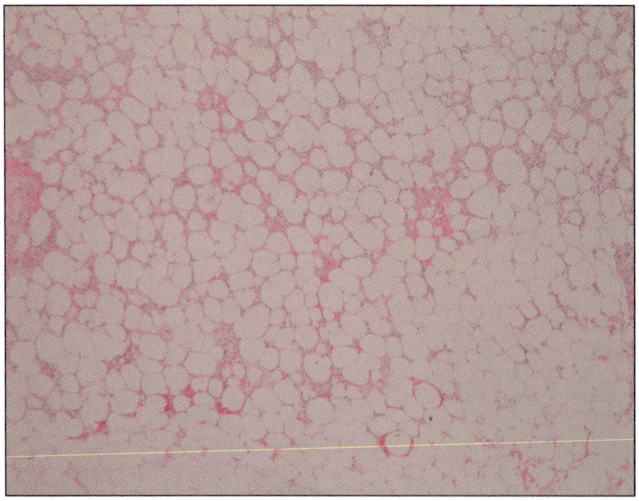

FIGURE 12.11 Early fat necrosis showing disruption of adipocytes associated with hemorrhage and histiocytes.

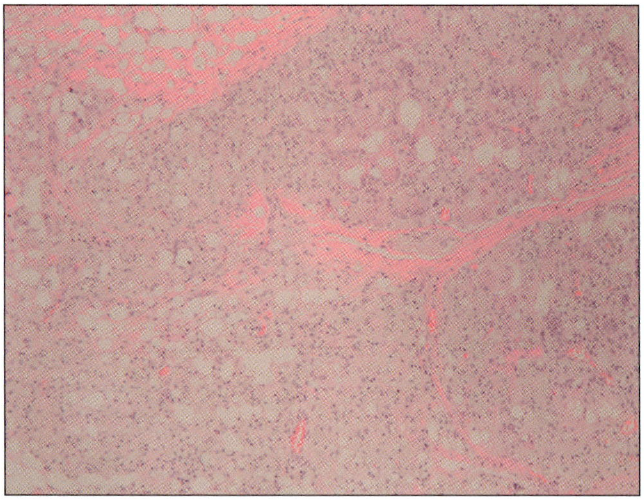

FIGURE 12.12 As fat necrosis organizes, the histiocytes coalesce to form multinucleated giant cells associated with chronic inflammatory cells.

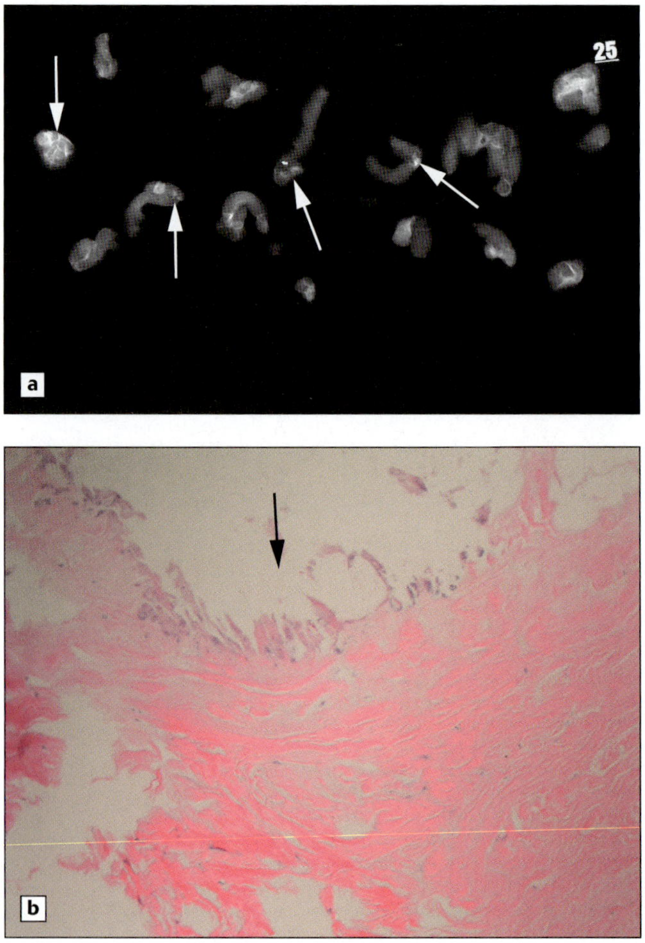

FIGURE 12.13 Specimen radiograph **(a)** of Fig. 12.5 shows several cores with pleomorphic coarse clustered calcifications (arrows). Histology **(b)** shows end stage fat necrosis that is fibrotic and calcified (arrow).

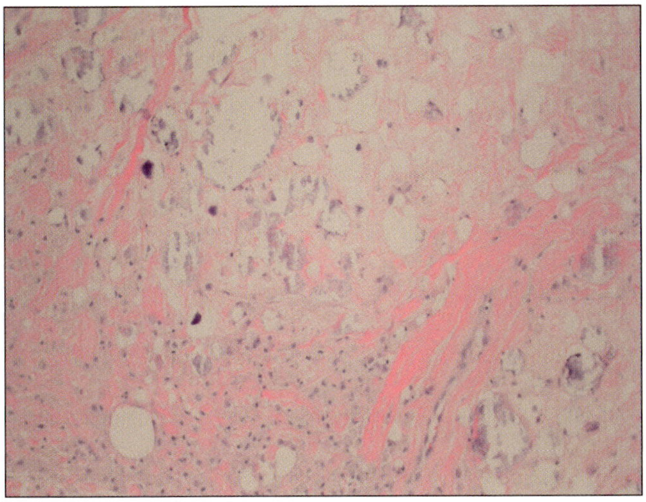

FIGURE 12.14 The calcifications associated with fat necrosis maybe found within histiocytes and disrupted adipocytes.

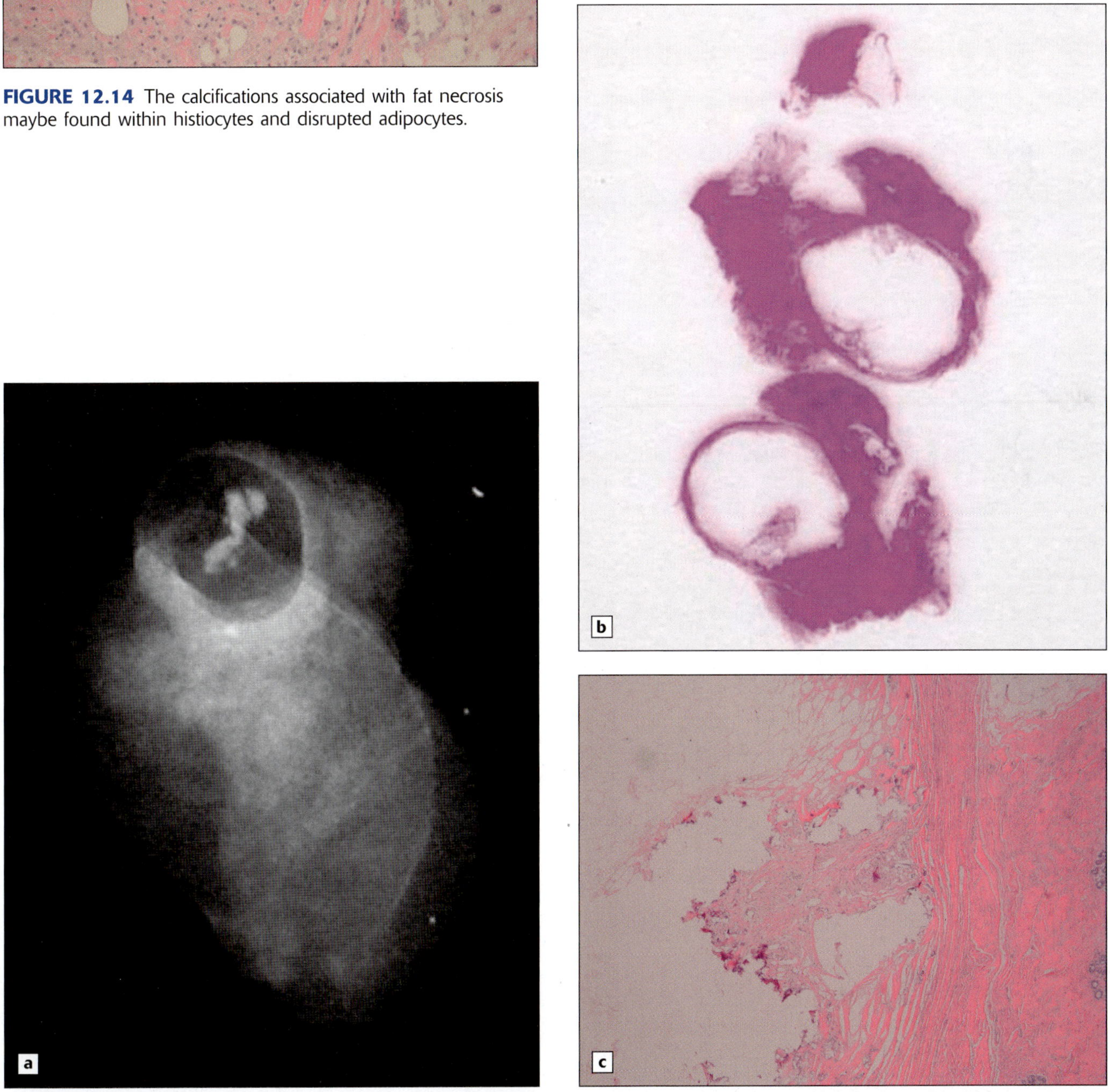

FIGURE 12.15 Magnified view of a core from a specimen radiograph **(a)** with rim-like calcifications correlating with calcifications in cystic fat necrosis, as seen on a whole mount histologic section **(b)** and at higher power **(c)**.

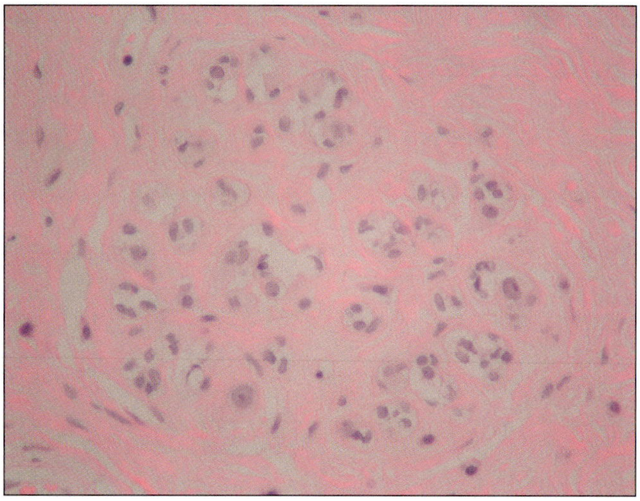

FIGURE 12.16 Radiation induced cytologic changes include epithelial atrophy, fibrosis and atypical cytological features limited to terminal duct lobular units.

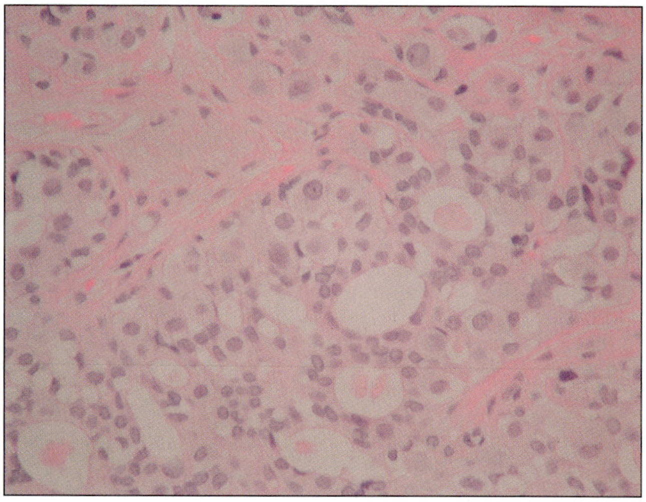

FIGURE 12.17 The distinction of radiation induced atypia from lobular spread of recurrent intraductal carcinoma can be challenging as seen in this case. However, in radiation induced cytologic changes as seen in this case the changes are limited to individual cells rather than the entire population of cells.

or inclusions and delicate irregularly folded nuclear membranes (Fig. 12.18).

Duct ectasia is defined as the leakage of proteinaceous contents of ducts into surrounding breast tissue secondary to localized rupture of the duct wall. Histologic changes often consist of intense reactive changes both within and outside the ruptured duct. On occasion the proteinaceous material may calcify, producing large, densely basophilic structures (Fig. 12.19) correlating to high density calcifications.

A few case reports have described the phenomenon of osseous metaplasia in the breast[4,5]. High-density branching type calcifications were described mammographically in one case.[5] The fibroblast, purported to have metaplastic potential and thus the capacity to differentiate into any type of mesenchymal cell, is hypothesized to be the cell of origin for this lesion. In one case report, it was noted to occur in response to chronic mastitis;[4] however, in our practice, we have seen instances of bony metaplasia in both surgically treated and radiated breasts as well as in breasts not previously biopsied or treated (Fig. 12.20).

Vascular calcifications are radiographically typically composed of two parallel partially continuous lines

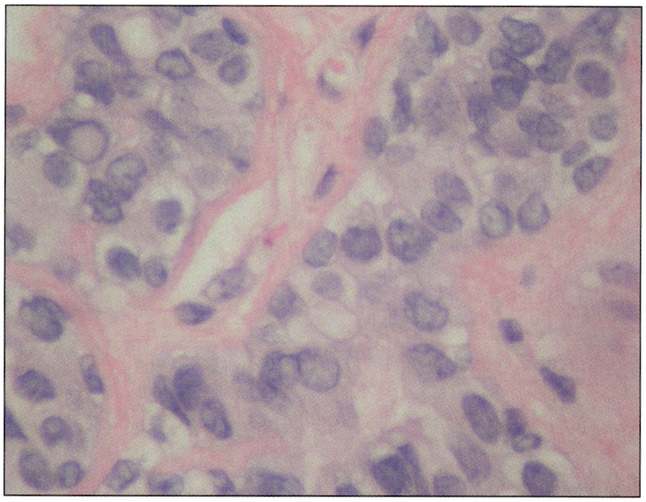

FIGURE 12.18 Radiation induced cytologic nuclear changes include intranuclear holes or inclusions and delicate irregularly folded nuclear membranes.

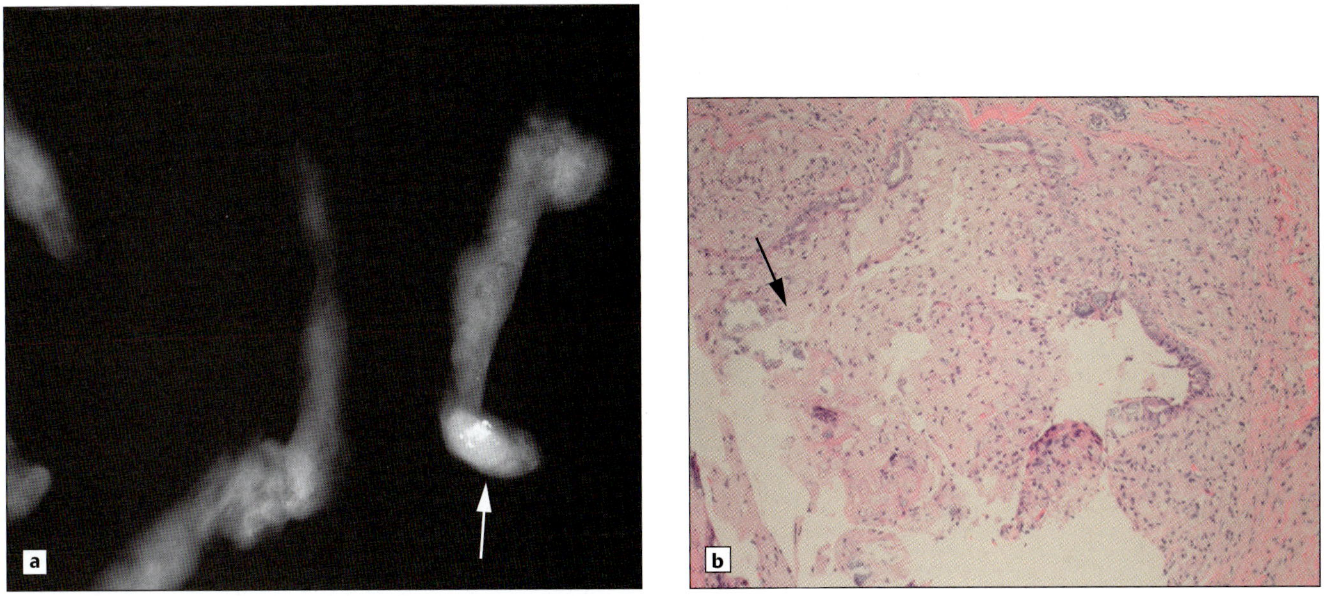

FIGURE 12.19 The calcifications (arrows) in duct ectasia may be dense as seen on the specimen radiograph **(a)** correlating with large, densely basophilic structures on H&E **(b)**.

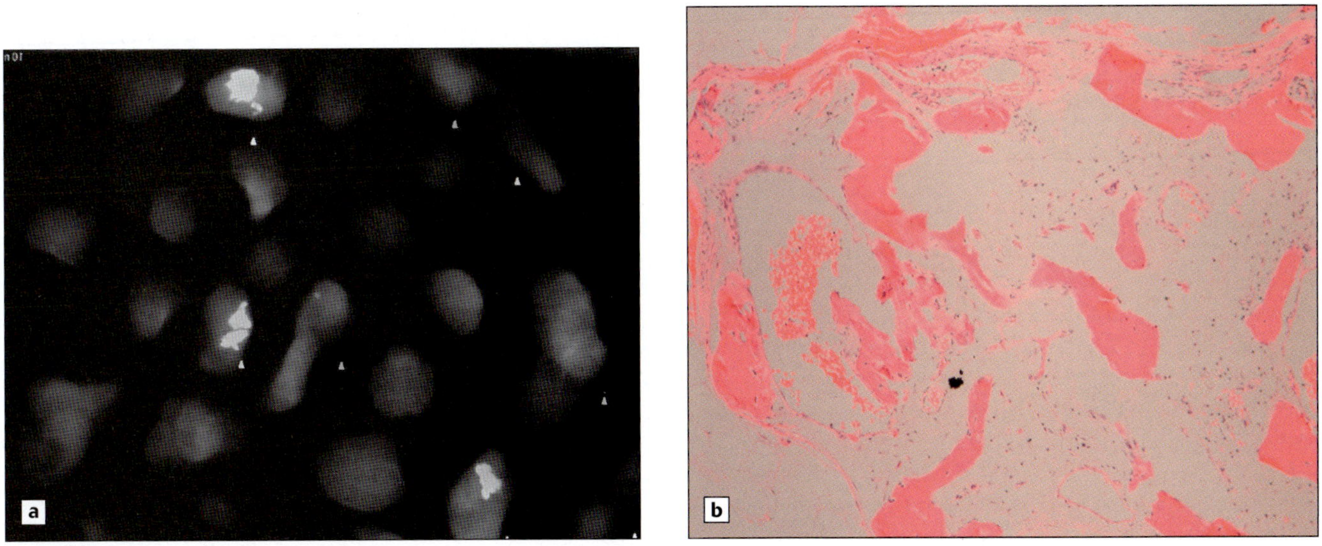

FIGURE 12.20 Specimen radiograph **(a)** showing obvious high density calcifications which correlate with mammary osseous metaplasia **(b)**.

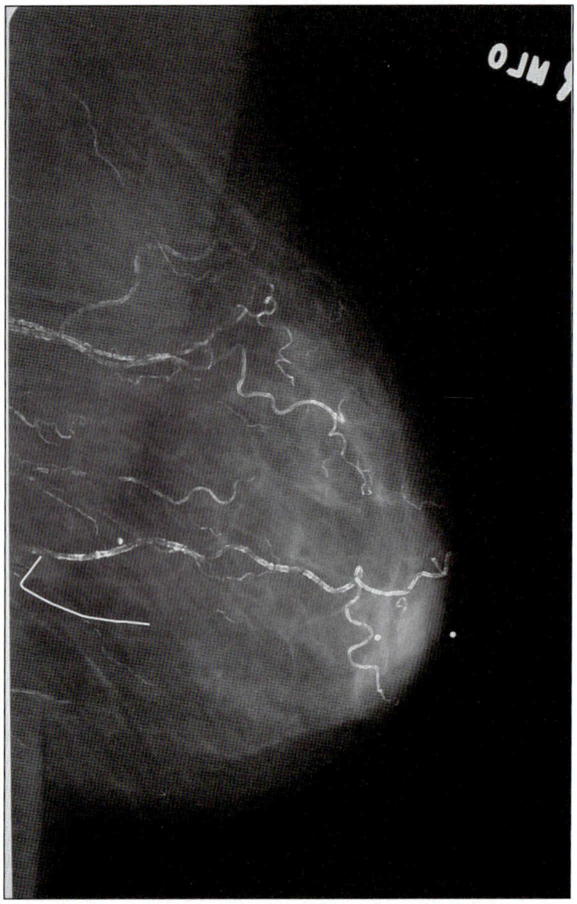

FIGURE 12.21 Typical mammogram of vascular calcifications characterized by two parallel partially continuous lines corresponding to calcifications along an arterial wall.

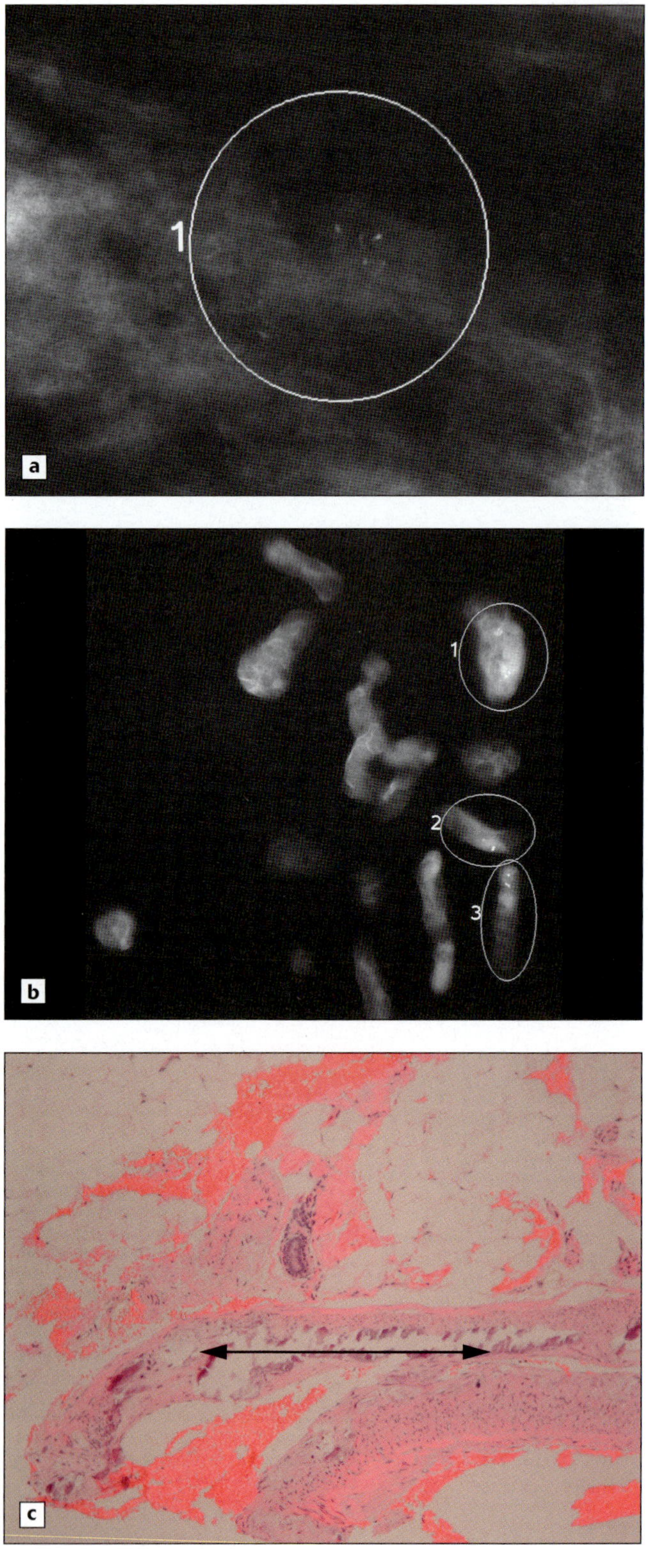

FIGURE 12.22 Rarely the calcifications associated with vessels may appear linear as seen on the mammogram **(a)** and specimen radiograph **(b)** and difficult to distinguish from comedo DCIS. Histologic sections **(c)** however show vascular calcifications (arrow).

corresponding histologically to an arterial wall (Fig. 12.21). While most cases are easily recognized as such on imaging and are therefore not biopsied, rarely the distinction from malignant linear calcifications may prove challenging (Fig. 12.22). In such instances, a large amount of blood will accompany and may outnumber the core biopsy fragments as the procedure has obviously and unfortunately resulted in hematoma formation (Fig. 12.22). Of course this may also occur if a non-calcified artery is accidentally broken and sampled by the procedure.

Finally, we have occasionally observed large calcium deposits in lactational change. They occur as a response to apoptosis and stasis of secretions that spontaneously involute or disappear with time. In lactational change, the calcifications are usually bilateral and diffuse, usually round and punctate (Fig. 12.23). Today, the incidence of lactational change associated with calcifications diagnosed on core biopsy has increased due to several reasons. As the modern woman delays motherhood, she is at an age when she is already undergoing annual mammograms. Thus, calcifications associated with lactational

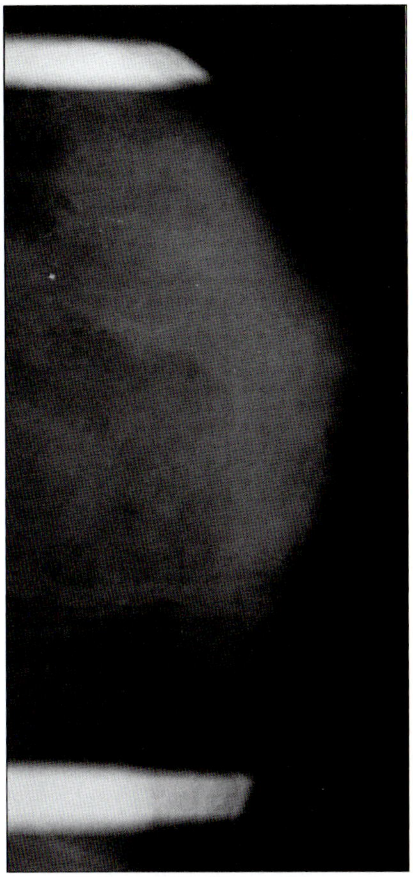

FIGURE 12.23 Typical mammogram of lactational changes showing bilateral and diffuse, round and punctate calcifications.

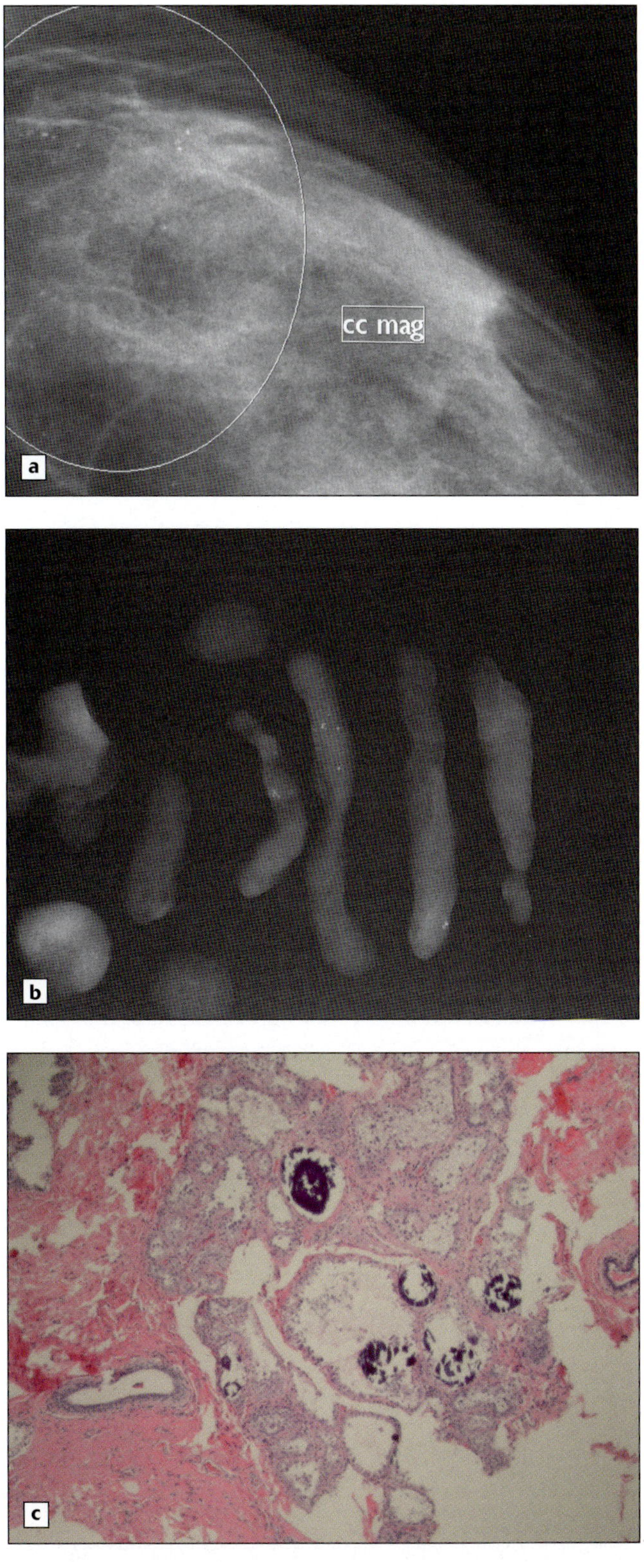

FIGURE 12.24 Mammogram **(a)** and specimen radiograph **(b)** showing coarse calcifications correlating with large, globular ones as seen on H&E **(c)** associated with pseudo lactational change.

changes which were undetected decades ago in the younger women who was not eligible for mammographic screening, are now detected in the older post partum mother. Given their transient nature, they are usually not appreciated at the time of the first screening mammogram of the younger mother. On the other hand, pseudo lactational change defined as lactational change in nonlactating nonpregnant women occurs at a frequency of 3%.[6] These changes may be related to selective susceptibility to estrogens, hormones, antipsychotics and antihypertensives or be idiopathic. As the modern postmenopausal women takes hormones, the incidence of lactational change and its association with calcifications will increase. In pseudolactational change, the calcifications can be large, globular and coarse (Fig. 12.24). In both lactational and pseudolactational change, the

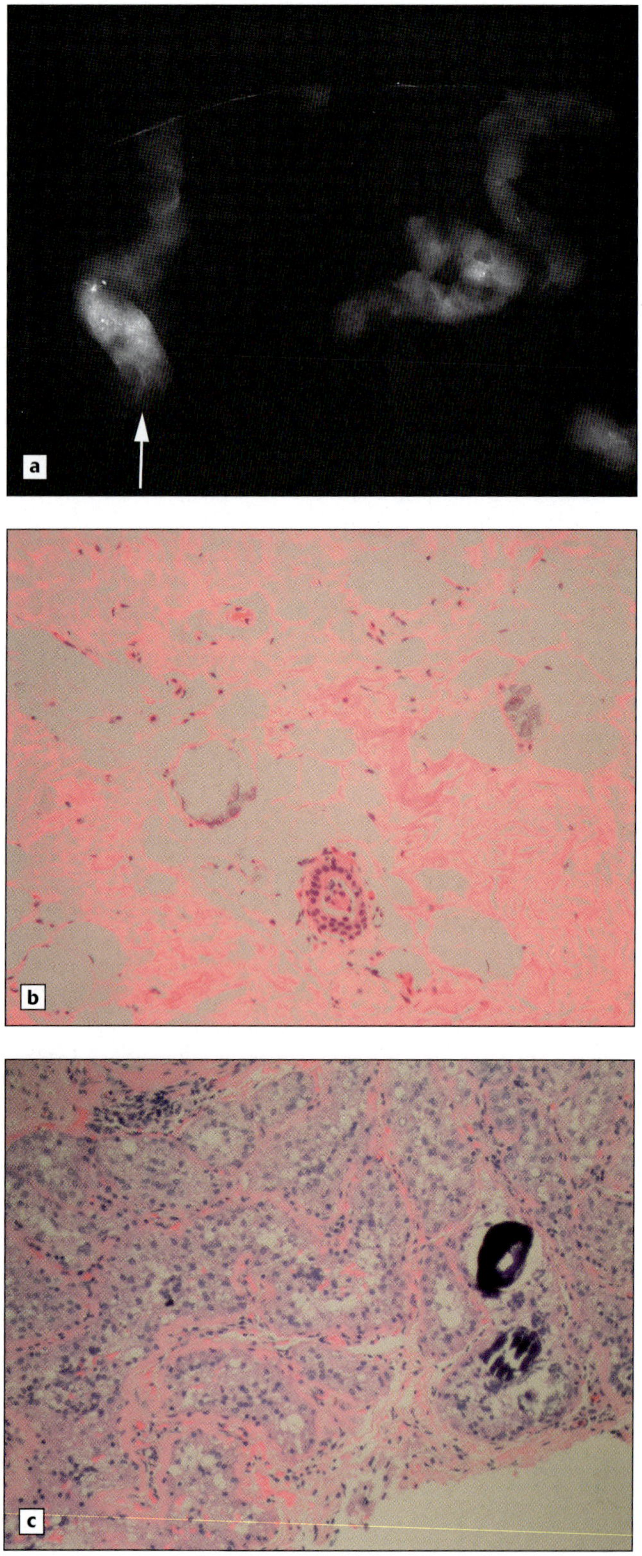

FIGURE 12.25 Specimen radiograph **(a)** showing coarse calcifications with rare linear forms (arrow) correlating with those found in adipose tissue adjacent to lactational changes **(b)** or in the lumina of terminal duct lobular units of breast which show lactational changes **(c).**

calcifications may occasionally present as high density calcifications that can rarely be linear (Fig. 12.25a). They maybe found in otherwise normal adipose tissue of breast (Fig. 12.25b) or in lumens of terminal duct lobular units of breast which show lactational changes (Fig. 12.25c) irrespective of the patient's age, or pregnancy. The calcifications have smooth rounded to lobulated contours with distinct unevenly spaced laminations (Figs 12.24 and 12.25).

Differential diagnoses of high-density possibly linear calcifications

- Recurrent breast carcinoma
- Hyalinized fibroadenoma
- Duct ectasia
- Fat necrosis
- Osseous metaplasia
- Vascular calcifications

POINTS TO REMEMBER

1. Fibroadenoma calcifications can fragment leaving minimal evidence of calcium.
2. Radiation changes (isolated nuclear atypia in terminal duct lobular units) need to be distinguished from recurrent intraductal carcinoma.

REFERENCES

1. Girling AC, Hanby AM, Millis RR. Radiation and other pathological changes in breast tissue after conservation treatment for carcinoma. J Clin Pathol 43:152–156,1990.
2. Meyer JE, Lester SC, DiPiro PJ, et al. Occult calcified fibroadenomas. Breast Dis 8:29–38,1995.
3. Schnitt SJ, Connolly JL, Harris JR, Cohen RB. Radiation-induced changes in the breast. Hum Pathol 15:545–550,1984.
4. France C, O'Connell J. Osseous metaplasia in the human mammary gland. Arch Surg 100: 100:238–239,1970.
5. Gal-Gombos EC, Esserman LE, Poniecka AW, et al. Osseous metaplasia of the breast: diagnosis with stereotactic core biopsy. Breast J 8:50–52,2002.
6. Shin SS, Rosen PP. Pregnancy-like (pseuodlactational) hyperplasia: A primary diagnosis in mammographically detected lesions of the breast and its relationship to cystic hypersecretory hyperplasia. Am J Surg Pathol 24:1670–1674,2000.

CHAPTER 13

Clustered low-density granular calcifications

The differential diagnoses of clustered granular low-density calcifications (Fig. 13.1) includes: fibrocystic changes with calcifications (Fig. 13.2a), florid duct hyperplasia with calcifications (Fig. 13.2b), atypical duct hyperplasia with calcifications (Fig. 13.2c) and intraductal carcinoma (low grade) with calcifications (Fig. 13.2d).

Atypical duct hyperplasia remains a difficult diagnosis despite well defined and accepted criteria, both at a qualitative and quantitative level. Beginning with the qualitative criteria, ADH is defined as a proliferative lesion that fulfills some but not all the morphological features of DCIS (Fig. 13.3), at both an architectural and cytologic level. By the quantitative criteria, the histologic features are consistent with DCIS but limited to a single duct space (Fig. 13.4) as proposed by Page et al.[1] or measuring <2 mm (Fig. 13.5), regardless of the number of ducts involved as proposed by Tavassoli et al.[2] In other words, by Page's criteria, it is a matter of whether the histologic features that are diagnostic of DCIS fill one space (and thus equivalent to ADH) or two or more spaces, the latter diagnostic of DCIS. The above criteria apply to core biopsies just as they do to excisional specimens.

The two most common patterns of atypical duct hyperplasia are cribriform and micropapillary. As its name suggests, the cribriform type is characterized by a proliferation of predominantly ductal epithelial cells forming uniform, rounded, rigid (so-called cookie cutter or punched out) spaces with few interspersed myoepithelial cells (Fig. 13.3). The micropapillary pattern is characterized by delicate avascular papillary structures projecting into the duct lumen and fusing to form "Roman bridges" (Fig. 13.6). When the micropapillae bud and break off such that they float in the luminal space, the histologic features are approaching the level of DCIS at least focally. In both patterns, the cytologic features are atypical comprised of cells with high nuclear to cytoplasmic ratio, enlarged hyperchromatic nuclei, irregular chromatin pattern, and prominent nucleoli (Fig. 13.7). Other less common variants of atypical duct hyperplasia include apocrine and columnar cell types to be described later.

The diagnosis of ADH conveys a four- to fivefold increased risk over that of the general population for the development of malignancy in either breast. The finding of ADH on core biopsy requires a subsequent excision largely because ADH and DCIS (usually of low nuclear grade) may coexist (Fig. 13.8) either in the same segment or even in different quadrants, probably due to a field effect. In other words, excision is necessary to exclude malignancy. Despite strict quantitative and qualitative criteria for distinguishing and diagnosing ADH and DCIS, their distinction may be particularly difficult on core biopsy material. Furthermore, the quantitative criteria for DCIS may not be met on the limited material of core biopsy, resulting in a diagnosis of ADH. Given the coexistence of ADH with DCIS and or invasive malignancy, it is questionable whether ADH diagnosed on core biopsy is truly representative of a heterogeneous target lesion. In many cases, ADH may be found geographically at the periphery of DCIS[3] (Fig. 13.9).

Studies correlating ADH on core biopsies with subsequent excision specimens reveal underestimation of malignancy (DCIS more often than invasive carcinoma) ranging from 11–88%,[4–6] primarily in cases investigating mammographic calcifications rather than a mass.[7,8] Adequate evaluation of calcifications requires extensive tissue removal and is greatly influenced by sampling. This has been facilitated by directional vacuum-assisted mammotome core biopsy that can retrieve multiple and larger tissue specimens (11-gauge) with one pass (Fig. 13.10). This enables contiguous sampling, leading to a lower underestimation rate (0–15% versus 41–44%) for automated core biopsy.[9–12] In addition, the overall sampling error is lower with vacuum assisted mammotome core biopsies (<1%) than automated core biopsy (6–14%).[13] Greater tissue retrieval by stereotactic[14] and, more recently, by ultrasound-guided[15] mammotome core biopsy may lead to removal of the entire target lesion, particularly when using a large needle to evaluate a small lesion. Various series in the literature report a frequency of this situation ranging from 13% to 93% using 11 to 14-gauge mammotome ranging from 5 to 12 mm.[13,16] Lesions most susceptible to this phenomenon were those <0.7 cm mammographically, with more than 14 cores removed, and showing complete removal of the mammographic abnormality.

These findings have provoked the question whether all cases of ADH need to be excised. In other words, if one could predict which cases of ADH on core needle biopsy

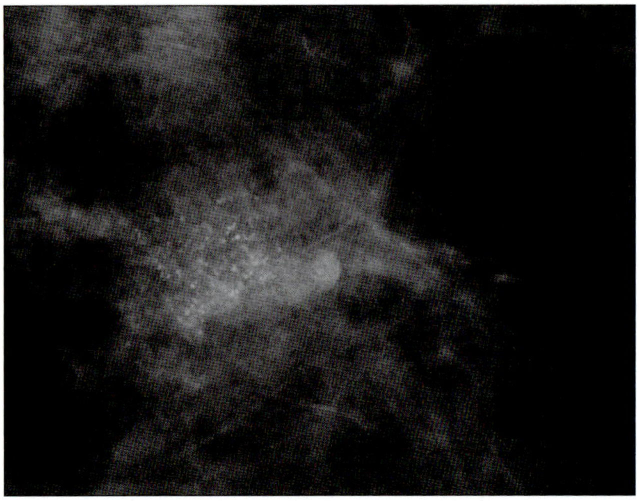

FIGURE 13.1 Mammogram showing clustered low-density granular calcifications.

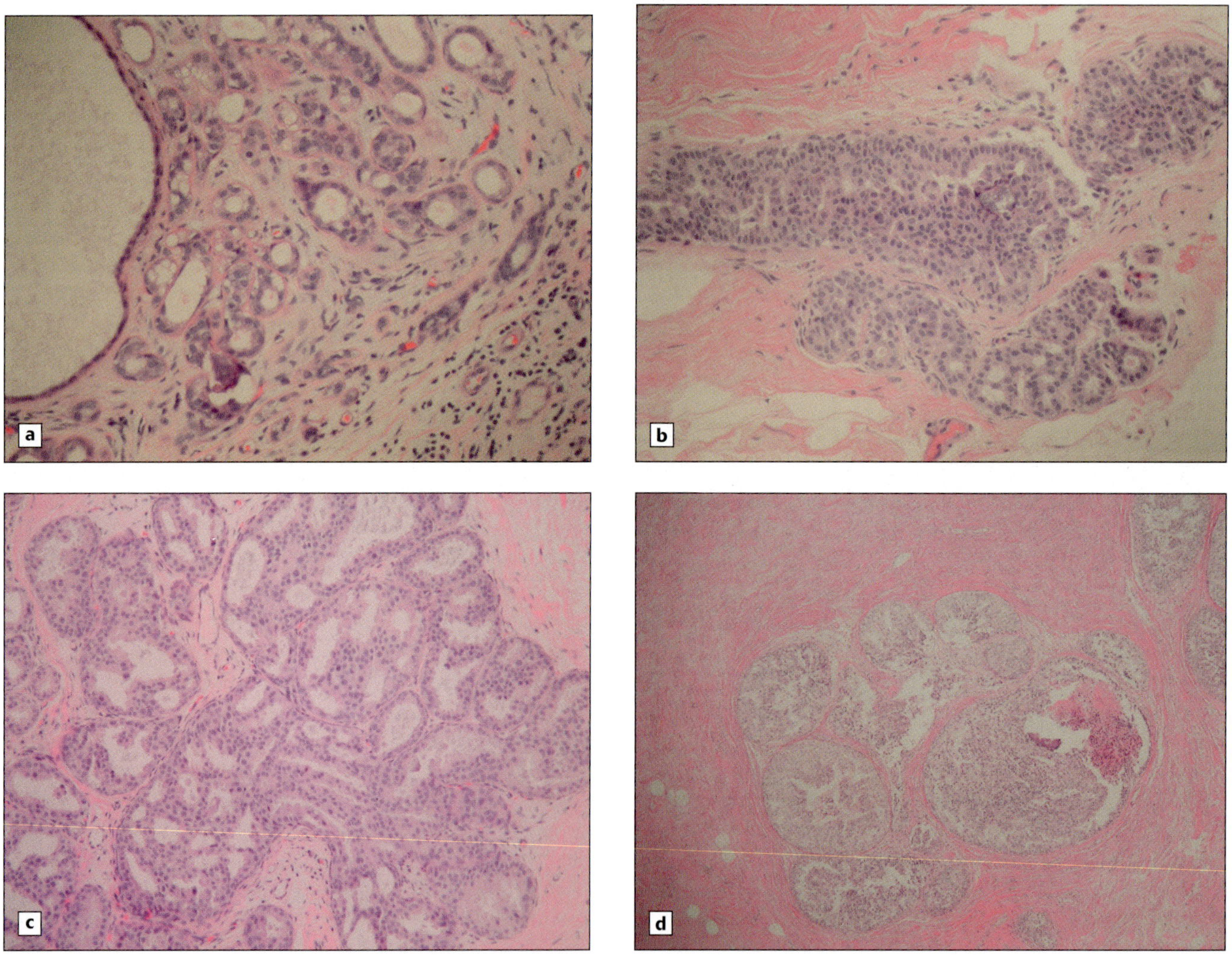

FIGURE 13.2 Histologic differential diagnosis of clustered low-density granular calcifications consisting of **(a)** fibrocystic changes, **(b)** florid duct hyperplasia, **(c)** atypical duct hyperplasia, **(d)** and DCIS.

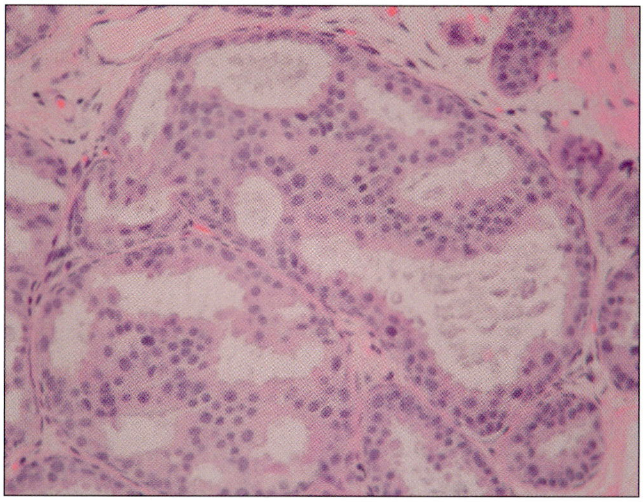

FIGURE 13.3 ADH is characterized by a proliferative lesion that fulfills some but not all the morphological features of DCIS.

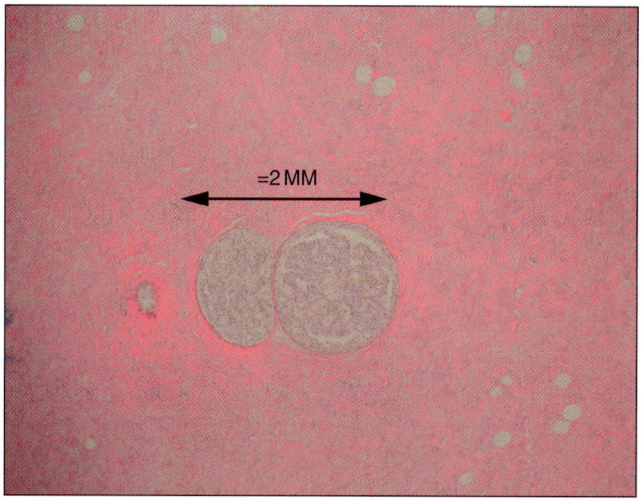

FIGURE 13.5 Qualitative criteria for ADH state that the histologic features are consistent with DCIS if >2 mm, but ADH if measuring <2 mm.

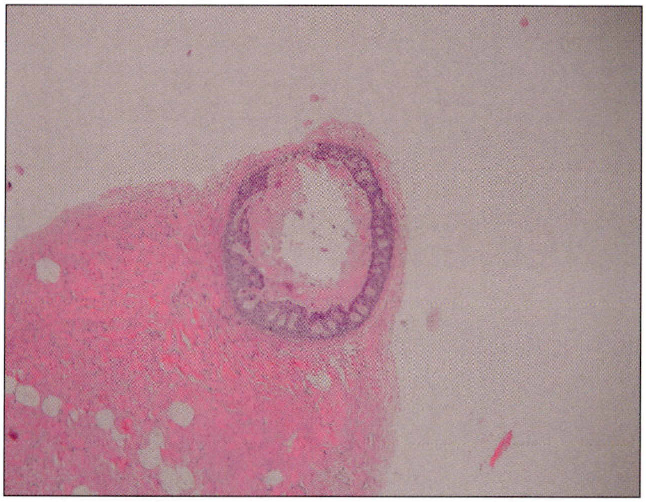

FIGURE 13.4 Quantitative criteria for ADH state that the histologic features are consistent with DCIS but limited to a single duct space.

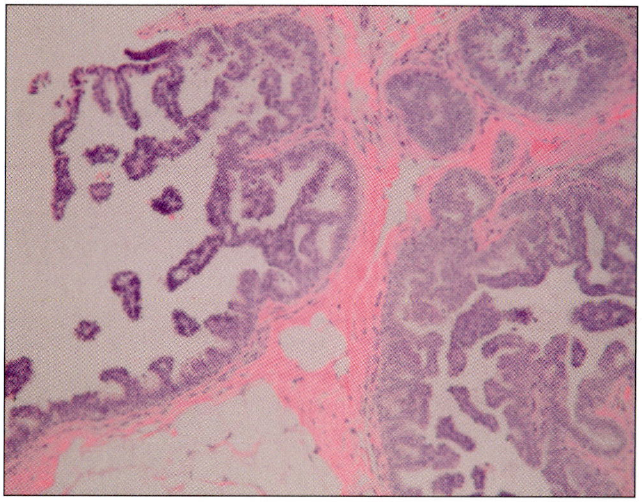

FIGURE 13.6 The micropapillary type of ADH is characterized by delicate avascular papillary structures projecting into the duct lumen and fusing to form "Roman bridges".

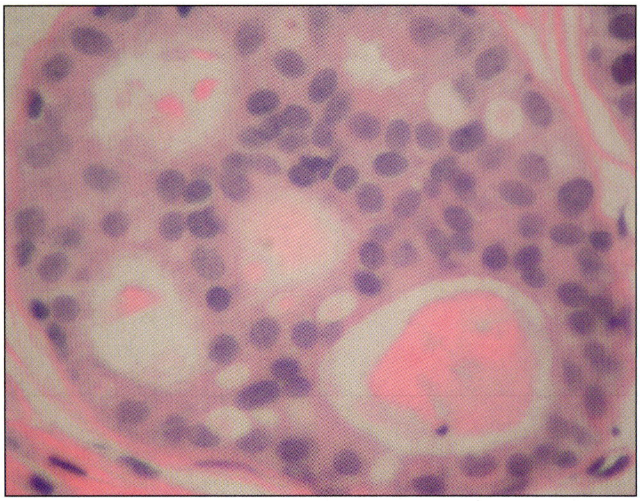

FIGURE 13.7 Atypical cytologic features of ADH.

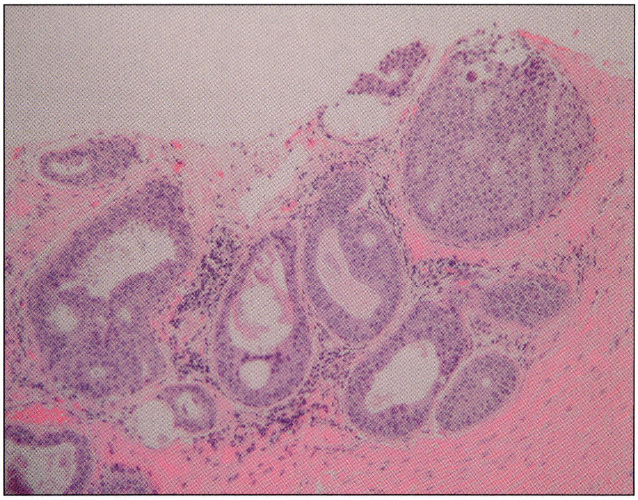

FIGURE 13.8 Co-existence of ADH and DCIS in a core biopsy makes the distinction of ADH from DCIS in limited material difficult, resulting in a diagnosis of ADH.

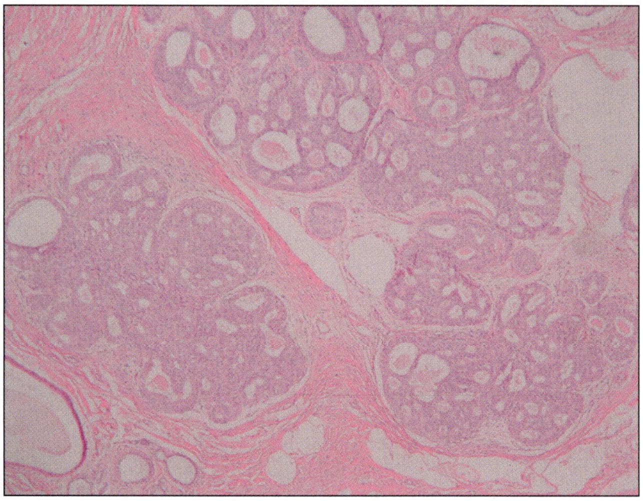

FIGURE 13.9 ADH presented at the periphery of DCIS.

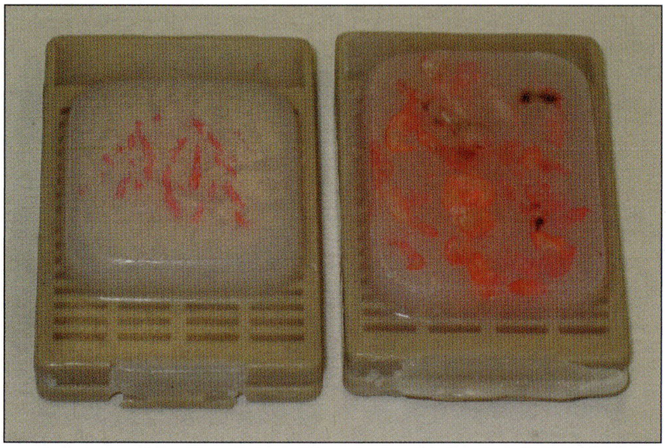

FIGURE 13.10 Comparison of tissue volume on paraffin blocks of USG (left) versus directional vacuum assisted mammotome core biopsy (right) that can retrieve multiple and larger tissue specimens.

will (or not) have atypia or malignancy on excision, excision would be spared in those cases with no residual disease on excision.

In an attempt to answer this question, various series have looked at specific morphologic features that maybe predictive of benignity, atypia and malignancy. Cases that had malignancy on excision after a core biopsy of ADH and thus worthy of excision included those with marked atypia, a history of breast cancer, and incomplete removal of calcifications.[17] Obviously, the greater the amount of calcifications removed, the smaller the risk of underestimation, such that if all of the calcifications are removed, underestimation is eliminated. The extent and morphological pattern (micropapillary) of ADH[11,18] also correlated with finding malignancy on excision, specifically DCIS. Ely et al[11] quantified the extent of ADH by the counting number of foci of large duct and individual terminal duct lobular unit involvement. By their criteria, carcinoma was present on excision specimens in those cases with more than four foci of ADH, whereas those with fewer than two foci had no subsequent malignancy. Lim et al[18] found that ADH involving less than three terminal duct lobular units did not require excision provided all of the calcifications were removed. By contrast, Liberman et al,[19] in their attempt to completely remove the mammographic abnormality by mammotome core biopsy, reported residual disease in 73% of cases. It should be stressed that these series searching for histologic features predictive of benignity, atypia and malignancy, were limited by the lack of radiologic–pathologic correlation. Clearly more studies with radiologic–pathologic correlation and larger numbers are needed before conclusions can be drawn regarding which cases of ADH diagnosed on cores might be spared excision.

Given the limited data available, we currently agree with those who recommend surgery for all such cases.[20–22] Instead, we find the differentiation of ADH from florid duct hyperplasia (Figs 13.2b,c) on core biopsies to be of greater clinical importance since the latter does not require excision. Actually, we see this type of misdiagnosis quite frequently in our consultation practice. Morphologically, in contrast to ADH, florid duct hyperplasia is composed of a mixed population of ductal and myoepithelial cells in a streaming pattern with slit like spaces. Unfortunately over diagnosing atypia on this end of the proliferative spectrum will result in unnecessary surgery rather than prevent it.

It is crucial for the pathologist to histologically identify the core biopsy site in the excision specimen in order to confirm excision of the correct area. This of course applies equally to excision of core-biopsied densities and/or calcifications. In studies utilizing preoperative wire localization of clips, clip placement accuracy has been documented showing average distances of 5–9 mm from clip to the biopsy site.[23,24] Nevertheless, in a small percentage of cases, localization distances measuring >24 mm from the biopsy cavity have been reported.[23] Clip migration has been attributed to release of breast compression after mammotome core biopsy. We have occasionally seen such cases in which the specimen radiography documents clip removal, yet reactive changes of the prior biopsy are not evident or are found only minimally, usually at the margin of the specimen (Fig. 13.11). Such cases require re-excision, as finding the histologic core biopsy site is of paramount importance, regardless of the location of the clip.

For the remainder of the chapter, we will discuss two variants of ADH, specifically columnar cell type and atypical apocrine adenosis. Beginning with the columnar cell lesions, these newly described lesions are increasingly being detected since the advent of screening mammography leading to an increased number of breast biopsies performed for mammographically detected calcifications. Consequently, pre-invasive proliferations such as columnar cell lesions are increasingly found. They usually occur in premenopausal women, are multifocal, and represent a spectrum ranging from benign entities with numerous overlapping appellations (columnar alteration of lobules,

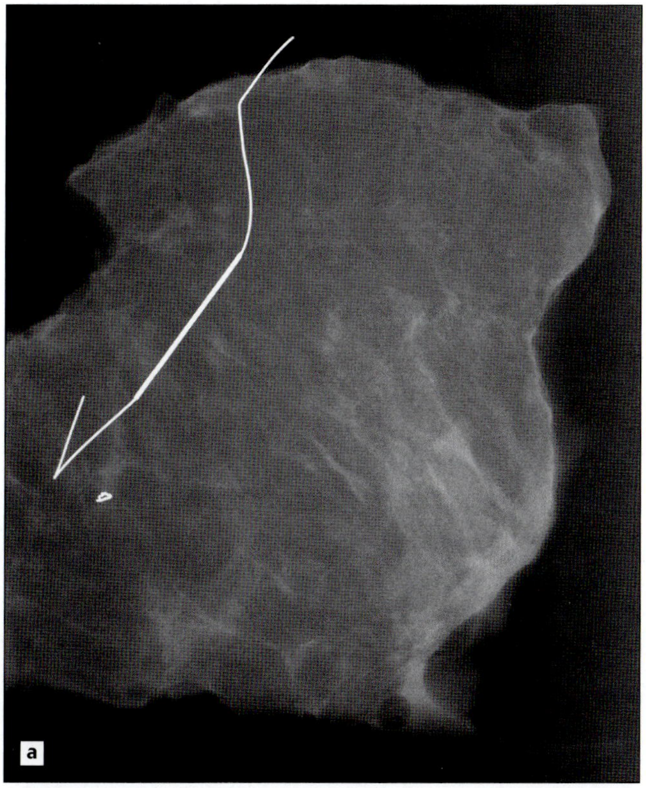

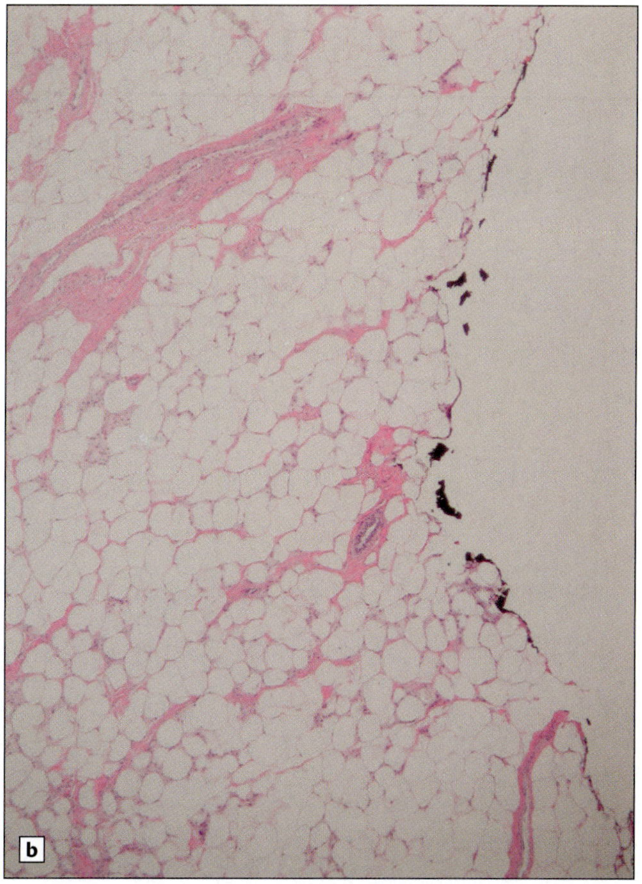

FIGURE 13.11 Although the specimen radiograph **(a)** documents clip removal, minimal reactive changes of the prior biopsy are found only at the **(b)** margin of the specimen (denoted by black ink).

blunt duct adenosis, metaplasie cylindrique, pretubular hyperplasia, columnar alteration with prominent apical snouts and secretions [CAPSS])[25] to atypical and malignant ones (DCIS; micropapillary, cribriform, and clinging types). Morphologically, the benign form may be flat or hyperplastic. The flat lesions are characterized by dilated ducts stratified by one to two layers of columnar epithelial cells with uniform, ovoid to elongated nuclei oriented perpendicular to the basement membrane, containing dispersed chromatin (Fig. 13.12). The cells have increased cytoplasm, apical blebs or snouts, hobnail cells and flocculent secretion (Fig. 13.13). Although columnar cells and apocrine cells have similar features such as apical cytoplasmic snouts, they are different in that the latter contains more abundant granular eosinophilic cytoplasm and a round nucleus that contains a prominent nucleolus (Fig. 13.14). Additionally, by immunohistochemistry, although they both express GCDFP15, columnar cells differ in that they also express estrogen receptor and bcl2.

Hyperplastic lesions have identical cytologic features as the benign lesions but are architecturally differentiated by small mounds, tufts or short micropapillations (Fig. 13.15). Both the flat and hyperplastic proliferations

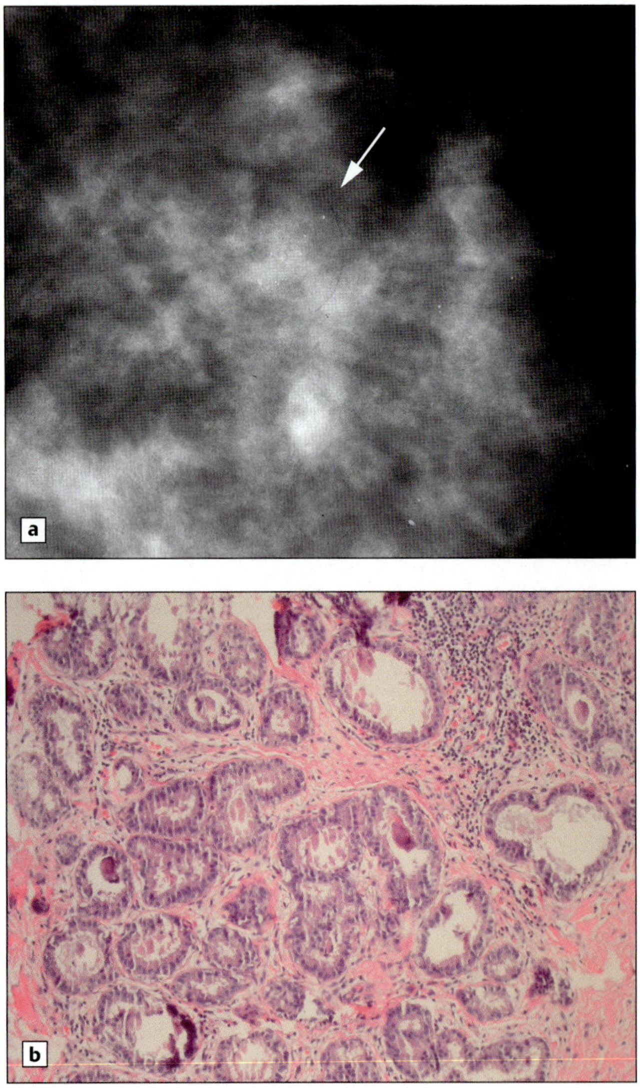

FIGURE 13.12 Mammogram **(a)** shows round non branching calcifications (arrow) correlating with benign columnar cell lesions characterized by dilated ducts stratified by one to two layers of columnar epithelial cells with uniform, ovoid to elongated nuclei containing dispersed chromatin, oriented perpendicular to the basement membrane, associated with flocculent secretions and luminal calcifications **(b)**.

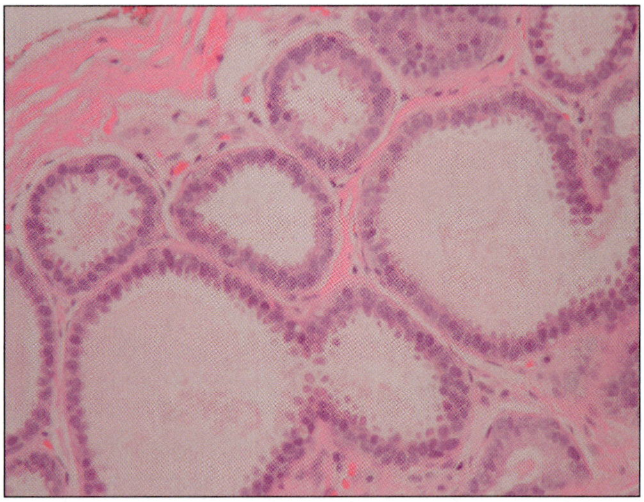

FIGURE 13.13 Higher power view of Fig. 13.12 showing cytologic features of benign columnar cell lesions characterized by increased cytoplasm, apical blebs or snouts and hobnail cells.

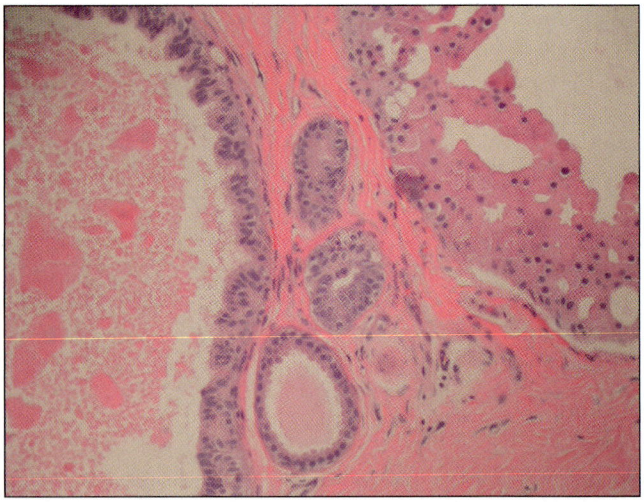

FIGURE 13.14 Contrasting morphologic features of apocrine cells (right) and columnar cells (left).

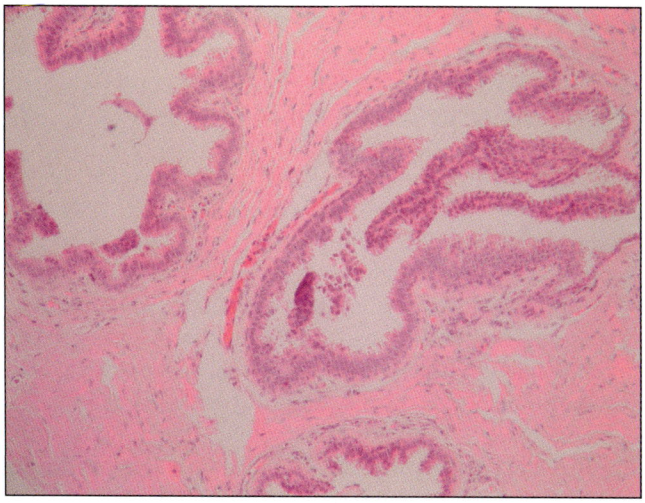

FIGURE 13.15 Hyperplastic columnar cell lesions characterized by small mounds, tufts or short micropapillations.

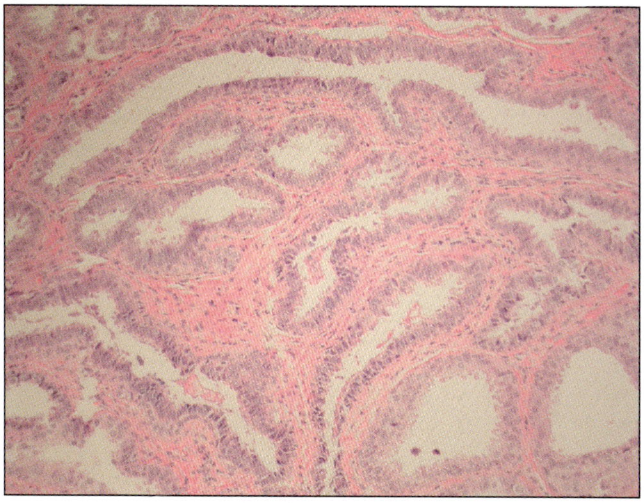

FIGURE 13.16 Low power of "columnar cell change with atypia" characterized by flat dilated ducts lined by atypical cells.

can be associated with luminal calcifications that may be either crystalline or ossifying, correlating with round non-branching calcifications on mammography (Fig. 13.12)

As with the benign proliferations, the atypical lesions can also be architecturally variable, ranging from flat epithelial lesions (Fig. 13.16) to more complex architectural forms. However, the flat atypical lesions designated as "columnar cell change with atypia", are cytologically distinguished by high nuclear to cytoplasmic ratio, prominent nucleoli and infrequent mitoses. In addition, the cells are morphologically characterized as columnar with round or ovoid rather than elongated nuclei that are not oriented perpendicular to the basement membrane

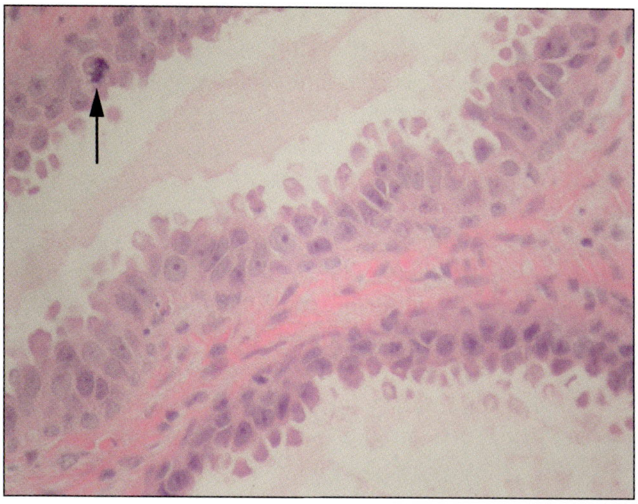

FIGURE 13.17 High power view of Fig. 13.16 showing cells with round or ovoid rather than elongated nuclei that are not oriented perpendicular to the basement membrane, with high nuclear to cytoplasmic ratio, prominent nucleoli and infrequent mitoses (arrow).

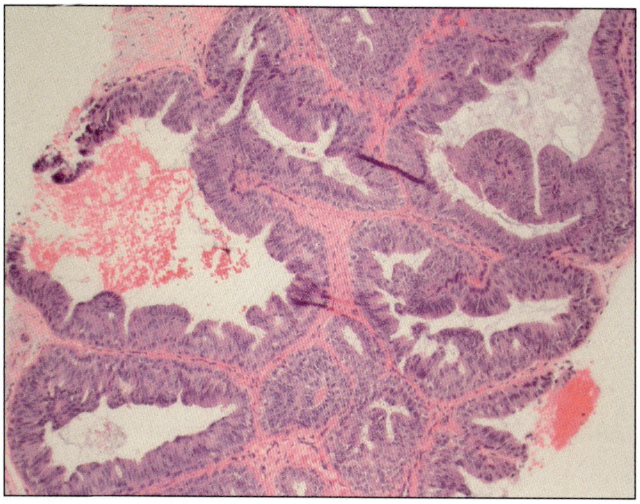

FIGURE 13.18 Columnar cells with complex architectural patterns such as increased number of cell layers that are disorderly, micropapillations, rigid cellular bridges and fenestrations.

(Fig. 13.17). Overall, they have subtle histologic features, simulating the cells lining the tubules in tubular carcinoma or in clinging carcinoma, and thus may be missed on low power. The hyperplastic lesion with atypia have identical cytologic features as the flat atypical lesions but acquire complex architectural patterns such as increased number of cell layers that are disorderly, micropapillations, rigid cellular bridges, arches and fenestrations (Fig. 13.18), features similar to conventional ADH.[26]

Columnar cell change with atypia and those with features of ADH are distinguished to better understand the clinical significance of these lesions. Although some feel that columnar cell change with atypia represents the earliest morphologic manifestation of low grade DCIS, follow up studies indicate a low risk of progression to invasive carcinoma.[27] While the diagnosis of these lesions on core needle biopsy warrants excision, their management on excision specimens is controversial because of their uncertain clinical significance. Long-term follow up studies are necessary to further assess these lesions. The treatment of hyperplastic atypical columnar cell proliferations is easier than the flat atypical lesions because their morphologic features are akin to those in ADH. Thus, they are best designated and managed as ADH. In addition, studies have shown not only geographic proximity but also cytologic, immunophenotypic and genetic similarities between atypical hyperplastic columnar lesions and low grade DCIS, suggesting that they represent an early phase in the development of low grade DCIS.[28] Follow-up studies indicate a more advanced lesion in one third of excision specimens.[27] Interestingly, these lesions may also be associated with atypical lobular hyperplasia and lobular carcinoma in situ, either in geographically distinct areas or in coexistence.[27,29–31]

Thus, based on these limited series, excision is currently recommended for both columnar cell change with atypia and those with features of ADH diagnosed on core needle biopsy.

Next, we will discuss another variant of ADH, namely atypical apocrine adenosis. As its name suggests, when apocrine metaplasia is superimposed on sclerosing adenosis, the resultant morphological pattern is called apocrine adenosis (Fig. 13.19). When the cells acquire significant cytologic atypia, it is known as atypical apocrine adenosis (Fig. 13.20). This lesion may mimic and be misdiagnosed as invasive carcinoma by the amateur, particularly on fine needle aspiration.[32] The precancerous significance of these lesions is currently unknown.[33] However, in one series, it was found to confer an increased risk of developing breast carcinoma in women over 60 years of age.[34] Furthermore, one study reported unusual overexpression of p53 and c-erb-B2 in these lesions.[35] In a single case report, monoclonality was detected in atypical apocrine adenosis.[36] Based on these limited studies, we recommend excision when the core biopsy shows atypical apocrine adenosis. In our experience, most of the excision specimens have shown adjacent apocrine DCIS (Fig. 13.21). Whether or not atypical apocrine adenosis represents a borderline lesion in the histologic spectrum between apocrine metaplasia and apocrine DCIS is currently speculative.

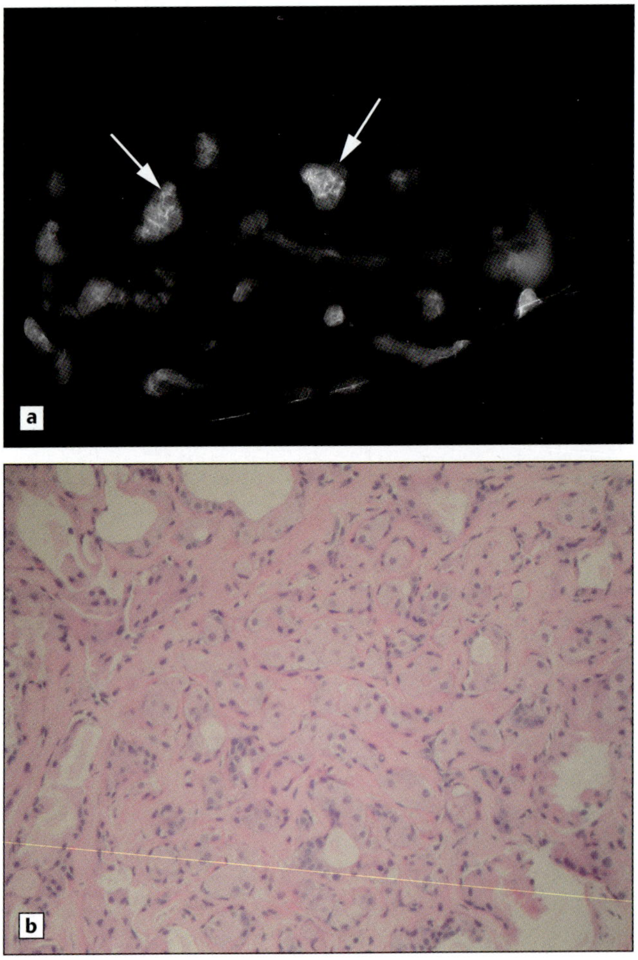

FIGURE 13.19 Specimen radiograph **(a)** shows clustered calcifications (arrows). **(b)** H&E shows sclerosing adenosis infused with apocrine cells, the result being apocrine metaplasia associated with calcifications (arrows).

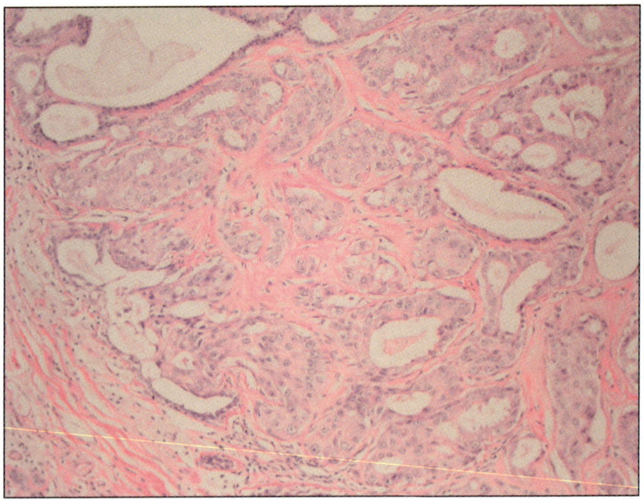

FIGURE 13.20 Apocrine metaplasia may acquire atypical cytologic and architectural features, resulting in atypical apocrine adenosis.

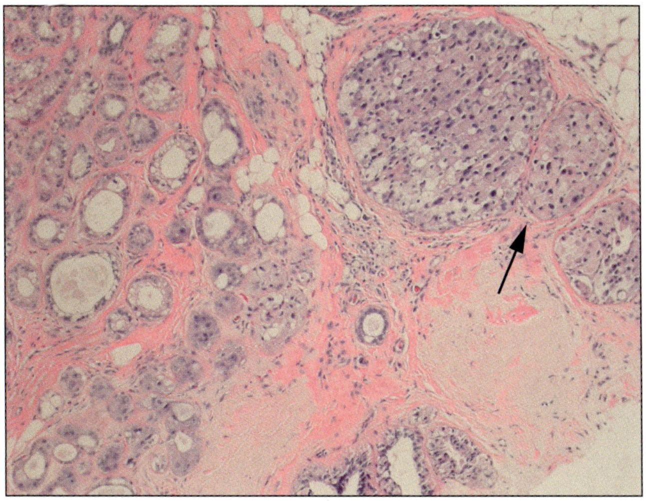

FIGURE 13.21 Atypical apocrine adenosis (left) associated with apocrine DCIS (right arrow).

Differential diagnoses of clustered granular low-density calcifications

- Fibrocystic changes with calcifications
- Florid duct hyperplasia with calcifications
- Atypical duct hyperplasia with calcifications
- Intraductal carcinoma (low grade) with calcifications

POINTS TO REMEMBER

1. The definition of ADH is based on the same quantitative and qualitative histologic features on cores as on excisional specimens.
2. ADH on core biopsy should be excised because of the high rate of subsequent DCIS due to sampling issues.
3. Over diagnosis of florid duct hyperplasia as ADH leads to unnecessary surgery.

REFERENCES

1. Page DL, Rogers LW. Combined histologic and cytologic criteria for the diagnosis of mammary atypical ductal hyperplasia. Hum Pathol 23:1095–1097,1992.
2. Tavassoli FA, Norris HJ. A comparison of the results of long-term follow-up for atypical intraductal hyperplasia and intraductal hyperplasia of the breast. Cancer 65:518–529,1990.
3. Lennington WJ, Jensen RA, Dalton LW, et al. Ductal carcinoma in situ of the breast: heterogeneity of individual lesions. Cancer 73:118–124,1994.
4. Moore MM, Hargett W, Hanks JB, et al. Association of breast cancer with the finding of atypical ductal hyperplasia at core breast biopsy. Ann Surg 225:726–733,1997.
5. Jackman RJ, Nowels KW, Rodriguez-Soto J, et al. Stereotactic, automated, large-core needle biopsy of nonpalpable breast lesions: false-negative and histologic underestimation rates after long-term follow-up. Radiology 210:799–805,1999.
6. Sneige N, Lim SC, Whitman GJ, et al. Atypical ductal hyperplasia diagnosis by directional vacuum-assisted stereotactic biopsy of breast microcalcifications. Am J Clin Pathol 119:248–253,2003.
7. Philpotts LE, Shaheen NA, Jain KS, et al. Uncommon high-risk lesions of the breast diagnosed at stereotactic core-needle biopsy: Clinical importance. Radiology 216:831–837,2000.
8. Jacobs TW, Connolly JL, Schnitt SJ. Nonmalignant lesions in breast core needle biopsies. To excise or not to excise? Am J Surg Pathol 26:1095–1110,2002.
9. Reynolds HE, Poon CM, Goulet RJ, et al. Biopsy of breast microcalcifications using an 11-gauge directional vacuum-assisted device. AJR Am J Roentgenol 171:611–613,1998.
10. Reynolds ••, Handel E. Core Needle Biopsy of Challenging Benign Breast Conditions: A Comprehensive Literature Review. AJR Am J Roentgenol 174:1245–1250,2000.
11. Ely KA, Carter BA, Jensen RA, et al. Core biopsy of the breast with atypical ductal hyperplasia. Am J Surg Pathol 25:1017–1021,2001.
12. Darling ML, Smith DN, Lester SC, et al. Atypical ductal hyperplasia and ductal carcinoma in situ as revealed by large-core needle breast biopsy: results of surgical excision. AJR Am J Roentgenol 175:1341–1346,2000.
13. Liberman L. Percutaneous image-guided core breast biopsy. Radiol Clin N Am 40:483–500,2002
14. Gajdos C, Levy M, Herman Z, et al. Complete removal of nonpalpable breast malignancies with a stereotactic percutaneous vacuum-assisted biopsy instrument. J Am Coll Surg 1189:237–240,1999.
15. Fine RE, Boyd BA, Whitworth PW, et al. Percutaneous removal of benign breast masses using a vacuum-assisted hand-held device with ultrasound guidance. Am J Surg 184:332–336,2002.
17. Adrales G, Turk P, Wallace T, et al. Is surgical excision necessary for atypical ductal hyperplasia of the breast diagnosed by mammotome? Am J Surg 180:313–315,2000.
18. Lim SC, Whitman GJ, Krishnamurthy S, et al. Directional vacuum-assisted stereotactic biopsy (DVAB) of breast microcalcifications with atypical ductal hyperplasia (ADH): surgical excision is not always necessary (Abstract). Mod Pathol 14:30A,2001.
19. Liberman L, Dershaw DD, Rosen PP, et al. Percutaneous removal of malignant mammographic lesions at stereotactic vacuum-assisted biopsy. Radiology 206:711–715,1998.
20. Jackman RJ, Nowels KW, Shepard MJ, et al. Stereotaxic large-core needle biopsy of 450 nonpalpable breast lesions with surgical correlation in lesions with cancer or atypical hyperplasia. Radiology 193:91–95,1994.
21. Liberman L, Cohen MA, Dershaw DD, et al. Atypical duct hyperplasia diagnosed at stereotaxic core biopsy of breast lesions: an indication for surgical biopsy. AJR Am J Roentgenol 164:1111–1113,1995.
22. Jackman RJ, Birdwell RL, Ikeda DM. Atypical ductal hyperplasia: can some lesions be defined as probably benign after stereotactic 11-gauge vacuum-assisted biopsy, eliminating the recommendation for surgical excision? Radiology 224:548–554,2002.
23. Burbank F, Forcier N. Tissue marking clip for stereotactic breast biopsy: initial placement accuracy, long-term stability, and usefulness as a guide for wire localization. Radiology 205:407–415,1997.
24. Kass R, Kumar G, Klimberg V, et al. Clip migration in stereotactic biopsy. Am J Surg 184:325–331,2002.
25. Fraser JL, Chorny RS, et al. Columnar alteration with prominent apical snouts and secretions: a spectrum of changes frequently present in breast biopsies performed for microcalcifications. Am J Surg Pathol 22:1521–1527,1998.
26. Brogi E, Tan LK. Findings at excisional biopsy (EBX) performed after identification of columnar cell change (CCC) of ductal epithelium in breast core biopsy (CBX) (Abstract). Mod Pathol 15:29A,2002.
27. Schnitt SJ,Vincent-Salomon A. Columnar cell lesions of the breast. Adv Anat Path 10:113–242,2003.
28. Simpson PT, Gale T, Reis-Filho JS, et al. Columnar cell lesions of the breast: The missing link in breast cancer progression? A morphologic and molecular analysis. Am J Surg Path 29:734–746,2005.
29. Sahoo S, Recant WM. Triad of columnar cell alteration, lobular carcinoma in situ, and tubular carcinoma of the breast. Breast J 11:140–143,2005.
30. Rosen PP. Columnar cell hyperplasia is associated with lobular carcinoma in situ and tubular carcinoma. Am J Surg Path 23:1561–1565,1999
31. Brogi E, Oyama T, Koerner FC. Atypical cystic lobules in patients with lobular neoplasia. Int J Surg Pathol 9:201–206,2001.
32. Kaufman D, Sanchez M, Mizrachy B, Jaffer S. Cytologic findings of atypical adenosis of the breast. Acta Cytol 46:369–372,2002.
33. Carter D, Rosen PP. Atypical apocrine metaplasia in sclerosing lesions of the breast: a study of 51 patients. Mod Pathol 4:1–5,1991.
34. Seidman J, Ashton M, Lefkowitz M. Atypical apocrine adenosis of the breast. Cancer 77:2529–2537,1996.
35. Selim AG, El-Ayat G, Wells CA. Expression of c-erbB2, p53, Bcl-2, Bax, c-myc and Ki-67 in apocrine metaplasia and apocrine change within sclerosing adenosis of the breast. Virchows Arch 441:449–455,2002.
36. Endoh Y, Tamura G, Kato N, Motoyama T. Apocrine adenosis of the breast: clonal evidence of neoplasia. Histopathology 38:221–224,2001.

CHAPTER 14

Linear and branching calcifications

Linear and branching calcifications are almost always pathognomonic of comedo DCIS (Fig. 14.1). Therefore if a specimen radiograph demonstrates these types of calcifications, it behooves the pathologist to find the DCIS or explain these findings. In a case with mixed worrisome appearing linear and branching calcifications and benign appearing calcifications (Figs 14.2a and 14.2b), if initial sections were to show only fibrocystic changes with calcifications (Fig. 14.2c), obviously a lack of correlation exists between the specimen radiograph and H&E, both in terms of the number and pattern of calcifications. If no apocrine metaplasia-lined cysts are present, there is no utility to view the slides under polarized light to search for calcium oxalate (Fig 14.3). The discrepancy can be resolved by x-raying the paraffin block which will most likely show residual linear calcifications (Fig. 14.2D). Deeper sections will enable finding the comedo DCIS on H&E (Fig. 14.2e). Comedo DCIS is characterized by a uniform proliferation of ductal cells with highly pleomorphic nuclei associated with central luminal necrosis and calcifications. Rarely, benign entities such as apocrine lined cysts with calcium oxalate (Fig. 14.4) and hyalinized fibroadenoma (See Chapter 12 Fig. 12.9) may present with linear but usually not branching calcifications.

Discrepant cases such as the one described above illustrate the importance and necessity of radiologic–pathologic correlation in the interpretation of mammotome core biopsies for calcifications. Lack of correlation can result in histologically missing the malignancy because it may remain hidden in the paraffin block as shown in the case above. In cases with highly suspicious calcifications, in spite of a benign histological diagnosis, it becomes incumbent upon the radiologist to recommend further work up because of seemingly discordant findings most likely due to sampling (Fig. 14.5). However, discordance may not always be due to sampling error on the part of the radiologist; rather, it maybe due to the pathologist who does not utilize the specimen radiograph to correlate with the H&E (Fig. 14.6). We utilize paraffin block radiography[1] for cases in which the number and pattern of histologic calcifications do not match those seen radiographically, especially when mammographic linear, branching forms are not found microscopically, since they are suspicious of comedo DCIS, as mentioned above[2].

In one study evaluating "exhaustive" searching for microcalcifications in stereotactic core needle biopsies, Grimes et al[3] found a discrepancy between the specimen radiograph and the H&E slide in 22% of cases. In less than half of these cases, complete sectioning provided the final diagnosis. They concluded that deeper levels provided additional specific diagnostic information in relatively few cases. Although accompanied by a high technical cost (414% per case), the additional information was crucial for appropriate patient management.

The heterogeneity of DCIS is reflected in its varied cytologic and architectural patterns.[4] Several proposed grading systems exist that vary in the relative value assigned to size, growth pattern, and presence or absence of necrosis. However, most agree on the importance of assessing nuclear pleomorphism. Currently, the grading of DCIS is a three-tiered system (low, intermediate and high), based on increasing pleomorphic cytologic features.

As all experienced surgical pathologists are aware, the distinction of high grade DCIS from lobular carcinoma in situ (LCIS) (Fig. 14.7) is straightforward. However, distinguishing low grade DCIS from LCIS may not always be feasible (Fig. 14.8). Morphologic overlap between these two proliferations can cause difficulty in classifying them as either DCIS or LCIS. The incidence of such problems has increased dramatically in the mammographic era, particularly with the advent of vacuum-assisted percutaneous biopsies which leads to greater tissue retrieval. Consequently the incidence of LCIS has increased due to its higher rate of detection on core biopsies[5] because classical LCIS does not produce a palpable abnormality, is multifocal, multicentric, and discontinuous in its distribution. Although LCIS may rarely be associated with calcifications (Fig. 14.9), it does not correspond to a specific radiologic finding.[6] Thus, at least in its classical form, it is an incidental finding seen in 0.5%[7,8] to more recently described 8% of breast biopsies,[9] discovered upon investigation of another palpable or radiologic abnormality, regardless of the technique used, i.e., excision or core biopsy (Fig. 14.10).

The cytological features of LCIS are similar to those in classical and signet ring cell invasive lobular carcinoma

Text continued on p. 144

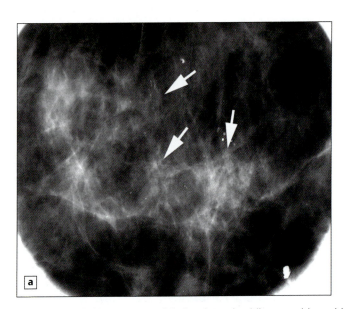

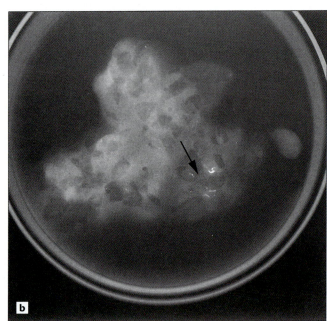

FIGURE 14.1 Mammogram showing linear and branching calcifications pathognomonic of comedo DCIS.

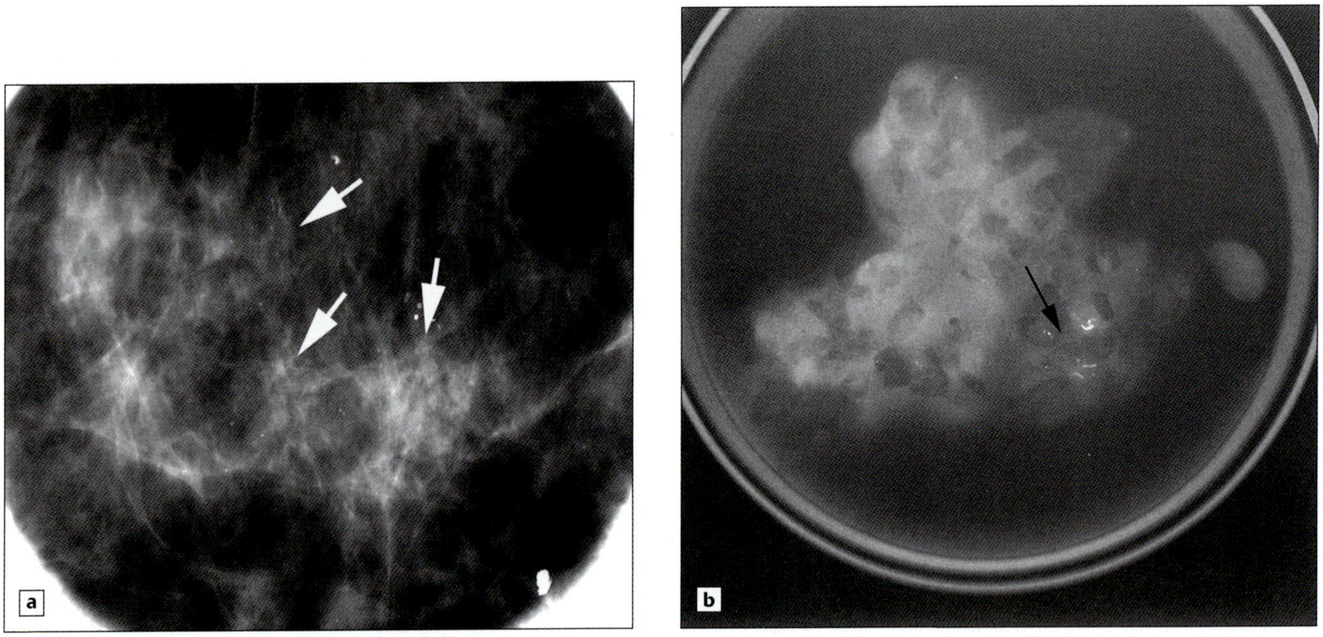

FIGURE 14.2 Mammogram **(a)** showing mixed linear and branching pleomorphic calcifications adjacent to punctate uniform ones (arrows). The specimen radiograph **(b)** also shows mixed calcifications.

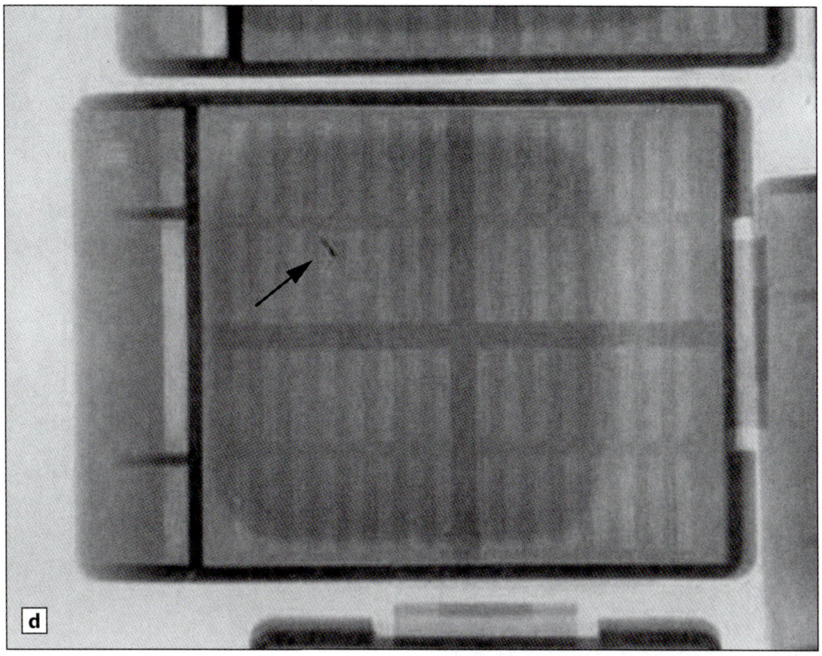

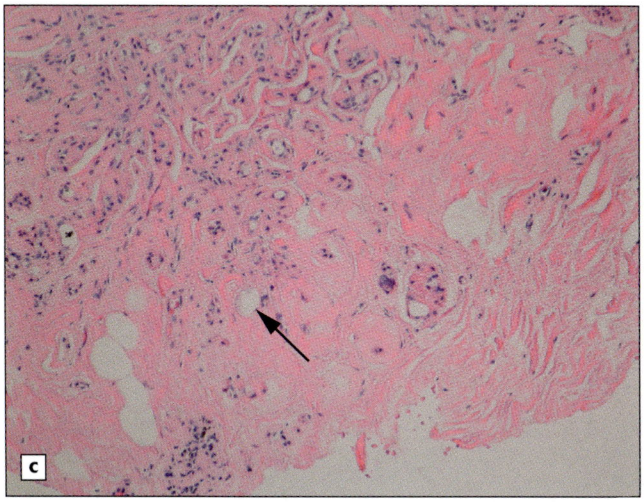

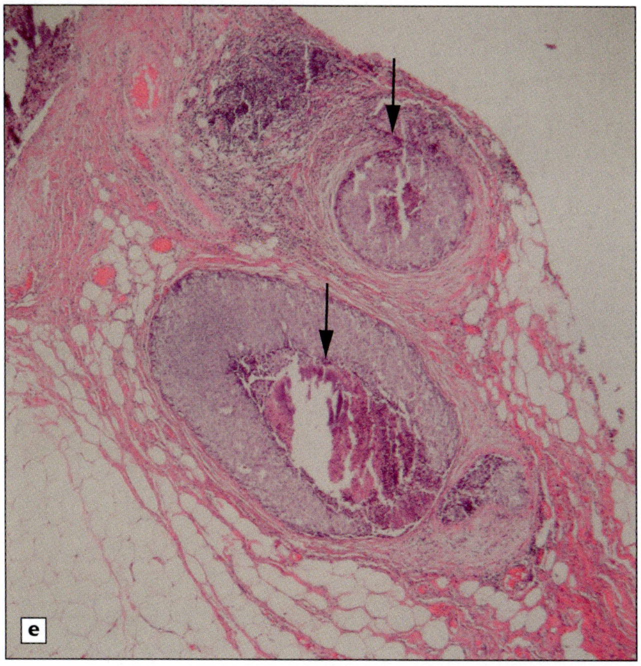

FIGURE 14.2—cont'd Initial H&E **(c)** sections show sclerosing adenosis with calcifications (arrow) which only correlated with the benign clustered ones but not the worrisome linear and branching forms. Paraffin block radiograph **(d)** was done due to the lack of correlation which showed residual linear calcification (arrow) which proved to be comedo DCIS with calcifications **(e)** (arrows).

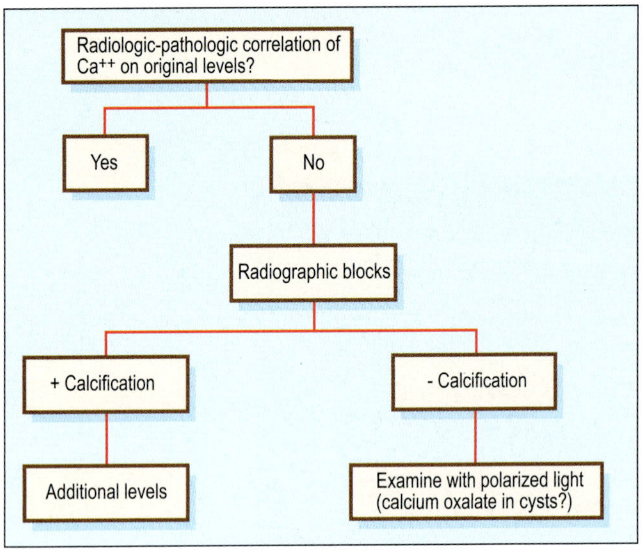

FIGURE 14.3 Flow chart for examination of calcifications in core biopsies.

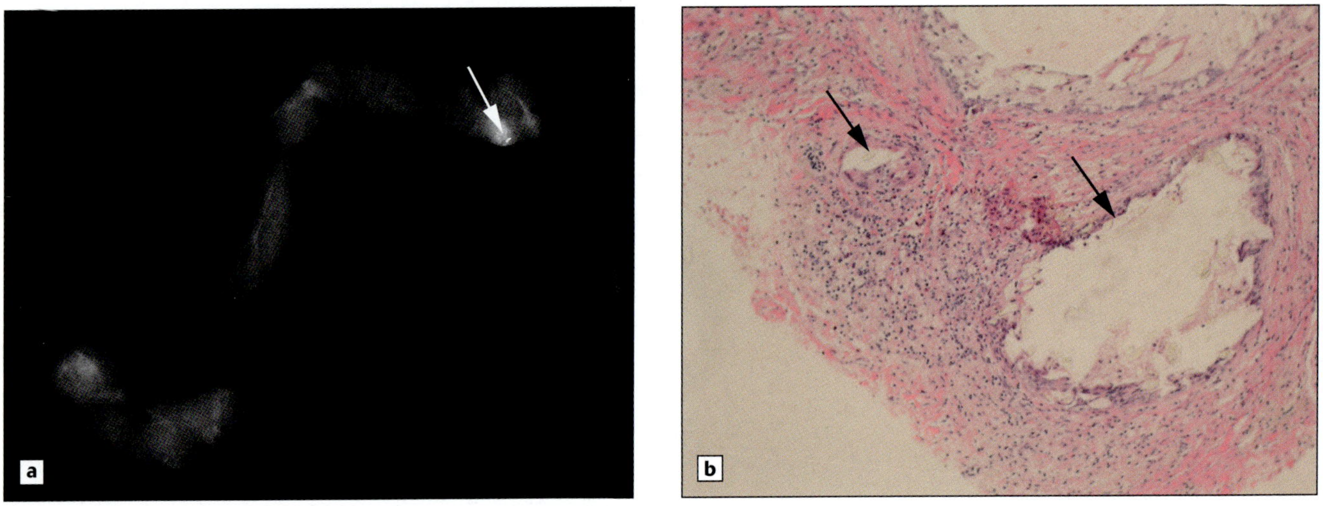

FIGURE 14.4 A rare case of linear calcification seen on specimen radiograph **(a)** (arrow) due to calcium oxalate **(b)** (arrows).

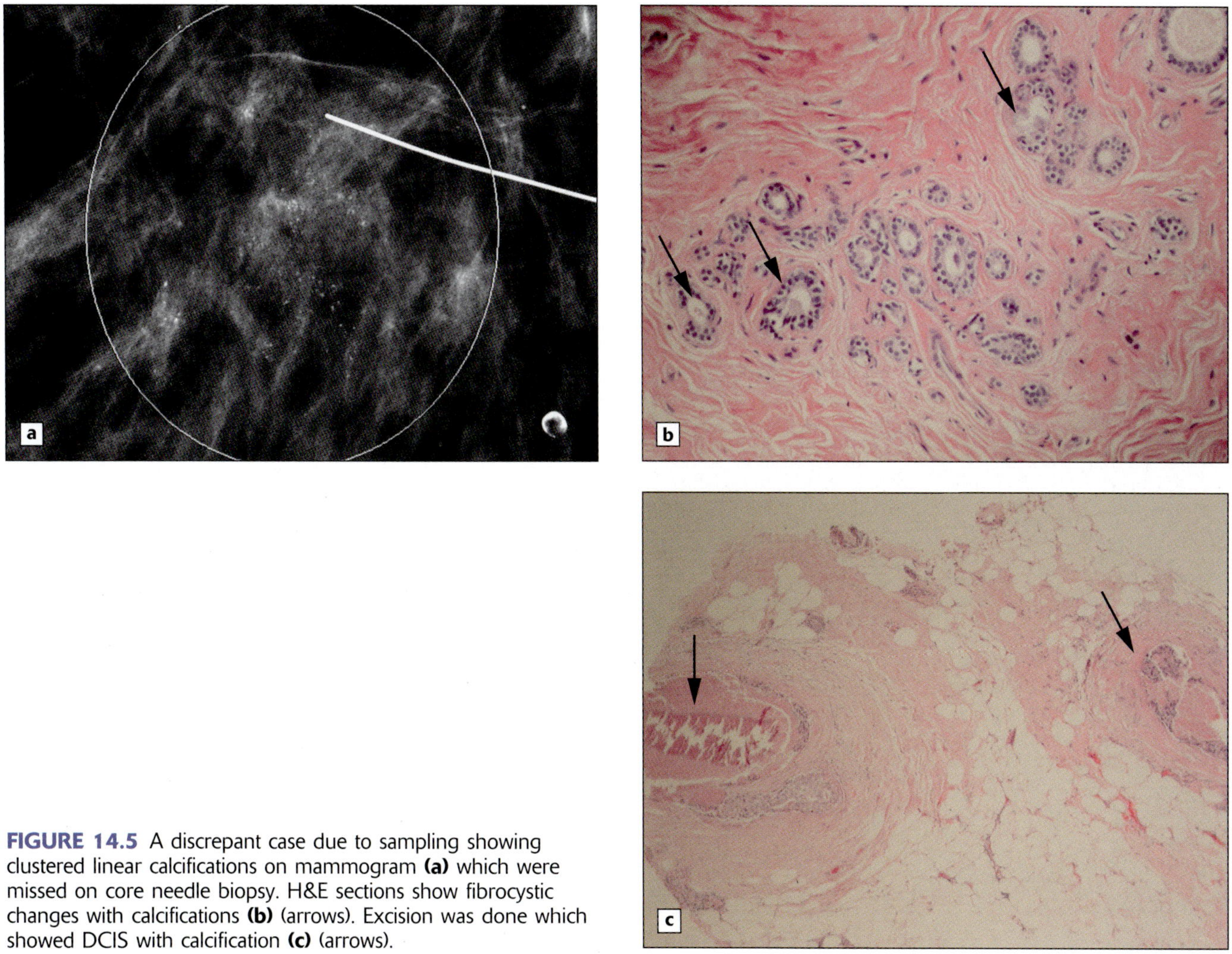

FIGURE 14.5 A discrepant case due to sampling showing clustered linear calcifications on mammogram **(a)** which were missed on core needle biopsy. H&E sections show fibrocystic changes with calcifications **(b)** (arrows). Excision was done which showed DCIS with calcification **(c)** (arrows).

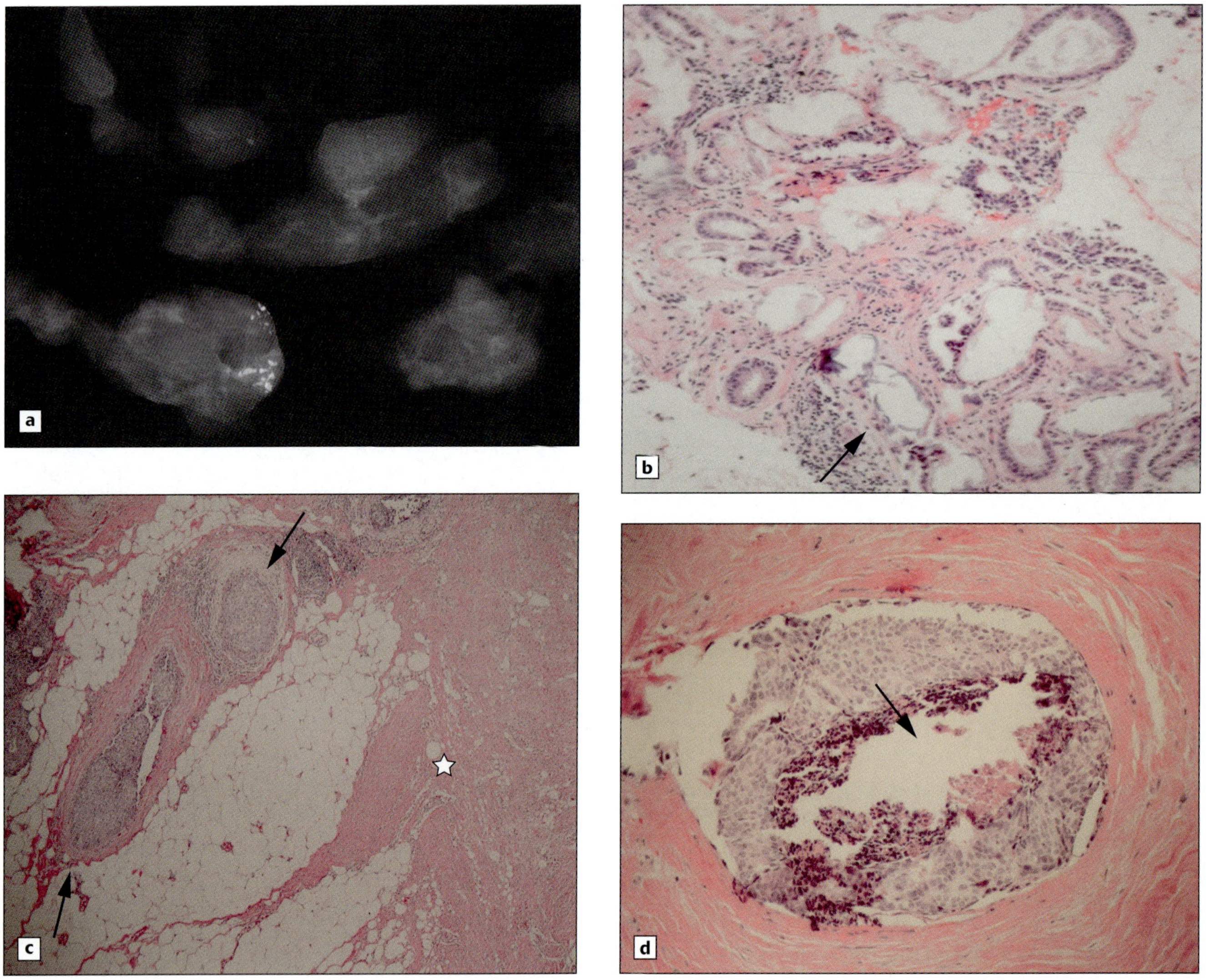

FIGURE 14.6 Specimen radiograph **(a)** shows linear calcifications suspicious for comedo DCIS. Histologic sections **(b)** showed fibrocystic changes with calcifications (arrow). The pathologist did not receive the specimen radiograph and was not aware of the linear quality of the calcifications. Radiograph of paraffin blocks was not performed at the outside institution. Instead due to radiologic–pathologic discordance, excision was recommended; this revealed DCIS, comedo type (arrow) **(c)**, at biopsy site changes (asterisk), with calcifications seen at higher power **(d)**.

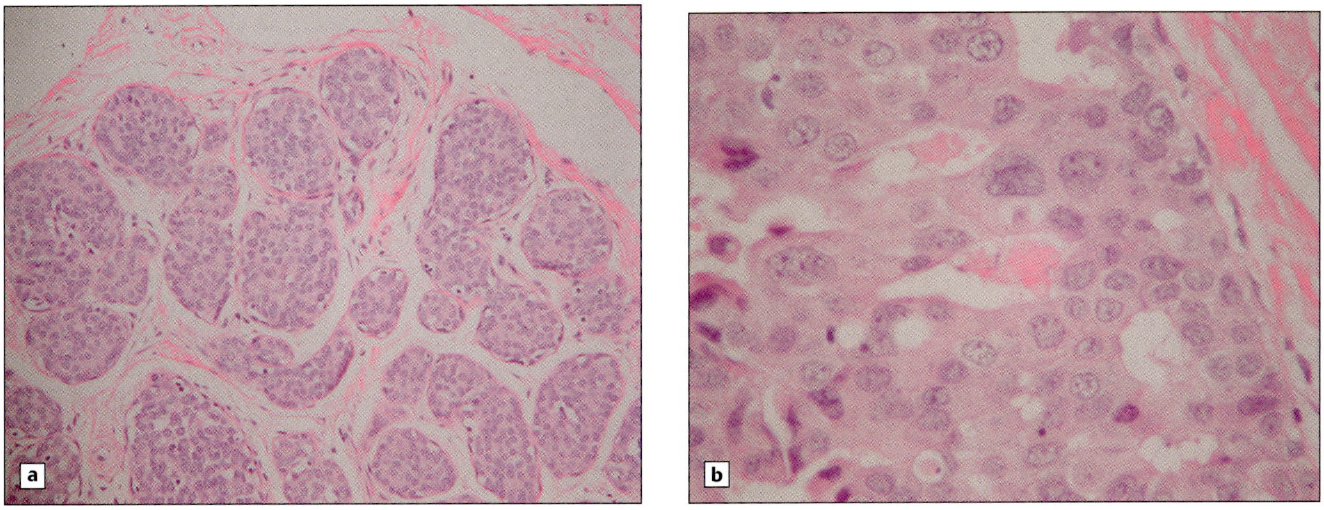

FIGURE 14.7 The distinction of LCIS **(a)** from high grade DCIS **(b)** is straightforward.

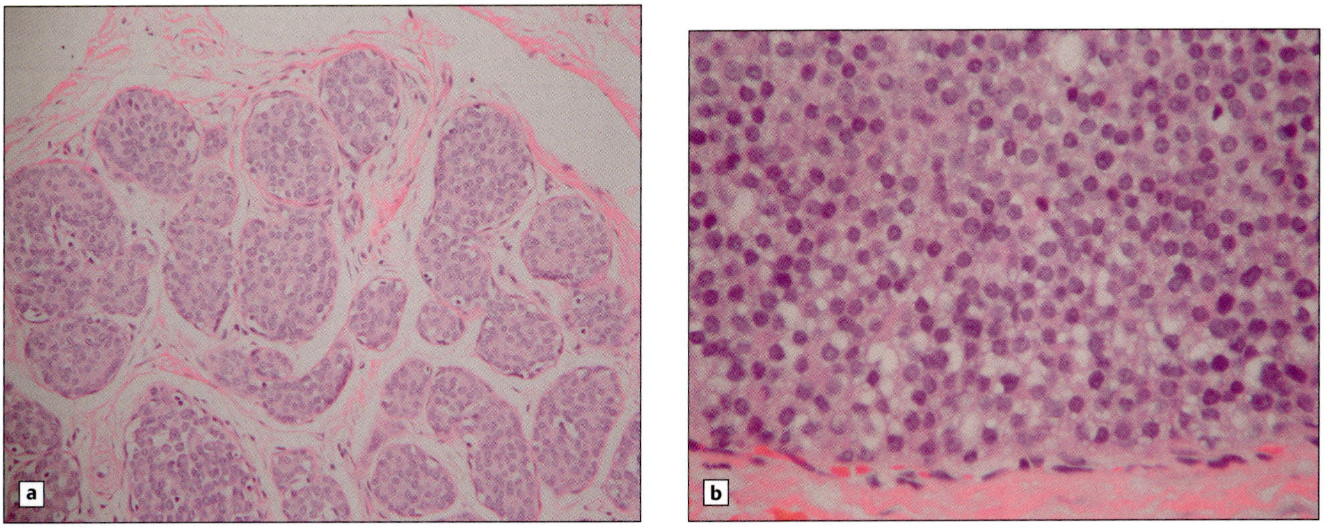

FIGURE 14.8 The distinction of LCIS **(a)** from low grade DCIS **(b)** can be challenging due to overlapping features.

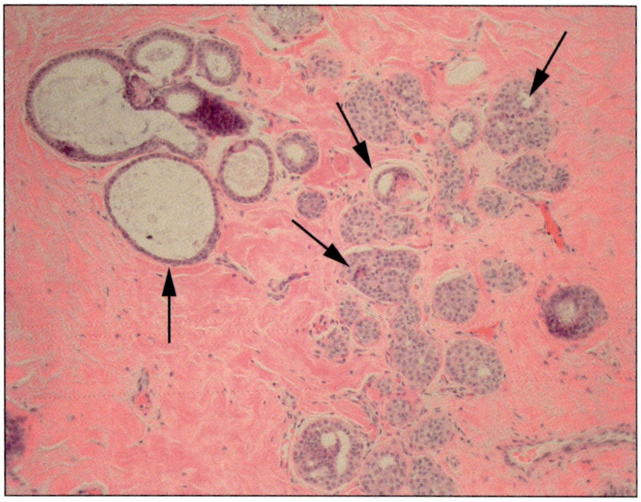

FIGURE 14.9 Calcifications within fibrocystic changes (left arrow) and LCIS (right arrows).

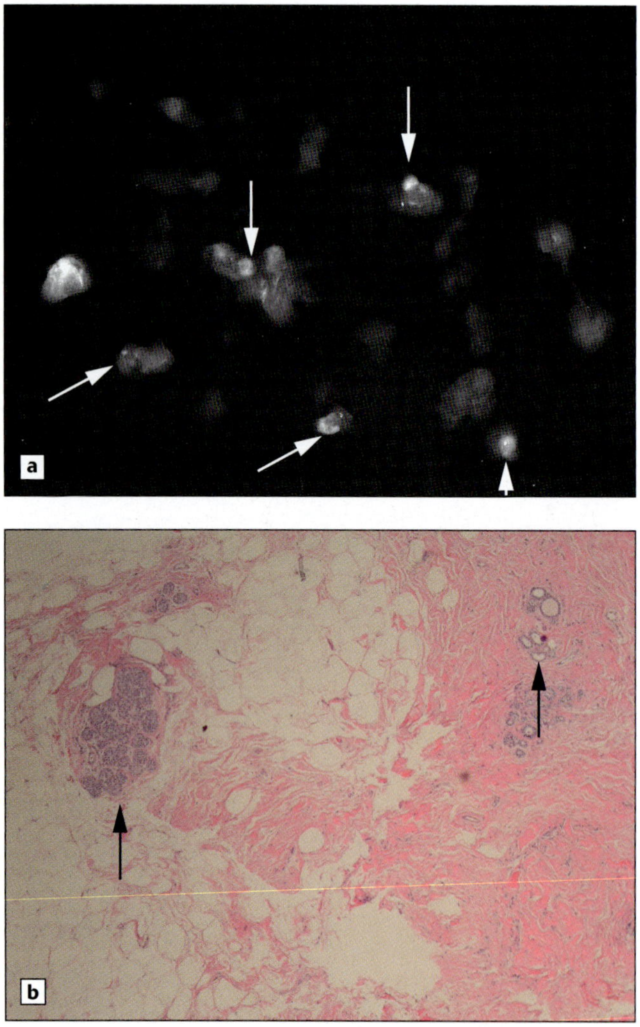

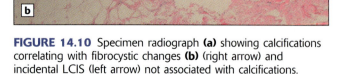

FIGURE 14.10 Specimen radiograph **(a)** showing calcifications correlating with fibrocystic changes **(b)** (right arrow) and incidental LCIS (left arrow) not associated with calcifications.

(see Chap. 9) (Fig. 14.11). LCIS is characterized by distended lobules confined by basement membrane, composed of a uniform population of small round blue dyscohesive cells with occasional signet ring cell forms (Figs 14.7–14.11). Less developed forms have been termed atypical lobular hyperplasia in which less than 50% of the acini of a TDLU dilated and filled by this proliferation (Fig. 14.12).[10] The uniform small cells of classical (also termed type-A) LCIS usually make the diagnosis quite straightforward, but when the cells become larger, with more pleomorphic nuclear size and shape with prominent nucleoli (Figs 14.13 and 14.14), occasional mitoses (Fig. 14.15a), single cell necrosis (Fig.

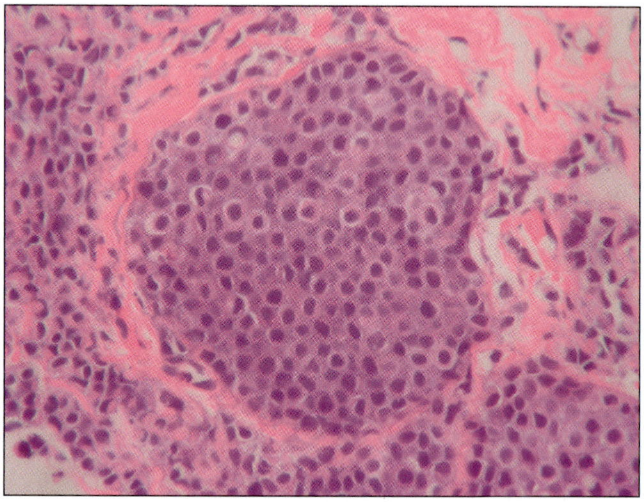

FIGURE 14.11 Note how the cytologic features of LCIS are similar to those in classical and signet ring cells of invasive lobular carcinoma (left).

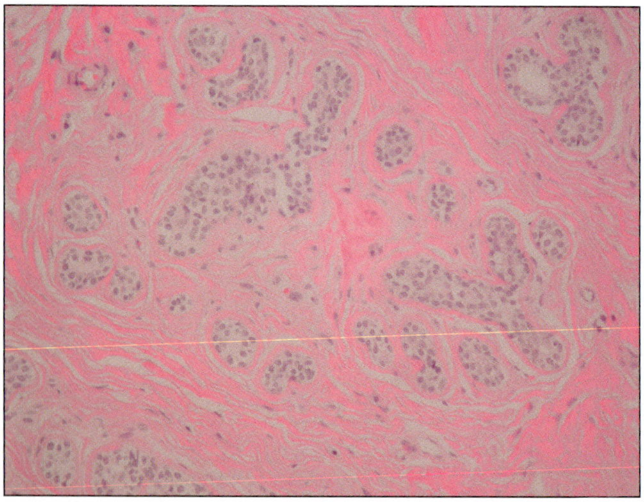

FIGURE 14.12 Atypical lobular hyperplasia characterized by less than 50% of the acini of a TDLU dilated and filled by a proliferation similar to LCIS.

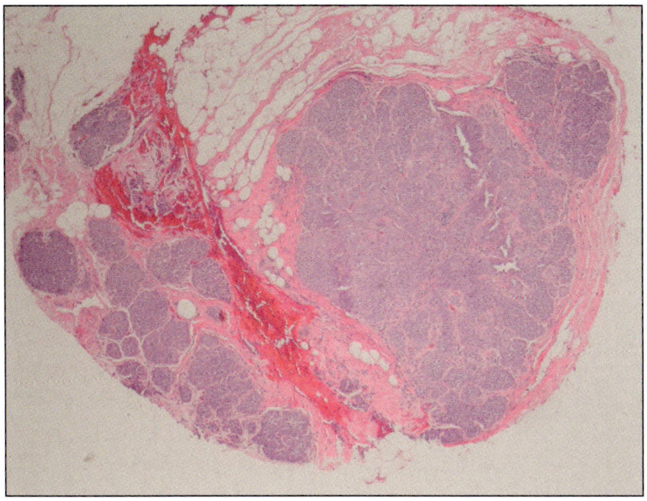

FIGURE 14.13 A lobulocentric growth pattern of this in situ proliferation is composed of dyscohesive cells.

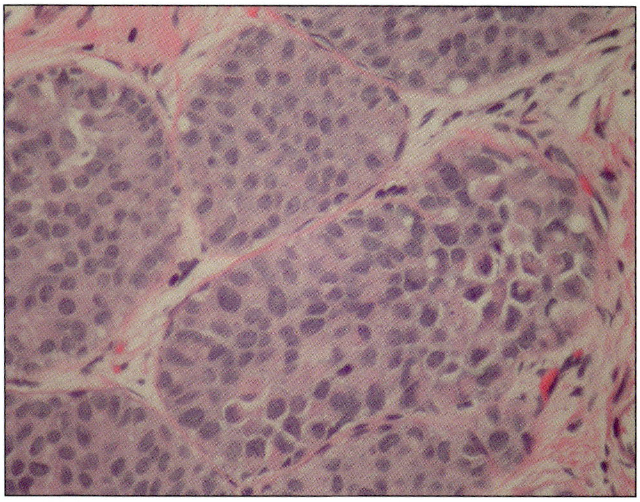

FIGURE 14.14 Higher power view of Fig. 14.13 showing pleomorphic nuclear features and prominent nucleoli.

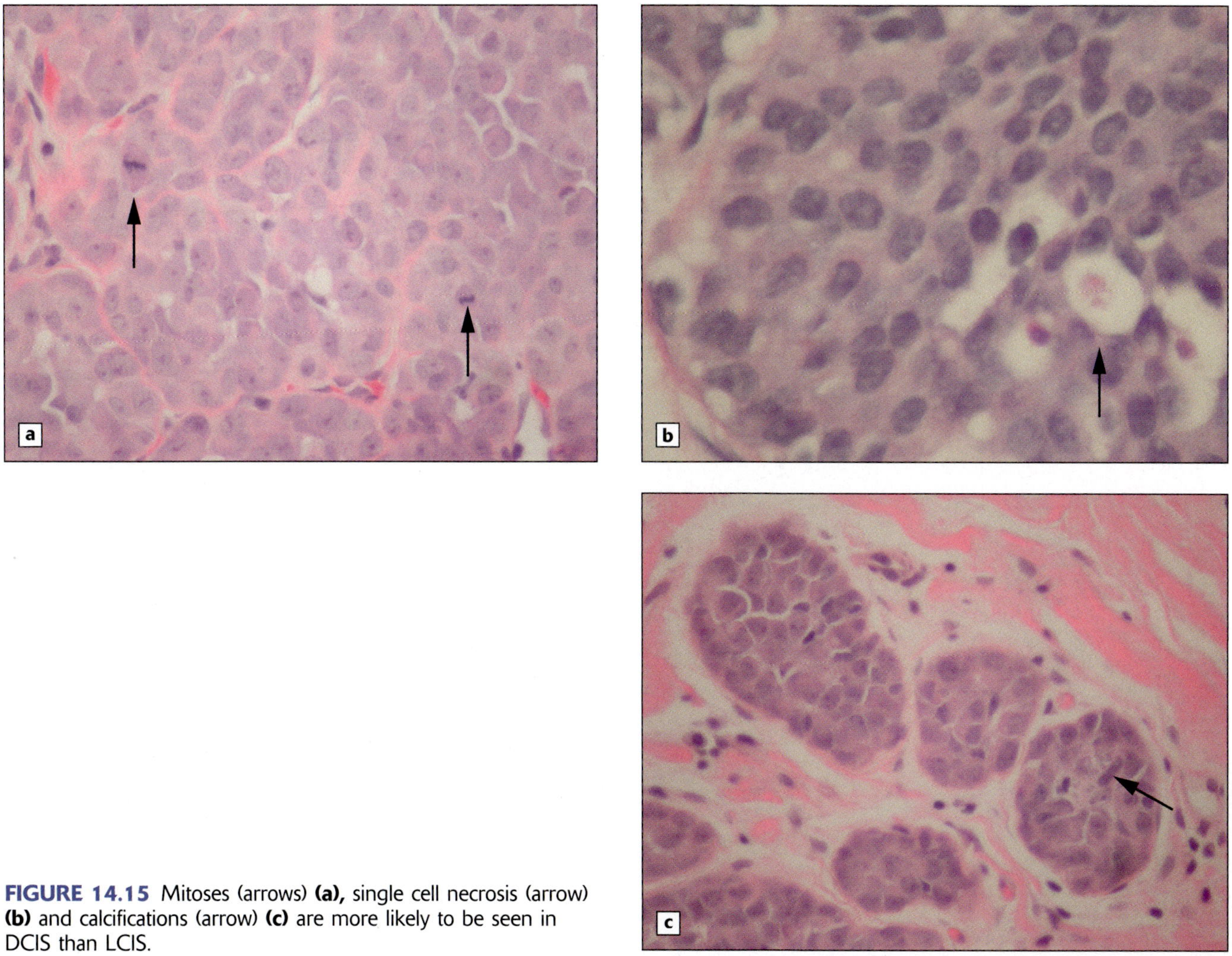

FIGURE 14.15 Mitoses (arrows) **(a),** single cell necrosis (arrow) **(b)** and calcifications (arrow) **(c)** are more likely to be seen in DCIS than LCIS.

14.15b) and calcifications (Fig. 14.15c), the distinction from intralobular extension of DCIS or solid type pattern of DCIS becomes difficult. Such in situ proliferations have been variably called LCIS "type-B," "pleomorphic" LCIS,[11,12] "florid" LCIS, low to intermediate grade signet ring cell DCIS (Fig. 14.16),[13] and indeterminate mixed ductal-lobular carcinoma in situ (Fig. 14.17).[14]

The proper distinction of DCIS from LCIS is of more than academic interest, since LCIS is currently regarded as a risk factor to development of invasive carcinoma in either breast (17–37% after 14–24 years of follow up).[15]

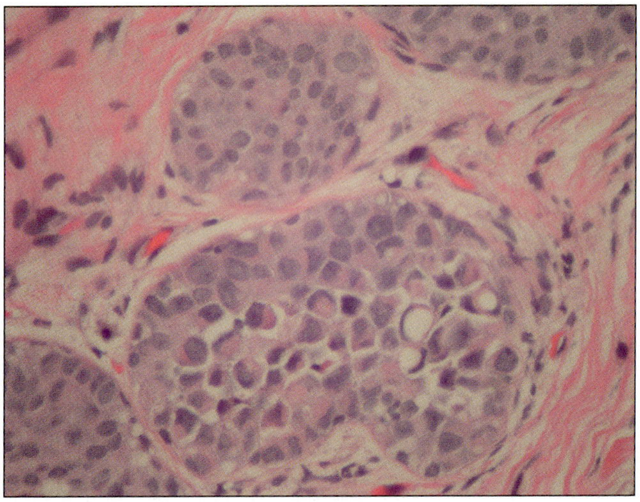

FIGURE 14.16 These in situ proliferations with mixed features usually have signet ring cell differentiation.

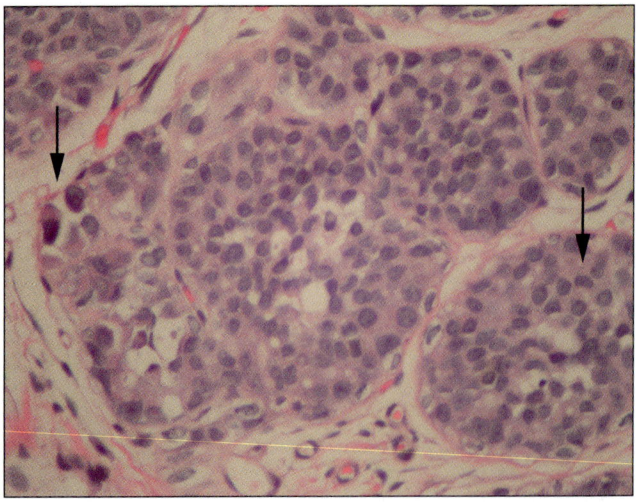

FIGURE 14.17 Mixed features of ductal (left arrow) and lobular carcinoma in situ (right arrow) may be present.

It is not typically surgically treated, bilateral simple mastectomy being the only real surgical option due to its multicentric, often bilateral nature. It is important to know that due to the low incidence of LCIS on excision specimens (0.5–8.0%), the above recommendations have been made based on few retrospective studies limited by small number of patients.[5] DCIS, on the other hand, is surgically treated, the goal being to achieve clear margins, since it is considered a true precursor to invasive carcinoma. Thus, if we apply the same logic to core biopsies as to excisions, a correct diagnosis of incidental LCIS on core should not provoke surgical excision. This, however, has become a matter of considerable controversy.[16–19] Some of the reported high risk of DCIS or invasive carcinoma on excision after a core needle biopsy of LCIS, may be due to discordant findings, i.e., an irregular mass was missed by the biopsy (Fig. 14.18), lack of correlation of radiologic and pathologic calcifications (DCIS still in the block) (Fig. 14.2), or classifying a lesion of the same histology as LCIS on core and DCIS on subsequent excision.

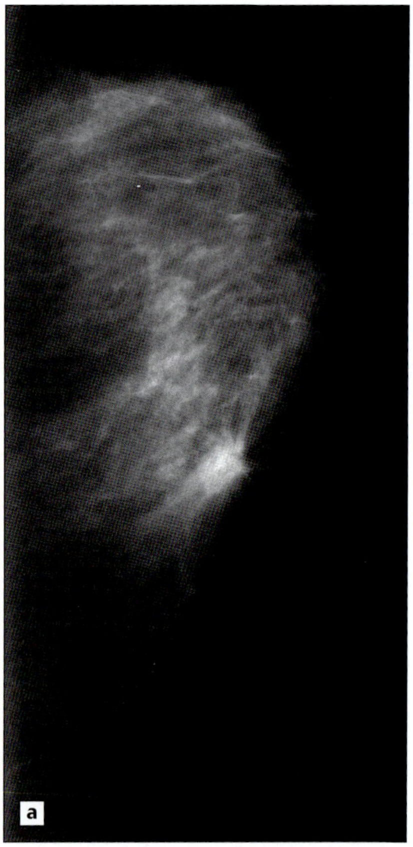

FIGURE 14.18 Mammogram **(a)** shows a spiculated lesion.

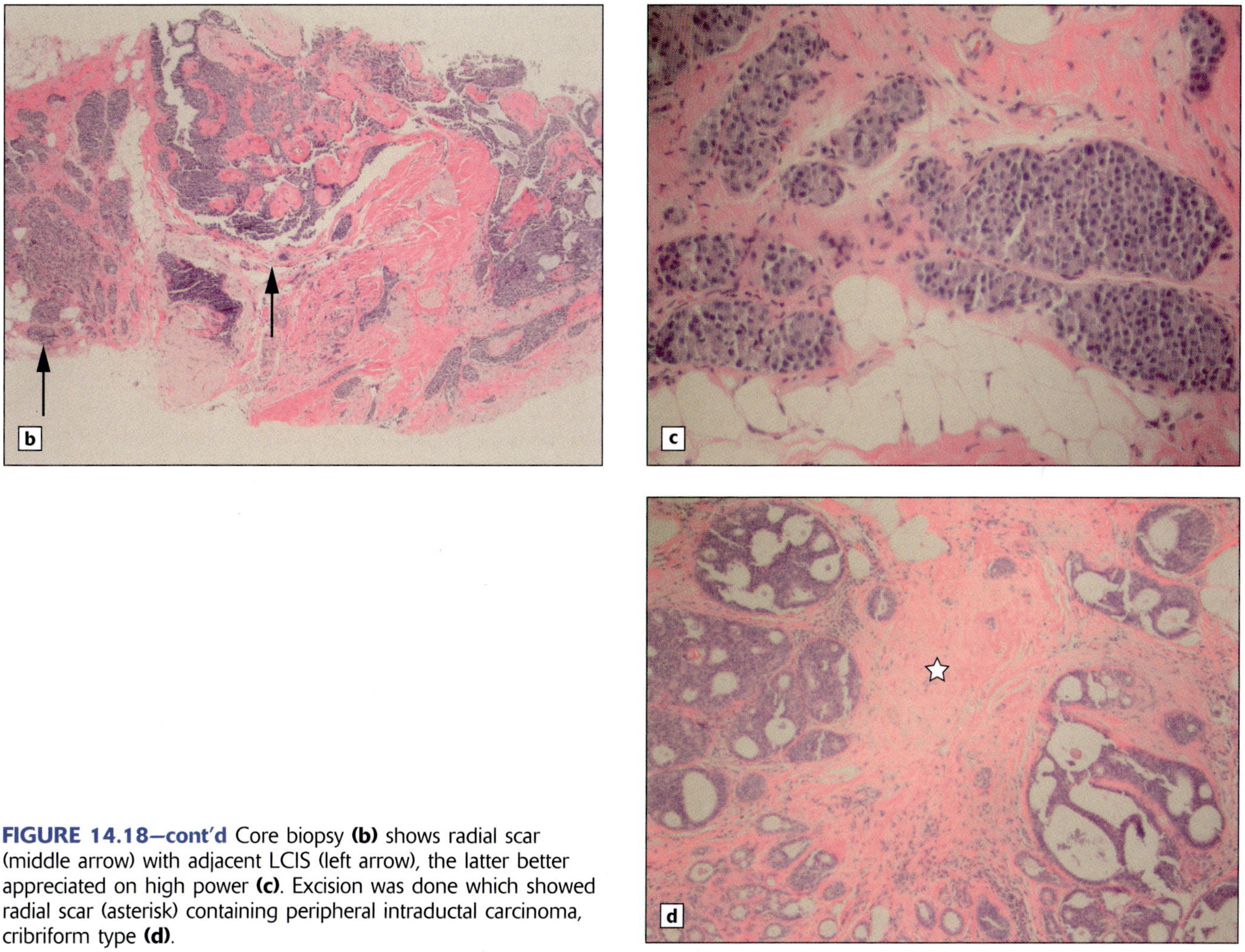

FIGURE 14.18—cont'd Core biopsy **(b)** shows radial scar (middle arrow) with adjacent LCIS (left arrow), the latter better appreciated on high power **(c)**. Excision was done which showed radial scar (asterisk) containing peripheral intraductal carcinoma, cribriform type **(d)**.

The need for objective differentiation of DCIS from LCIS has led to a search for novel immunohistochemical markers. E-cadherin, a transmembrane glycoprotein, is a molecule crucial for the formation of intercellular junctional complexes. Its inactivation has a key role in the dispersed and dyscohesive growth patterns of LCIS and invasive lobular carcinoma (ILC). Thus, whereas DCIS usually expresses an intense continuous pattern of E-cadherin staining (Fig. 14.19), this is reportedly absent in LCIS.[20,21] In the in situ proliferations with ductal and lobular features described above, E-cadherin has been found to be consistently negative,[22,23] but mutational alteration of E-Cadherin has also been demonstrated; however, we have noted occasional mixed staining patterns and occasional bona fide DCIS cases which are E-cadherin negative. While these results suggest a closer relationship of these lesions to LCIS than DCIS, morphologic features such as cell size and nuclear pleomorphism

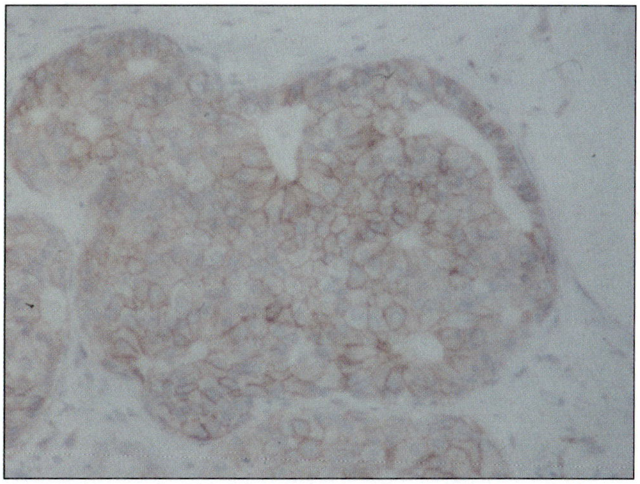

FIGURE 14.19 DCIS showing strong membranous staining with E-cadherin.

are more akin to DCIS. In fact, when such areas are occasionally accompanied by central necrosis and calcifications, they typically have a continuous geographic distribution similar to DCIS and have an associated mammographic abnormality[12] (Fig. 14.20). In our experience, we have observed these lesions admixed with classical LCIS (Fig. 14.17), suggesting origin from a terminal duct lobular unit with simultaneous bimodal expression or differentiation. In many of these cases we have also noted either in the initial biopsy or on excision, subtle areas of invasive lobular carcinoma, with aggressive phenotypes such as signet ring cell, pleomorphic and histiocytoid types (Fig. 14.21). Therefore, we feel these mixed proliferations most likely represent aggressive variants of LCIS which paradoxically typically have a unifocal DCIS type distribution. Logically, they should also be treated more aggressively than LCIS. Thus, we are more comfortable in designating these lesions DCIS, solid type, rather than a variant of LCIS, especially when associated with necrosis and calcifications (Fig. 14.22) on core biopsy, so that they are not inappropriately under treated as LCIS. We agree with Georgian-Smith & Lawton[12] that they should be treated like DCIS, with wide excision with or without radiation. We similarly recommend excision for core biopsies in which the distinction between LCIS and DCIS is unclear and is incidental to the biopsied calcifications. We do not believe that excision is necessary for classical LCIS diagnosed as incidental to the calcifications. Other authors also subscribe to this view.[18]

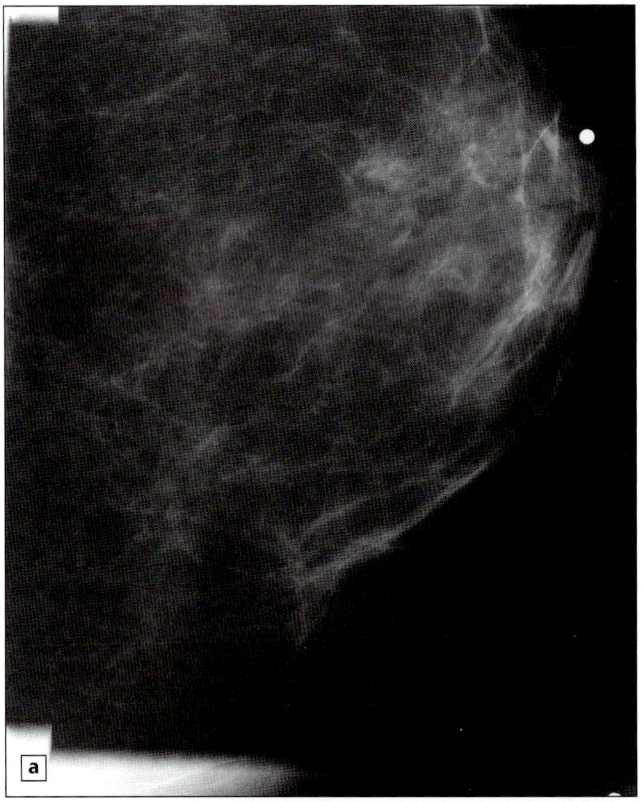

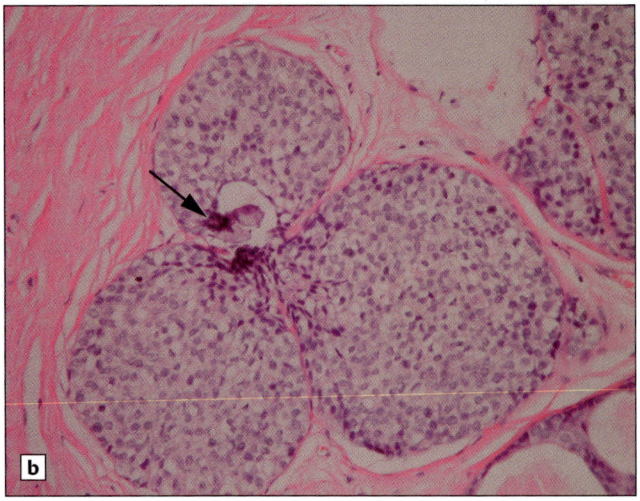

FIGURE 14.20 Mammogram **(a)** shows clustered calcifications which correlate with an in situ proliferation **(b)** accompanied by central necrosis and calcifications (arrow) which typically has a continuous geographic distribution typical of DCIS but not LCIS.

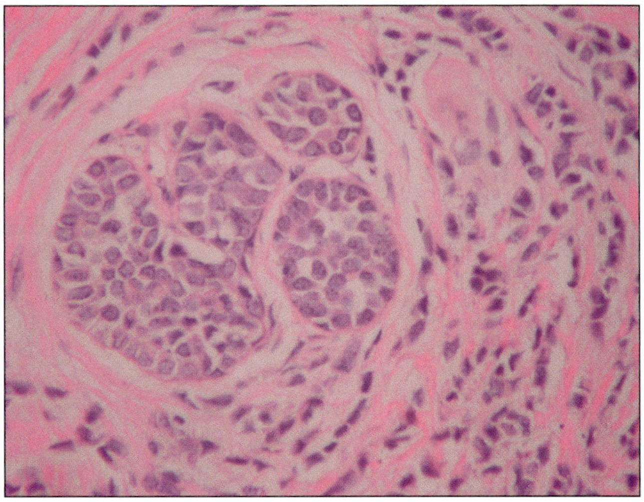

FIGURE 14.21 These in situ proliferations are also associated with subtle areas of invasive lobular carcinoma.

Differential diagnoses of linear branching calcifications

- Intraductal carcinoma (comedo type with calcifications)
- Hyalinized fibroadenoma with calcifications

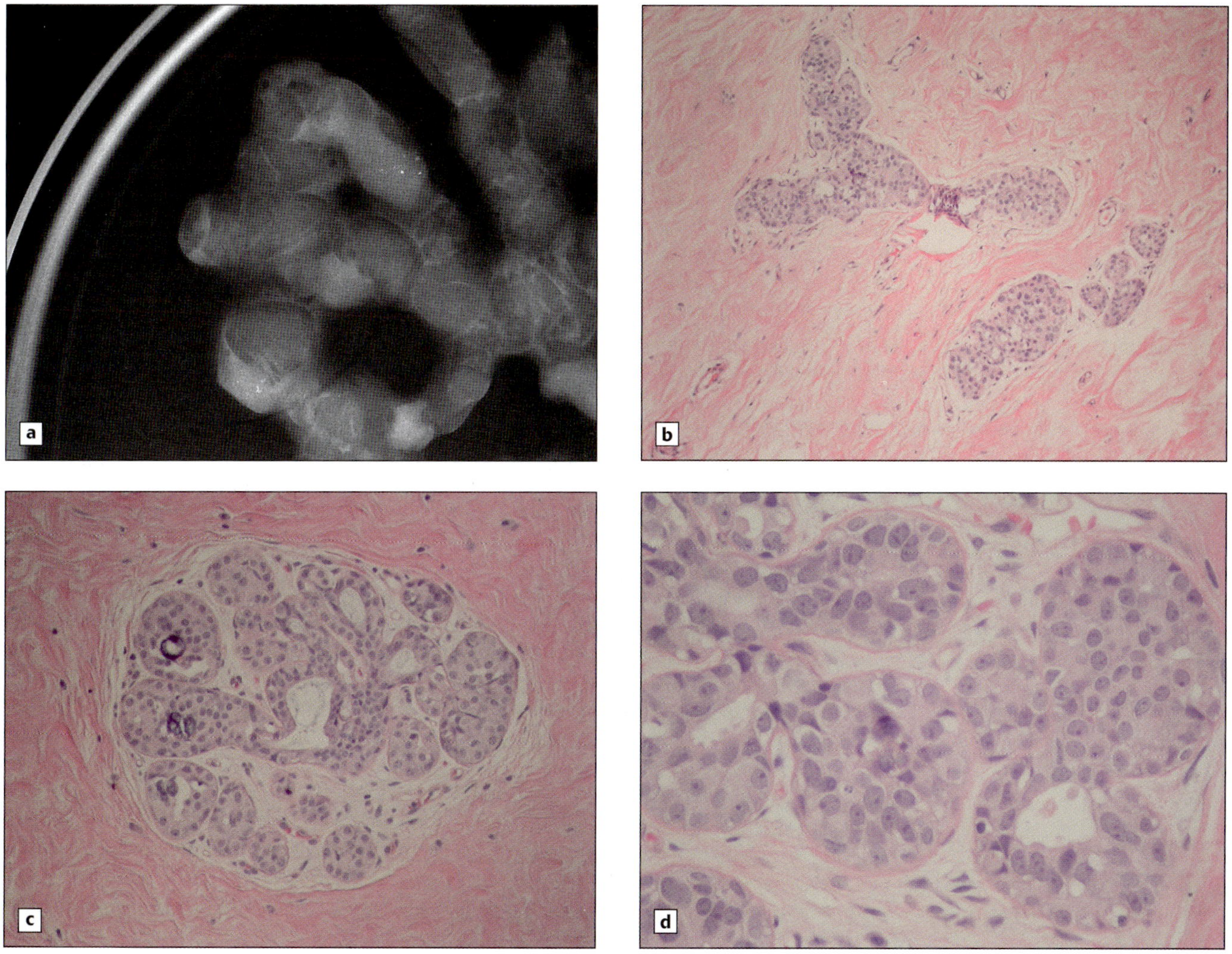

FIGURE 14.22 A challenging case in which the specimen radiograph **(a)** showed a few punctate calcifications. Histologic sections at low power **(b)** and high power **(c)** showed LCIS with larger cells suggestive but not diagnostic of DCIS with calcifications (in c). Excision specimen showed low grade solid DCIS **(d)**.

POINTS TO REMEMBER

1. Linear, branching calcifications must be explained microscopically and may represent DCIS hidden in the paraffin blocks.
2. DCIS can be distinguished from LCIS by its larger more atypical cells, prominent nucleoli, necrosis, and associated calcifications.
3. Excision is recommended after a core biopsy diagnosis of LCIS only if:
   a. Another pathologic diagnosis on the core biopsy is absent (radiologic-pathologic discordance), highly suggestive of a missed lesion
   b. The features overlap with DCIS
   c. It coexists with another lesion such as ADH or radial scar

REFERENCES

1. Rebner M, Helvie MA, Pennes DR, et al. Paraffin tissue block radiography: Adjunct to breast specimen radiography. Radiology 173:695–696,1989.
2. Hermann G, Keller RJ, Drossman S, et al. Mammographic pattern of microcalcifications in the preoperative diagnosis of comedo ducal carcinoma in situ: histopathologic correlation. Can Assoc Radiol J 50: 235–240,1999.
3. Grimes MM, Karageorge LS, Hogge JP. Does exhaustive search for microcalcifications improve diagnostic yield in stereotactic core needle breast biopsies. Mod Pathol 14:350–353,2001.
4. Jaffer S, Bleiweiss IJ. Histological classification of ductal carcinoma in situ. Microsc Res Techn 59:92–101,2002.
6. Hermann G, Keller R, Tartter P, et al. Lobular carcinoma in situ as a nonpalpable breast lesion: Mammographic features and pathologic correlation. Breast Dis 6:269–276,1993.
7. Foster MC, Helvie MA, Gregory NE, et al. Lobular carcinoma in situ or atypical lobular hyperplasia at core needle biopsy: is excisional biopsy necessary? Radiology 231:617–621,2004.
8. Middleton LP, Grant S, Stephens T, et al. Lobular carcinoma in situ diagnosed by core needle biopsy: When should be it excised? Mod Pathol 16:120–129,2003.
9. Elsheikh TM, Silverman JF. Follow up surgical excision is indicated when breast core needle biopsies show atypical lobular hyperplasia or lobular carcinoma in situ. Am J Surg Pathol 29:534–543,2005.

10. Page DL, Dupont WD, Rogers LW, Rados MS. Atypical hyperplastic lesions of the female breast. A long-term follow-up study. Cancer 55:2698–2708, 1985.
11. Frost AR, Tsangaris TN, Silverberg SG. Pleomorphic lobular carcinoma in situ. Pathol Case Rev 1:27–31,1996.
12. Georgian-Smith D, Lawton TJ. Calcifications of lobular carcinoma in situ of the breast: Radiologic–pathologic correlation. AJR Am J Roentgenol 176:1255–1259,2001.
13. Fisher ER, Brown R. Intraductal signet ring carcinoma. A hitherto undescribed form of intraductal carcinoma of the breast. Cancer 55:2533–2537,1985.
14. Sneige N, Wang J, Baker BA, Krishnamurthy SK and Middleton LP. Clinical, histopathologic, and biologic features of pleomorphic lobular (ductal-lobular) carcinoma in situ of the breast: A report of 24 cases. Mod Pathol 15:1044–1050,2002.
15. O'Driscoll D, Britton P, Bobrow L, et al. Lobular carcinoma in situ on core biopsy – what is the clinical significance? Clin Radiol 56: 216–220,2001.
16. Berg WA, Mrose HE, Ioffe OB. Atypical lobular hyperplasia or lobular carcinoma in situ at core-needle breast biopsy. Radiology 218:503–509,2001.
17. Liberman L, Sama M, Susnik B. Lobular carcinoma in situ at percutaneous breast biopsy: Surgical biopsy findings. AJR Am J Roentgenol 173:291–299,1999.
18. Renshaw AA, Cartagena N, Derhagopian RP, Gould EW. Lobular neoplasia in breast core needle biopsy specimens is not associated with an increased risk or ductal carcinoma in situ or invasive carcinoma. Am J Clin Pathol 117:797–799,2002.
19. Rosen PP and Shin SJ. Excisional biopsy should be performed if lobular carcinoma in situ is seen on needle core biopsy. Arch Pathol Lab Med 126:697–701,2002.
20. Vos CB, Cleton-Jansen AM, Berx G, et al. E-cadherin inactivation in lobular carcinoma in situ of the breast: an early event in tumorigenesis. Br J Cancer 76:1131–1133,1997.
21. Gupta SK, Douglas-Jones AG, Jasani B, et al. E-cadherin (E-cad) expression in duct carcinoma in situ (DCIS) of the breast. Virchows Arch 430:23–28,1997.
22. Jacobs TW, Pliss N, Kouria G, et al. Carcinoma in situ of the breast with indeterminate features; role of E-cadherin staining in categorization. Am J Surg Pathol 25:229–236,2001.
23. Acs G, Lawton TJ, Rebbeck TR, et al. Differential expression of E-cadherin in lobular and ductal neoplasms of the breast and its biologic and diagnostic implications. Am J Clin Pathol 115:85–98,2001.

CHAPTER 15

Miscellaneous unusual and rare lesions

While the preceding chapters discussed the vast majority of lesions and situations that will be commonly encountered in routine breast imaging and breast pathology practice, other entities will occasionally be seen. This chapter will present examples of the imaging and core biopsy characteristics of less common diagnoses. In many, an awareness of the imaging findings, particularly when they are characteristic to the particular entity, can help the pathologist to arrive at the proper diagnosis. Likewise, by keeping rare entities in the back of his or her mind, the radiologist can assist the pathologist by suggesting the possibility of such a lesion. Some diagnoses, as will be seen, lack specific imaging features. Thus, the format of this chapter and the one to follow will differ from previous chapters as they are organized by diagnosis rather than specific imaging findings. Note that this chapter is not meant to be an exhaustive review of all the rare entities that might be encountered in the breast; it is more of a pot-pourri of the more interesting cases we have seen.

ADENOID CYSTIC CARCINOMA

Adenoid cystic carcinoma (Fig. 15.1) of the breast is a rarely encountered tumor which has an excellent prognosis when found in pure form.[1] A shared histologic appearance is its only relationship to the aggressive and insidiously infiltrative carcinoma of the same name that is more commonly seen in the head and neck region. The mammographic and sonographic imaging characteristics are nonspecific and can be those of a well-circumscribed mass or one with irregular margins.[2] Histologically the classical low grade lesion is composed of quite variably sized nests of two types of cells arranged around rigid gland-like microcystic spaces that contain basophilic or eosinophilic material. Higher grade lesions are characterized by more solid proliferations but still may not have a more aggressive clinical course.[3] Because the tumor's growth pattern is so difficult to differentiate from intraductal carcinoma, some authors have questioned whether an in situ form of the lesion even exists. In our experience the extent of invasive tumor tends to be greater than that seen radiologically since, as is the case with invasive lobular carcinoma, there is a relative lack of desmoplastic reaction peripherally. Even at relatively large size, pure tumors show a distinctive tendency to be associated with negative lymph nodes, no doubt accounting for their excellent prognosis. Sampling can be an issue, however, since cases of invasive duct carcinoma can occasionally have focal features of adenoid cystic carcinoma. The diagnosis can be made on core biopsy with enough confidence, however, that the next surgical procedure should be lumpectomy (or mastectomy) with sentinel lymph node sampling only, since lymph node metastasis is highly unlikely.

ADENOMYOEPITHELIOMA

Adenomyoepithelioma (Fig. 15.2) is an aptly titled benign tumor composed of a proliferation of both ductal epithelial cells and intimately associated myoepithelial cells which show a distinctive clear cytoplasm.[4,5] It is characteristically a well-circumscribed round to oval solid nodule, and the knowledge of the imaging characteristics can greatly assist the pathologist in reaching a diagnosis, since the main differential, invasive well-differentiated duct carcinoma or tubular carcinoma, typically is an ill-defined lesion or architectural distortion (see Chap. 8). In fact, a diagnosis of well-differentiated malignancy in the face of a well-circumscribed mass is discordant and should cause the radiologist to question the diagnosis. That being said, adenomyoepithelioma is an extremely rare tumor that we have encountered only once in routine core biopsy practice and once in consultation. Awareness of the entity is important, however, since it can be a difficult lesion particularly prone to overdiagnosis with resulting unnecessary axillary surgery and/or potentially unnecessary mastectomy. Some authors have described a relationship to intraductal papilloma, and others have reported a premalignant potential. Thus conservative excision would seem to be the logical approach given a diagnosis on core biopsy.

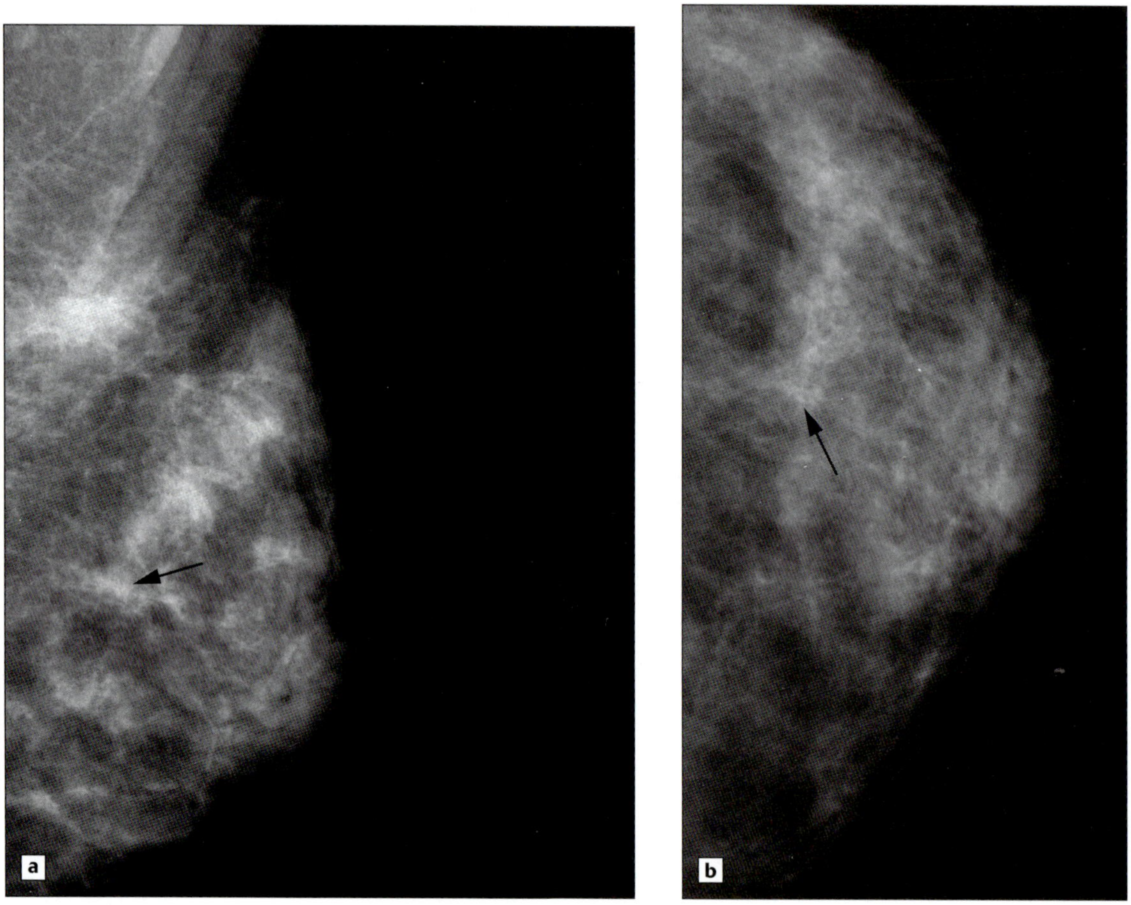

FIGURE 15.1 Adenoid cystic carcinoma. MLO **(a)** and CC **(b)** views demonstrate a new vague density (arrows) in the superior right breast of a 58-year-old woman.

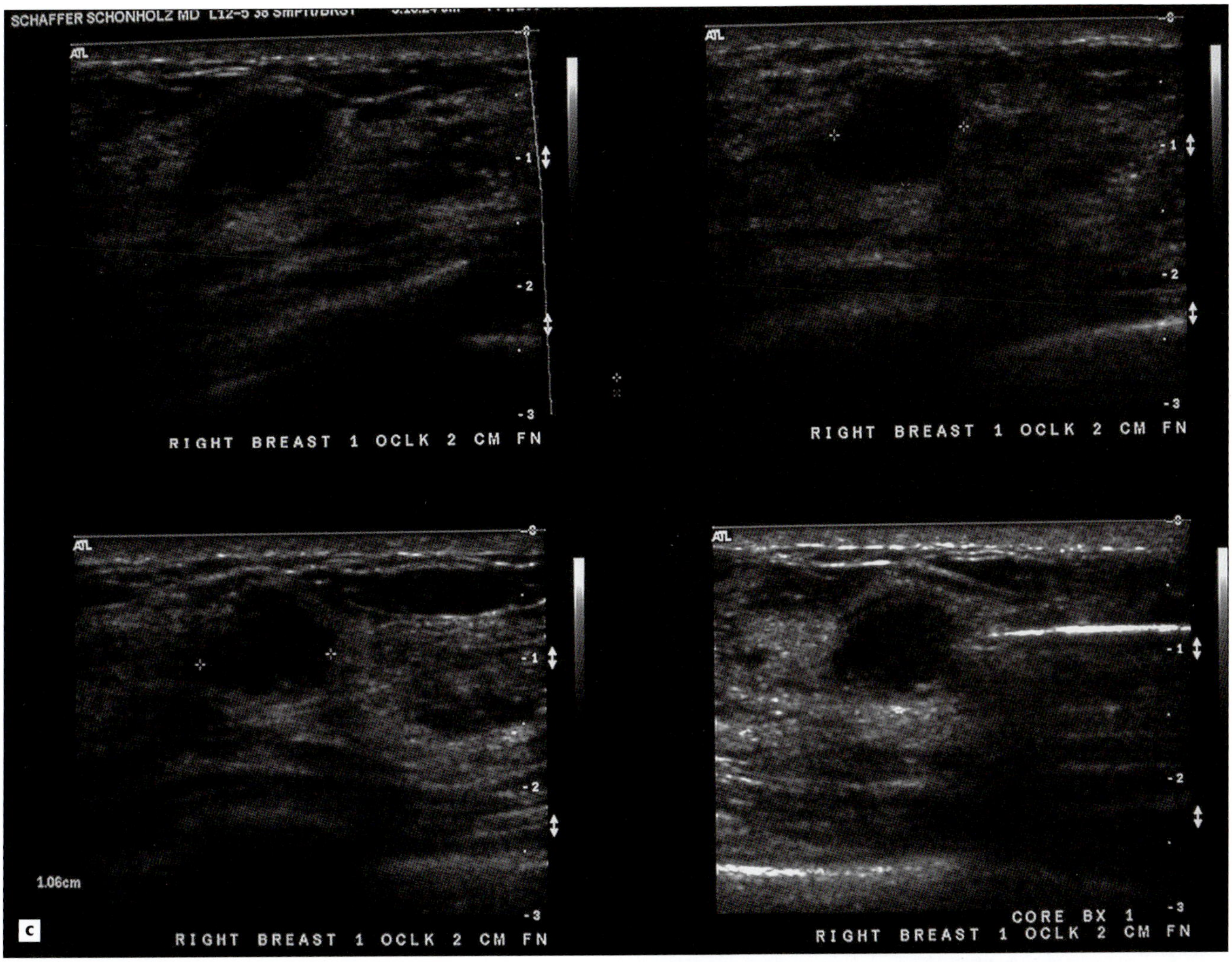

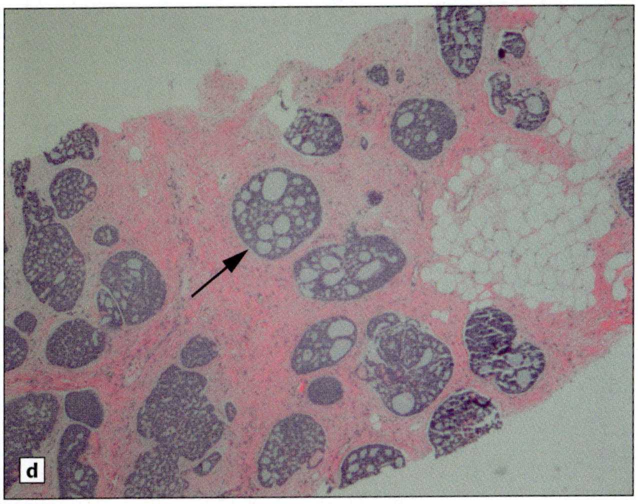

FIGURE 15.1—cont'd (c) Sonography demonstrates a microlobulated solid mass with irregular margins. The lower right image shows the lesion being biopsied. **(d)** core biopsy reveals a classical appearance of adenoid cystic carcinoma with variably sized nests of hyperchromatic cells creating sieve-like rigid cribriform spaces (arrow) haphazardly infiltrating the parenchyma.

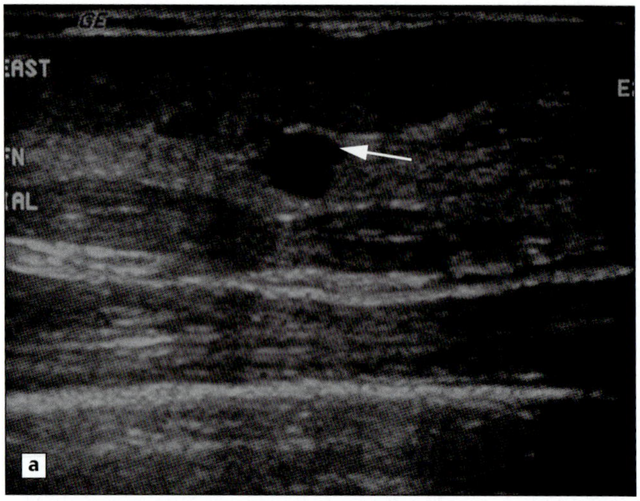

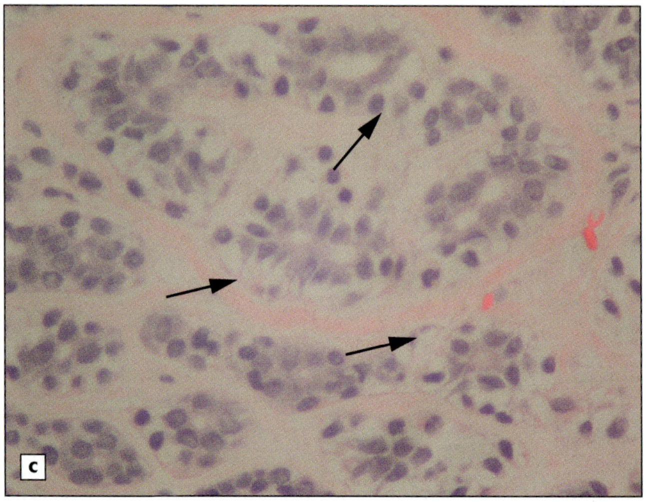

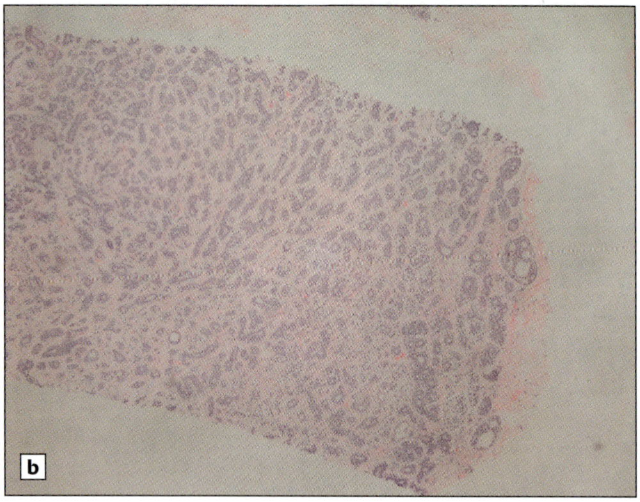

FIGURE 15.2 Adenomyoepithelioma. **(a)** Sonography of the right breast of a 67-year-old woman reveals a 0.55 cm hypoechoic circumscribed mass with a slightly angulated border (arrow). **(b)** Core biopsy shows a monotonous proliferation of well formed glands with a sharply defined border. **(c)** Higher power examination, however, reveals that the glands are composed of two intimately associated cell types: the inner epithelial cells which here are nearly devoid of cytoplasm and the outer myoepithelial cells which have a distinctive and abundant clear cytoplasm (arrows).

ANGIOLIPOMA

Angiolipoma (Fig. 15.3) of the breast is an uncommon benign circumscribed nodule composed of clusters of delicate blood vessels and adipose tissue lined by a thin fibrous capsule. Typically angiolipomas are radiodense well-circumscribed nodules that are slightly hyperechoic in sonography.[6,7] On core biopsy it may be difficult to distinguish angiolipoma from capillary hemangioma. This distinction is obviously not as important as differentiating this entity from low grade angiosarcoma.

ANGIOSARCOMA

In the current era of breast conservation, angiosarcoma (Fig. 15.4) can be seen as a sequela of radiation therapy, typically occurring in the skin and secondarily involving the underlying breast tissue; however, de novo angiosarcoma of the breast still occurs, both situations being rare.[8] The imaging findings are nonspecific, and we have encountered one case that presented as architectural distortion. The histology of such lesions can be deceptively bland, as low grade lesions can behave aggressively. A typical histologic feature is the presence of endothelial atypia in interanastomosing vessels with or without glomeruloid structures. The distinction from capillary hemangioma rests on angiosarcoma's disorganized structure and invasion of adjacent adipose tissue and terminal duct-lobular units.

CAPILLARY HEMANGIOMA

Perilobular hemangiomas (Fig. 15.5) are typically incidental findings as they are too small to be detected radiologically. Occasionally capillary hemangiomata will be large enough to be seen on imaging studies.[9] Such cases

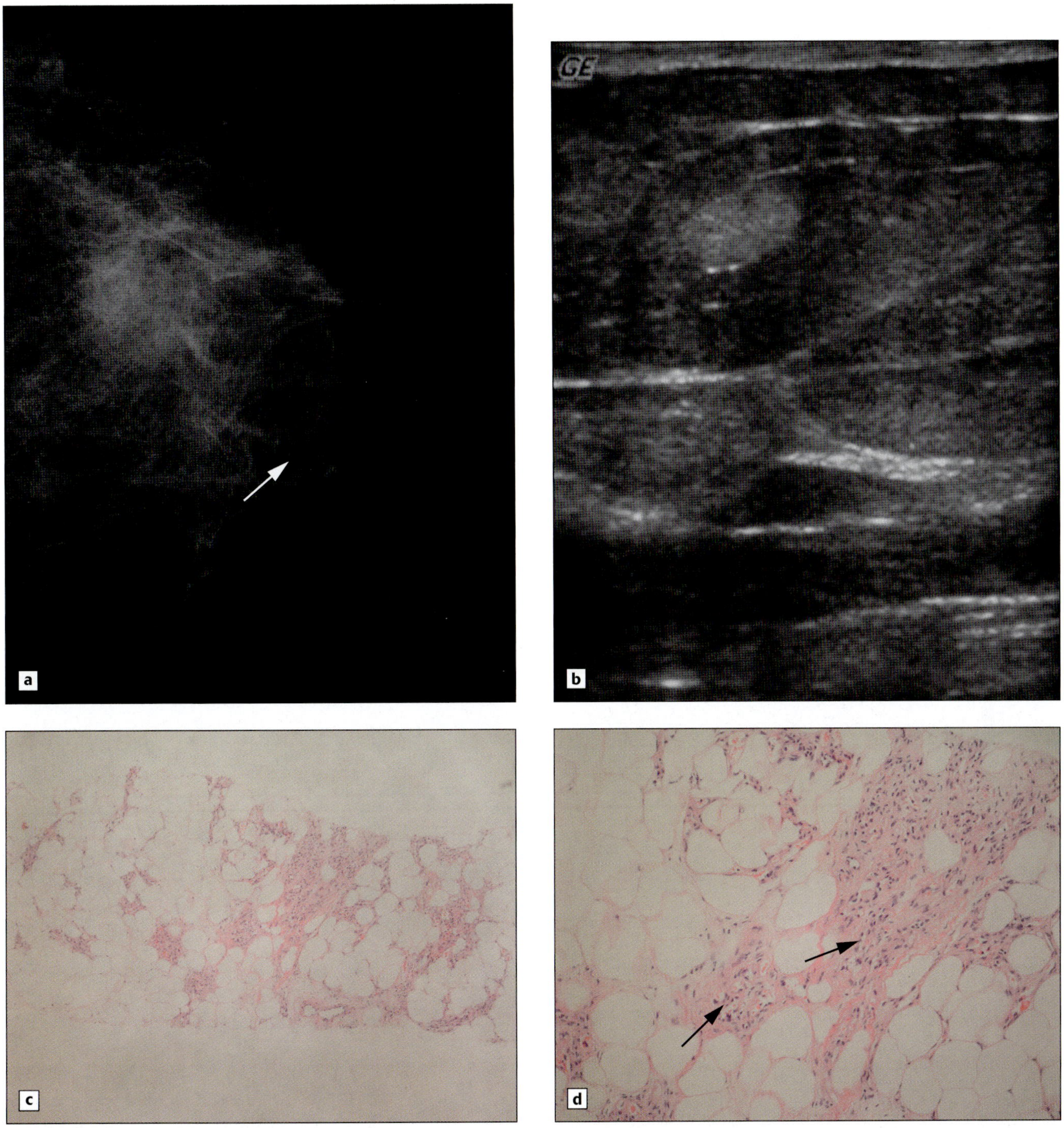

FIGURE 15.3 Angiolipoma. Screening mammogram in a 70-year-old woman. **(a)** CC view demonstrates a new 1 cm mass (arrow) in the medial right breast. **(b)** An oval well-circumscribed echogenic mass corresponds sonographically to the mammographic lesion. **(c)** Core biopsy shows that the lesion is composed of adipose tissue with an admixed proliferation of capillaries. **(d)** At higher power the capillaries are tightly compacted and lined by flat endothelial cells (arrows) lacking nuclear atypia. The histologic appearance is identical to that of angiolipoma seen in other soft tissue locations.

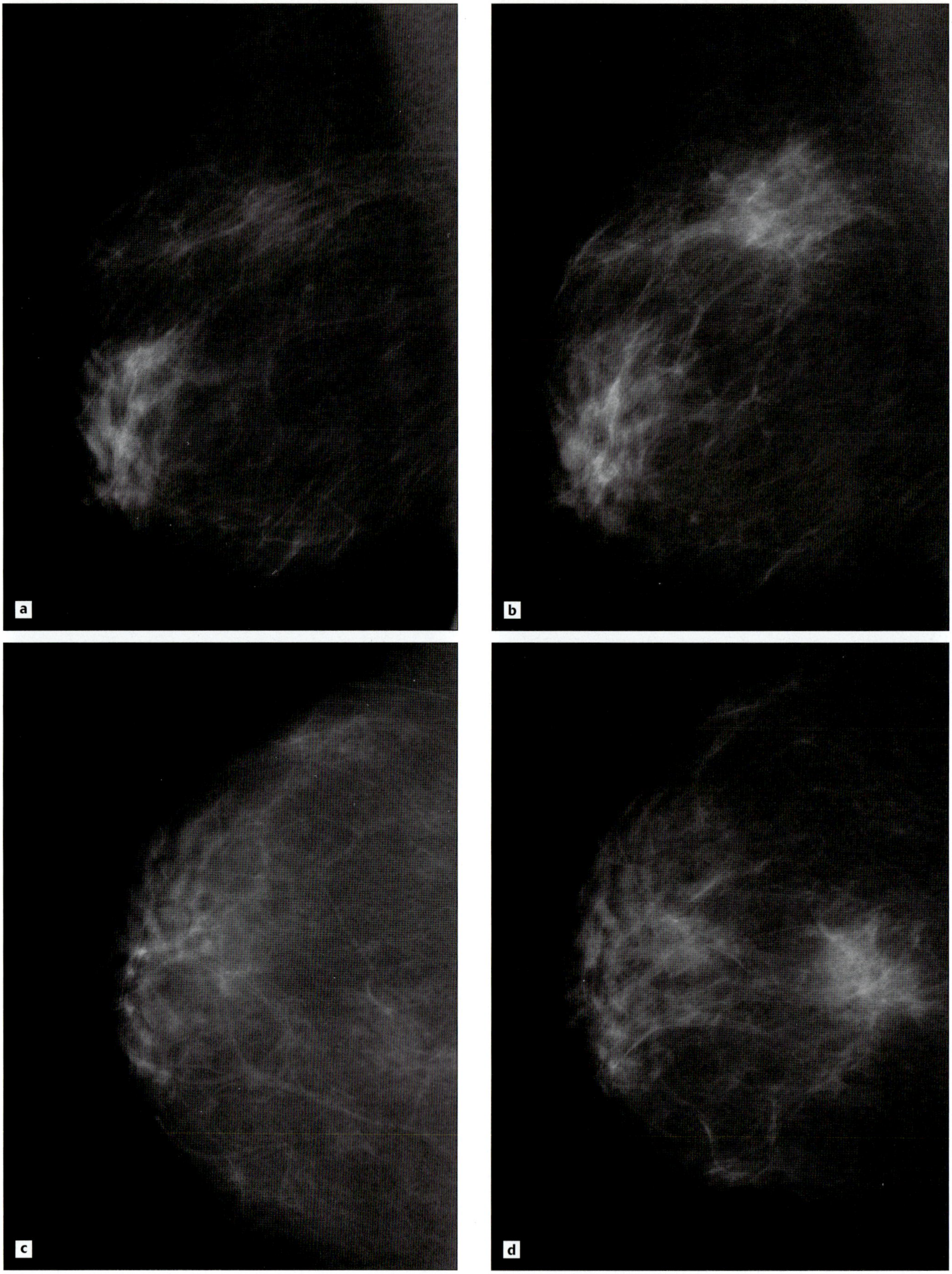

FIGURE 15.4. Angiosarcoma. Mammography in a 75-year-old woman: MLO **(a,b)** and CC **(c,d)** views in 2001 and 2002 reveal interval development of an asymmetric mass with irregular margins.

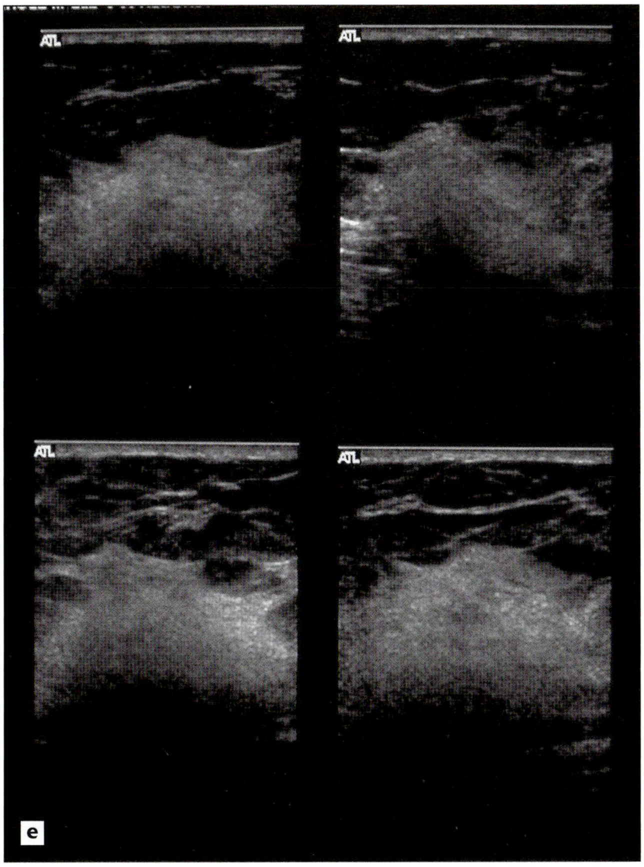

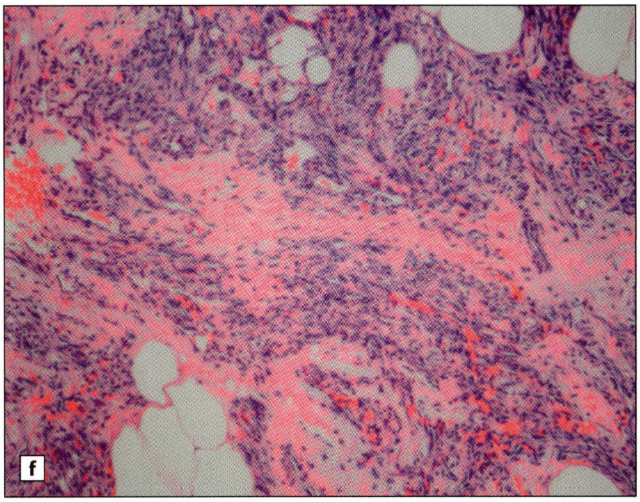

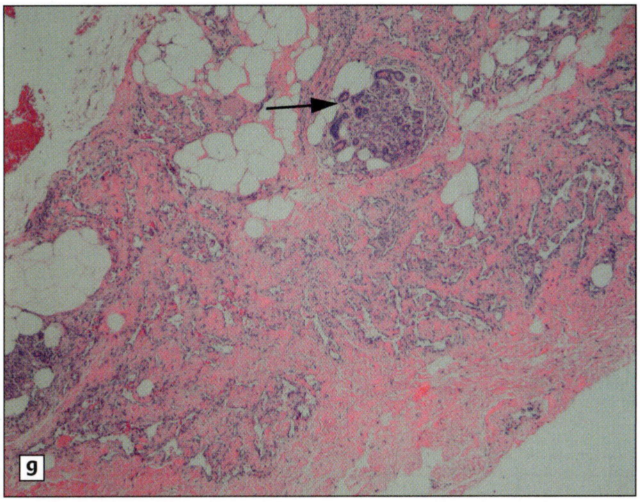

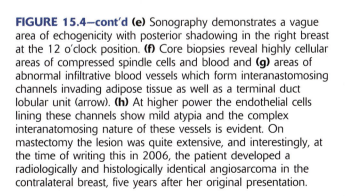

FIGURE 15.4—cont'd (e) Sonography demonstrates a vague area of echogenicity with posterior shadowing in the right breast at the 12 o'clock position. **(f)** Core biopsies reveal highly cellular areas of compressed spindle cells and blood and **(g)** areas of abnormal infiltrative blood vessels which form interanastomosing channels invading adipose tissue as well as a terminal duct lobular unit (arrow). **(h)** At higher power the endothelial cells lining these channels show mild atypia and the complex interanatomosing nature of these vessels is evident. On mastectomy the lesion was quite extensive, and interestingly, at the time of writing this in 2006, the patient developed a radiologically and histologically identical angiosarcoma in the contralateral breast, five years after her original presentation.

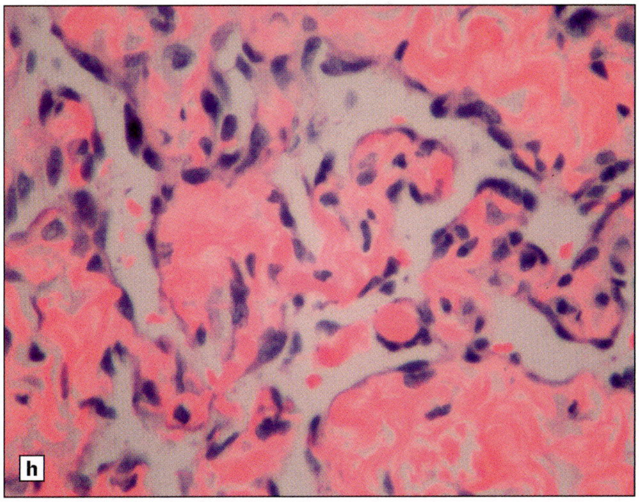

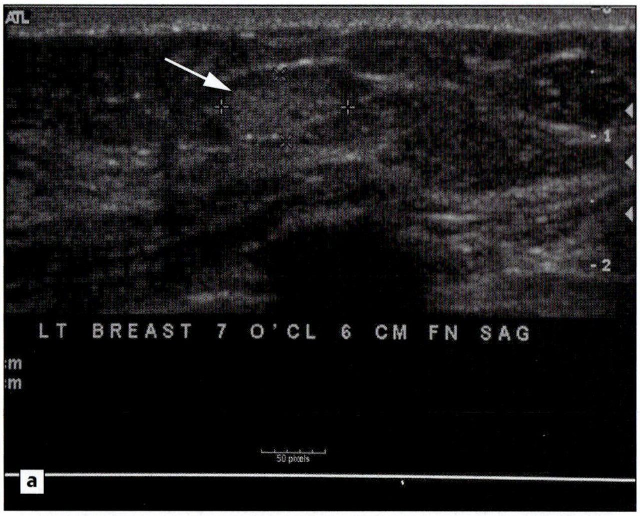

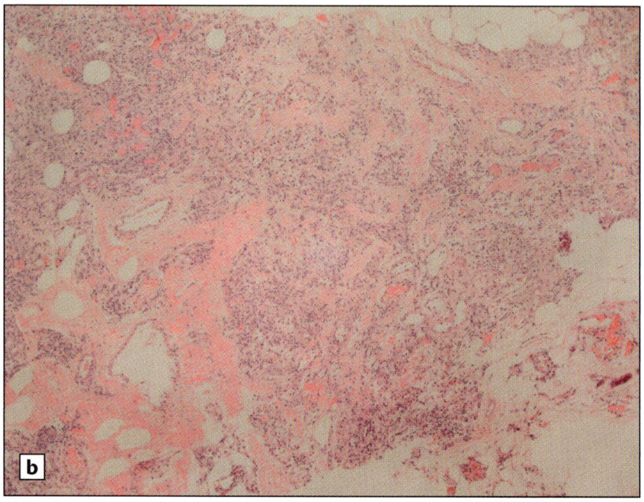

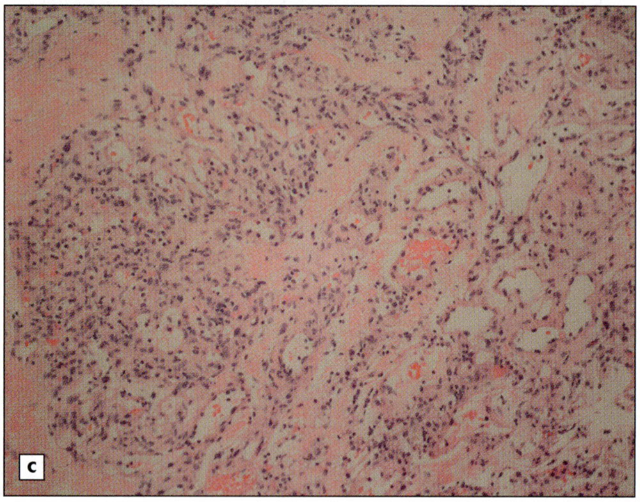

FIGURE 15.5 Capillary hemangioma. **(a)** Breast sonography in a 55-year-old woman shows a hyperechogenic mass (arrow) that is ovoid and fairly well circumscribed. **(b)** Core biopsy is nearly entirely composed of compact capillaries similar to those in Fig. 15.3, but without the admixture of adipose tissue. **(c)** At higher power the endothelial cells appear benign, there are a few dilated capillary spaces, and the growth pattern is rather nodular and organized.

should be evaluated histologically with great caution. Any amount of cytologic atypia or suspicion of invasion of adipose tissue should prompt a recommendation for excision. In our view one should have a low threshold for such a recommendation in order to avoid the underdiagnosis of low grade angiosarcoma.

DIABETIC MASTOPATHY

Both the radiologic and pathologic findings (Fig. 15.6) of this entity are nonspecific and require the correct clinical history for diagnosis. Imaging may reveal asymmetry or an irregular mass.[10,11] The most characteristic histologic findings, although by no means pathognomonic, are the combination of perilobular and perivascular chronic inflammation with nodular aggregates of dense keloid-like bundles of collagen. The diagnosis can only be suggested on core biopsy, but it is more important in the clinical context to diagnose the core biopsies as benign, since surgical excision is generally unwarranted.

FIBROADENOMA WITH FIBROMATOSIS LIKE PERIPHERY

As discussed in Chapter 2, the great majority of fibroadenomas are readily diagnosable on core biopsy. While typically sharply circumscribed, some cases have slight border irregularities usually corresponding to fatty infiltration

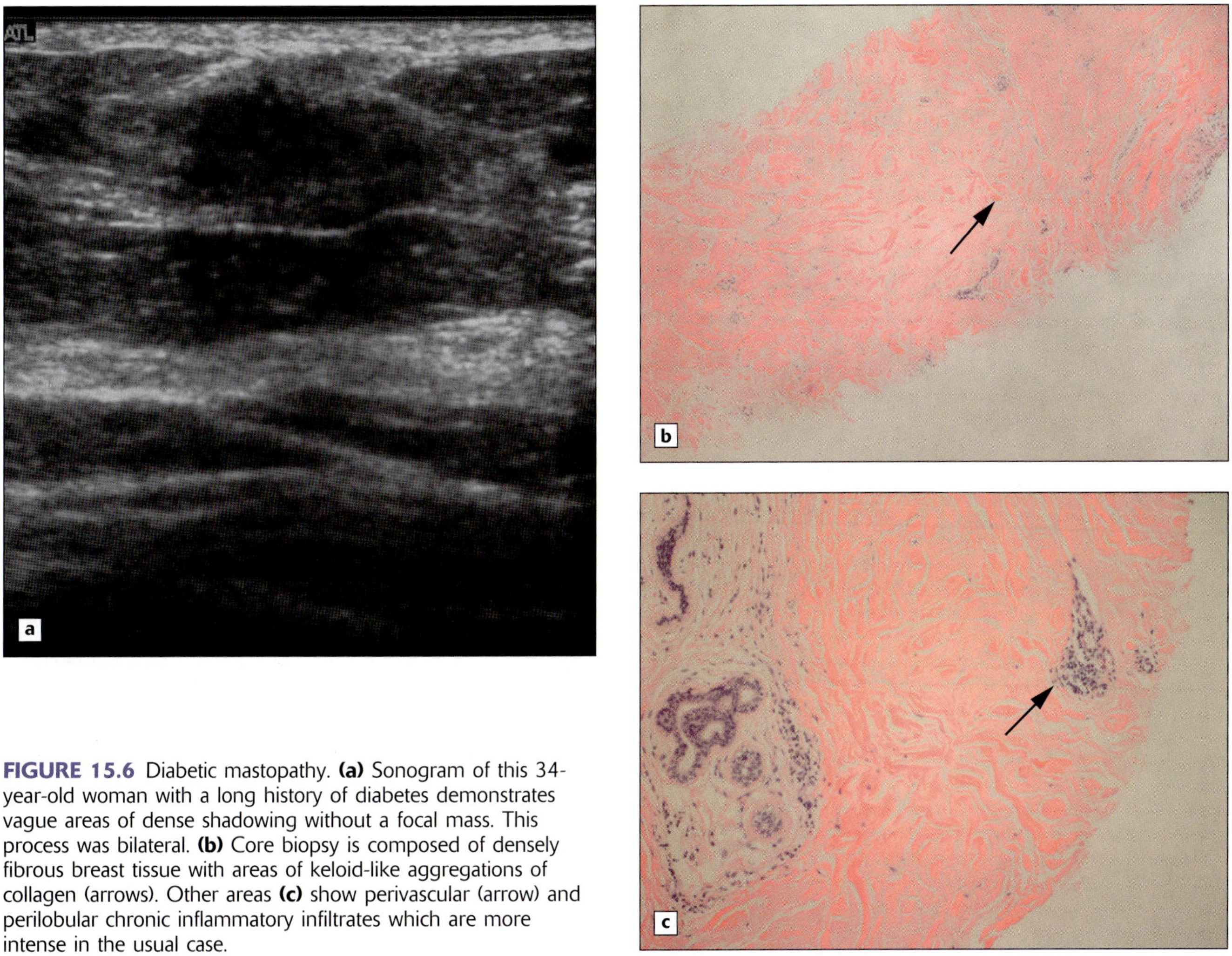

FIGURE 15.6 Diabetic mastopathy. **(a)** Sonogram of this 34-year-old woman with a long history of diabetes demonstrates vague areas of dense shadowing without a focal mass. This process was bilateral. **(b)** Core biopsy is composed of densely fibrous breast tissue with areas of keloid-like aggregations of collagen (arrows). Other areas **(c)** show perivascular (arrow) and perilobular chronic inflammatory infiltrates which are more intense in the usual case.

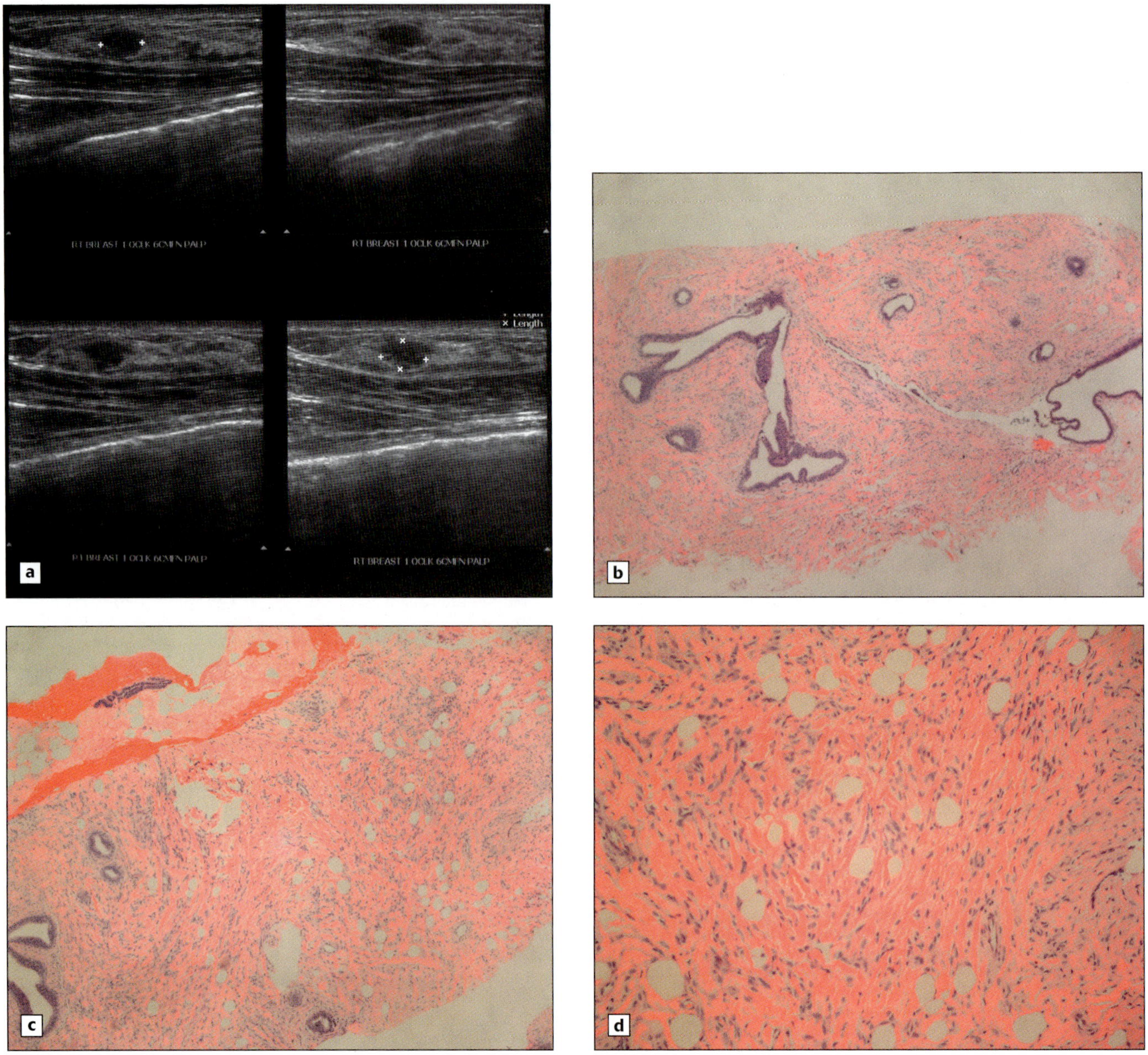

FIGURE 15.7 Fibroadenoma with fibromatosis like periphery. **(a)** Sonogram of a 43-year-old patient shows a sharply demarcated hypoechoic mass with slight border irregularities. **(b)** Core biopsy is composed of glands and slightly cellular stroma in a pattern typical of fibroadenoma. **(c)** The periphery of the lesion, however, shows haphazard infiltration of adipose tissue by small bundles of spindle cells and collagen. The benign cytology of the spindle cells is evident **(d)**.

(Fig. 15.7). Rarely these peripheral irregularities are seen histologically as fibromatosis-like areas. The sharp border of the fibroadenoma may be interrupted by outgrowth of variably dense fibrous tissue growing into fat a short distance from the main lesion. These areas are not cause for alarm, do not convey the local recurrence risk of fibromatosis, and therefore do not require excision.

FIBROMATOSIS

Fibromatosis of the breast (Fig. 15.8) is histologically similar to its more common counterpart found in soft tissue of the extremities. Variably cellular accumulations of benign spindle cells are found amidst a collagenous background. The collagen can be dense, and the key histologic feature is the invasion of usually fatty surrounding breast tissue by odd finger-like projections of the collagenous stroma.[12] Although metastatic behavior has not been reported, the lesion can persist and/or recur locally. Therefore complete excision is advised. In our view both the imaging and histologic features are nonspecific enough[13] that the diagnosis can only be suggested on the basis of core biopsy alone, although most radiologic reports describe irregular, high density lesions, suspicious for malignancy.[9–11] When such a diagnosis is entertained,

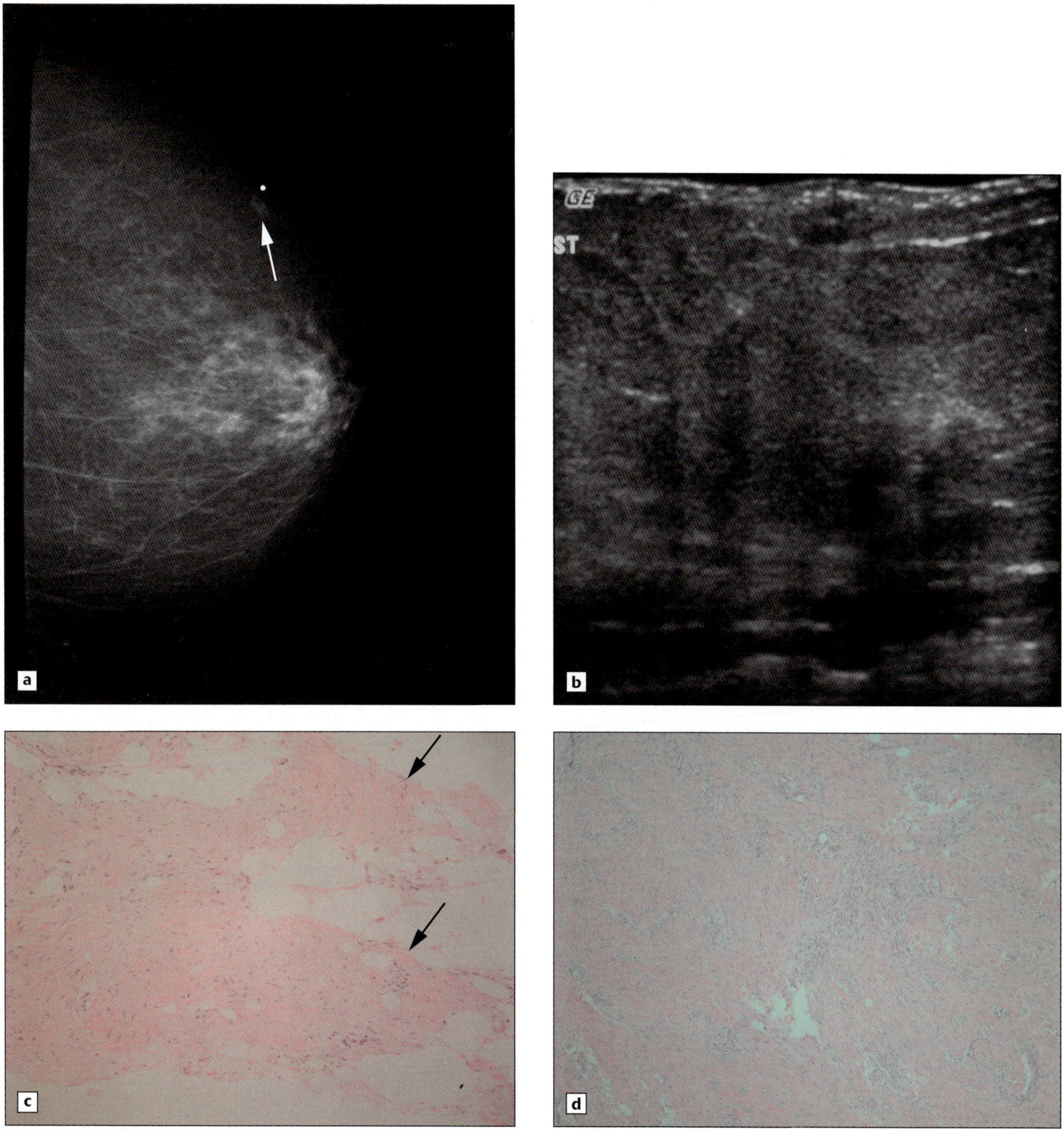

FIGURE 15.8 Fibromatosis. **(a)** A 3 mm marker was placed on a new palpable mass (arrow) in the outer right breast of a 71-year-old woman. The mammogram shows a 0.8 cm low density mass with indistinct borders. **(b)** The corresponding sonogram demonstrates a heterogeneous oval mass, causing elevation of the skin surface superficial to it. **(c)** On core biopsy the lesion is composed entirely of variably dense fibrous tissue with relatively little cellularity. The fibrous areas infiltrate into surrounding fat in so-called finger-like projections (arrows). We generally recommend excision of these lesions without much delay since extended delay produces difficulty in distinguishing scarring as healing progresses from the lesion itself, thus, potentially hampering accurate margin assessment. **(d)** In this re-excision specimen of fibromatosis, it is impossible to ascertain the relative contributions of fibrosis due to the lesion versus reactive fibrosis (compare also with Fig 16.1c,d).

however, excision should be performed without extensive delay since, with greater amounts of time, the healing process will progress to the point where it will become impossible to distinguish scar tissue fibrosis from that innate to the tumor, possibly interfering with correct interpretation of margins, particularly in smaller lesions (see also Chap. 16).

GALACTOCELE

While not particularly uncommon amongst pregnant or lactating women, only rarely is such a lesion biopsied or excised. On imaging studies galactocele is composed of dilated main lactiferous ducts.[14] Microscopically one finds cystically dilated ducts or strips of duct wall containing acellular proteinaceous material in the lumen and freely (Fig. 15.9), since the procedure disrupts the duct in a manner analogous to other cystic lesions. Secondary acute and chronic inflammation may also be seen.

GRANULAR CELL TUMOR

Perhaps no other lesion of the breast is such a perfect radiologic, clinical, and, to some extent pathologic, mimic of invasive breast carcinoma. A granular cell tumor presents as an irregular, ill-defined, solid mass[9] which, if large enough, can be palpable and hard, retracting tissue around it and even skin if it is superficial in location. Pathologically the infiltrative nature is also evident, but in addition to having a characteristic pink granular cytoplasm, the tumor cells lack cytologic atypia or mitotic activity and have normal nuclear/cytoplasmic ratios (Fig. 15.10). The differential diagnosis is obviously invasive duct carcinoma with apocrine differentiation, and such

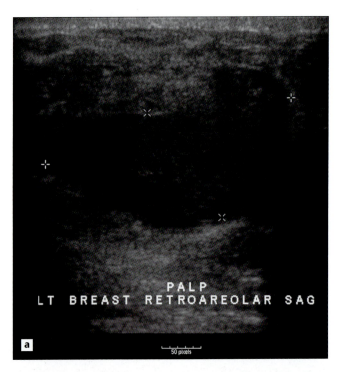

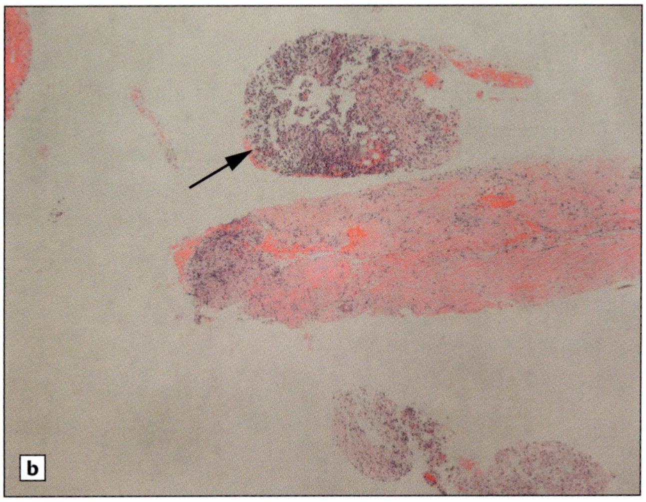

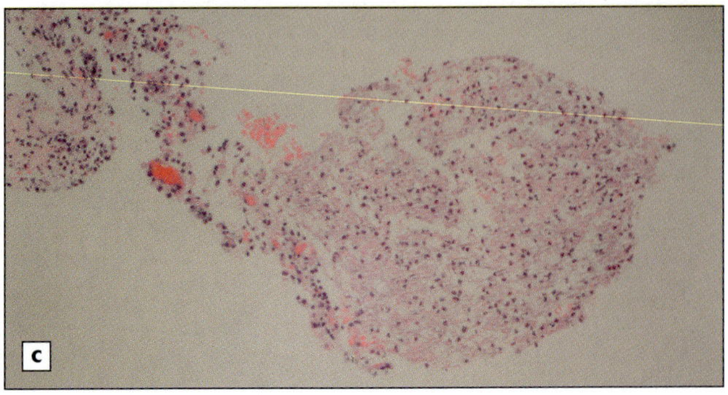

FIGURE 15.9 Galactocele. **(a)** Sonography in a lactating 30-year-old woman reveals a huge retroareolar elongated hypoechoic mass with mixed cystic and solid contents in the subcutaneous area. **(b)** Core biopsy shows fibrous tissue with inflammatory cells at the tip, typical of cyst walls, and detached fragments of mixed inflammatory infiltrate (arrow). Some of the loose fragments **(c)** contain proteinaceous debris with acute inflammatory cells.

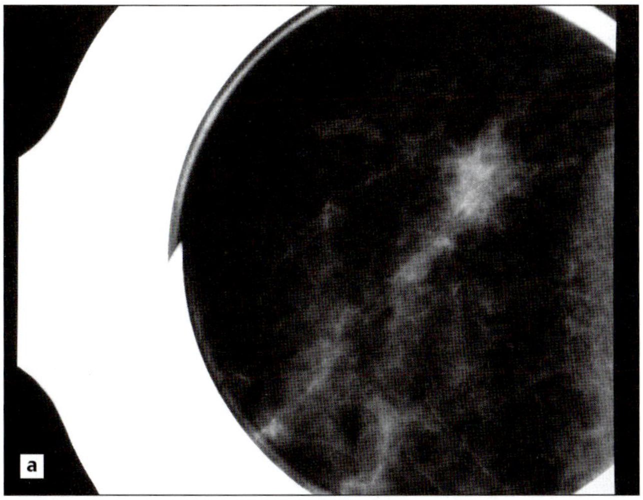

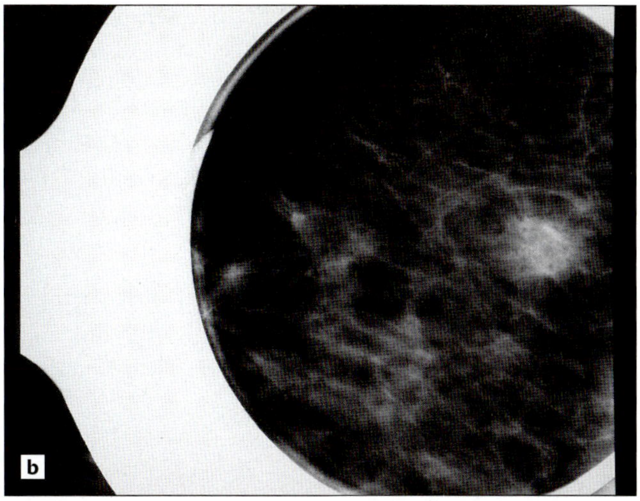

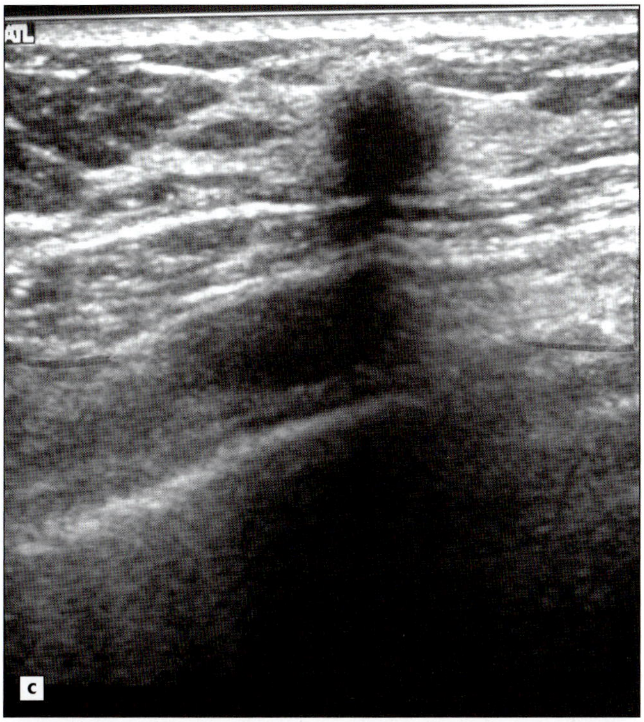

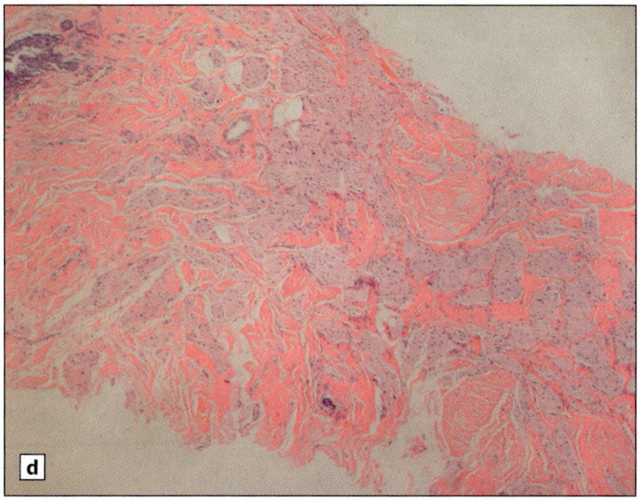

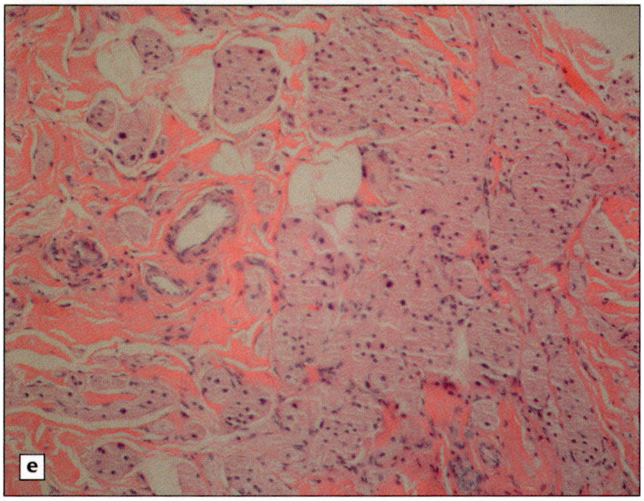

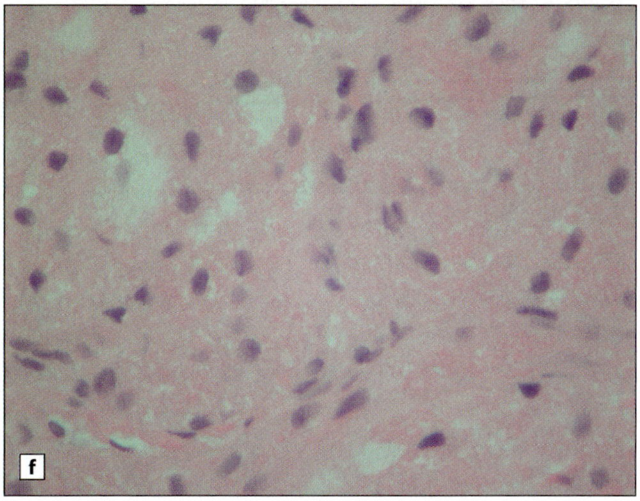

FIGURE 15.10 Granular cell tumor. **(a,b)** Routine mammogram in a 43-year-old woman revealed a spiculated density seen here in spot compression views. **(c)** Sonogram shows an 8 mm ill-defined, hypoechoic nodule with spiculated borders. **(d)** The classical appearance of granular cell tumor is evident on this core biopsy, composed of infiltrative nests and bundles of cells which have huge amounts of granular eosinophilic cytoplasm **(e)** and essentially no nuclear atypia **(f)**.

cases on core biopsy should be confirmed immunohistochemically by performing cytokeratin stains as well as S-100 protein. Granular cell tumors are characteristically positive for S-100 protein[15,16] and negative for cytokeratin, whereas the reverse is true for most carcinomas, although some invasive breast carcinomas can express S-100. Clearly this distinction must be made, since it will determine whether or not axillary sampling/dissection will be performed. Malignancy is exceptionally rare,[17] although the lesion's unpredictability in other primary sites has led most authors to agree that granular cell tumors of the breast probably deserve excision.

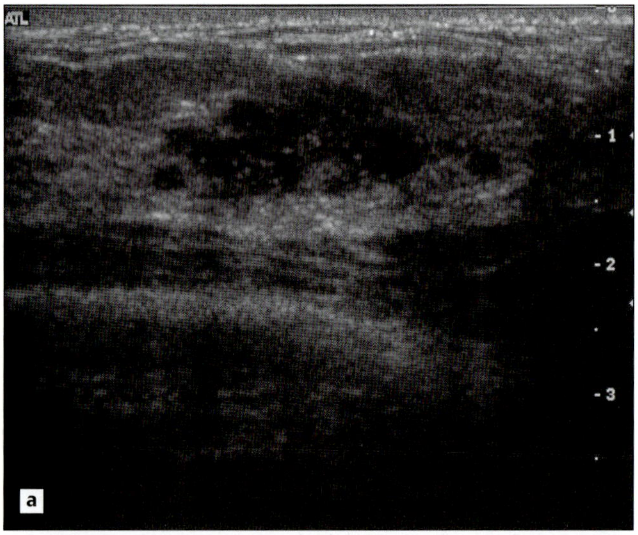

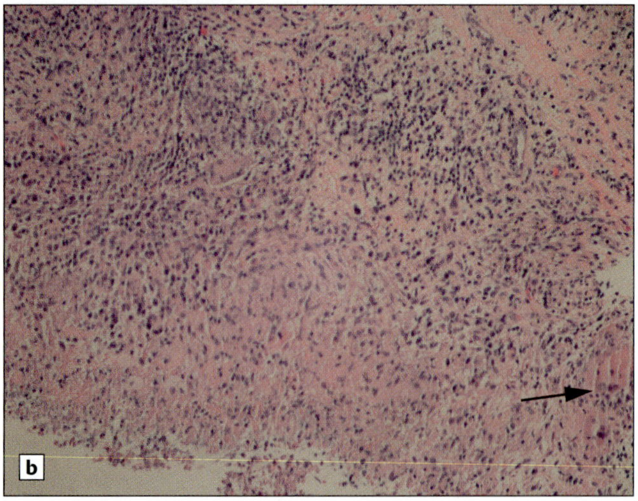

FIGURE 15.11 Granulomatous mastitis. Sonography of a palpable mass in a 22-year-old woman **(a)** reveals a hypoechoic mass with mixed echogenic structures in the subcutaneous area. The margins are microlobulated. **(b)** Core biopsy shows chronic inflammation with aggregates of histiocytes and occasional multinucleated giant cells (arrow). The lower portion of the photo shows focal necrosis, an unusual feature in idiopathic granulomatous mastitis.

GRANULOMATOUS MASTITIS

Granulomatous mastitis (Fig. 15.11), as the name implies, is composed of a mixed chronic inflammatory infiltrate that focally shows clusters of histiocytes and multinucleated giant cells (granulomata). Such lesions only rarely show necrosis,[18] in contrast to mammary tuberculosis, an extremely rare manifestation of systemic tuberculosis. The main differential diagnosis is sarcoidosis (see below). In the absence of these two disease entities, the default diagnosis is idiopathic granulomatous mastitis, as the etiology is unknown.[19] Imaging findings are nonspecific but usually consist of asymmetric radiodensity.[20]

METASTATIC CARCINOMA

Although the situation is exceedingly uncommon, the breast can be a site for metastasis of malignancies arising elsewhere (Fig. 15.12). Melanoma and carcinoma of the lung are the most frequently reported primaries[21] after lymphoma; however, other organs have also been reported. Regardless of the site of origin, metastases to the breast may be suspected radiologically when there are multiple, well circumscribed radiodensities, solid on ultrasound, in a patient with an appropriate clinical

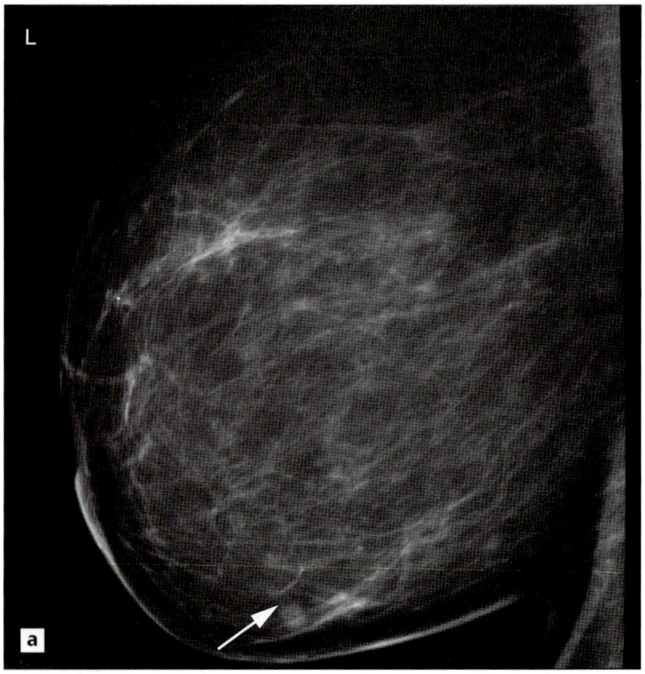

FIGURE 15.12 Metastatic carcinoma (of thyroid). Routine screening mammography was performed in this 65-year-old woman with a history of metastatic follicular thyroid carcinoma to the lung as well as right breast lumpectomy and radiation. **(a)** A 90° lateral-medial mammogram of the left breast and

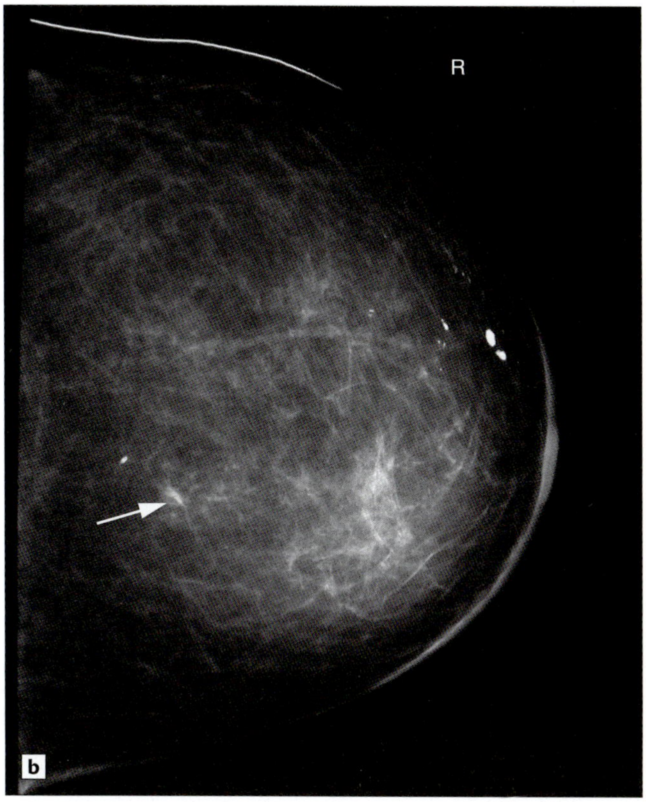

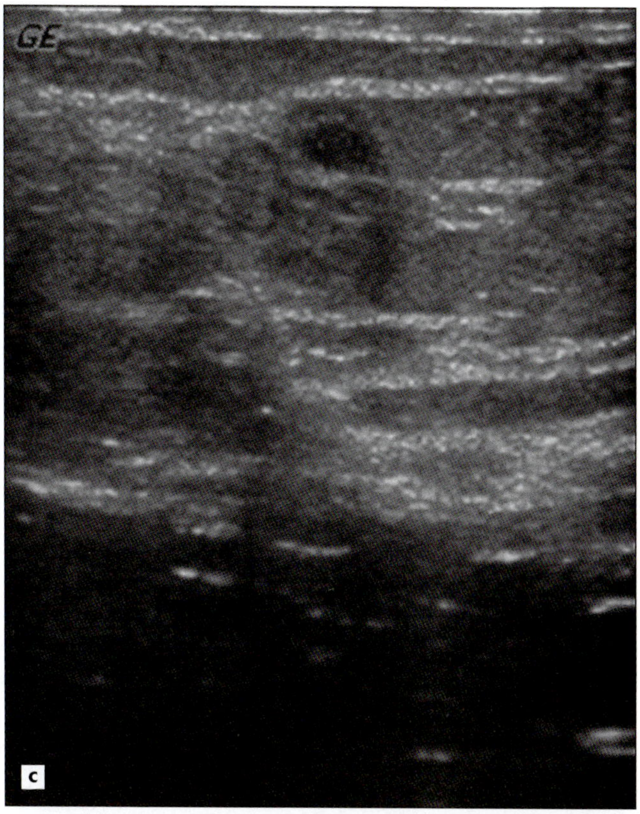

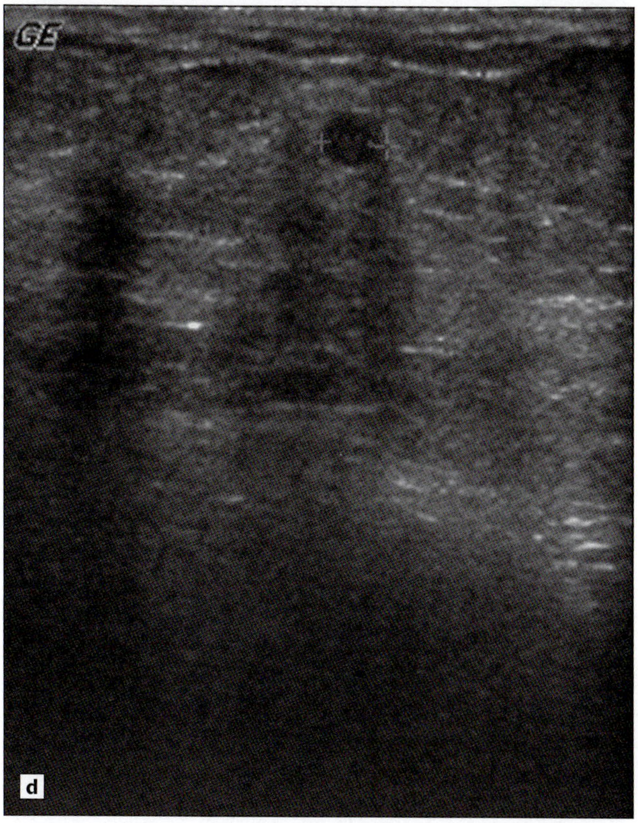

FIGURE 15.12—cont'd (b) CC view of the right breast both show small oval and round densities (arrows), respectively. Directed sonography of both breasts reveals **(c)** a 0.8 cm oval hypoechoic mass on the left and **(d)** a 0.5 cm round hypoechoic mass on the right.

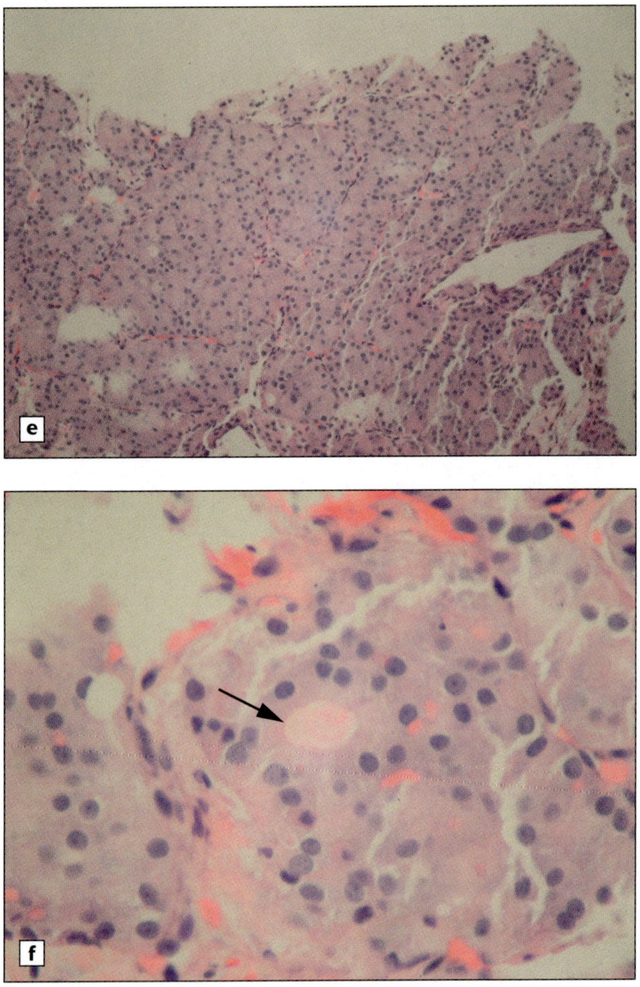

FIGURE 15.12—cont'd **(e)** Core biopsies reveal a proliferation of uniform epithelial cells arranged in rosette-like patterns without true gland formation. **(f)** Rarely the cells form follicles surrounding colloid (arrow), suggestive of thyroid tissue. Without the history, the diagnosis would not have been immediately apparent; however, the likely alternative diagnosis of infiltrating well differentiated duct carcinoma would have been discordant with a well-circumscribed mass and would have raised a red flag for additional workup.

history. Communication of this history to the pathologist is crucial to avoid the reflexive diagnosis of invasive mammary duct carcinoma.

MUCOCELE-LIKE LESION WITH CALCIFICATIONS

The incidence of mucocele-like lesions of the breast (Fig. 15.13) is approximately 2%.[22] The lesion can correspond to a well-circumscribed lobulated mass or an asymmetric density; however, in the current mammographic era, it usually presents as calcifications that have been variably described as clustered, pleomorphic, coarse, indeterminate to suspicious, or even occasionally linear.[23] Histologically, mucocele-like lesion is characterized by cystically

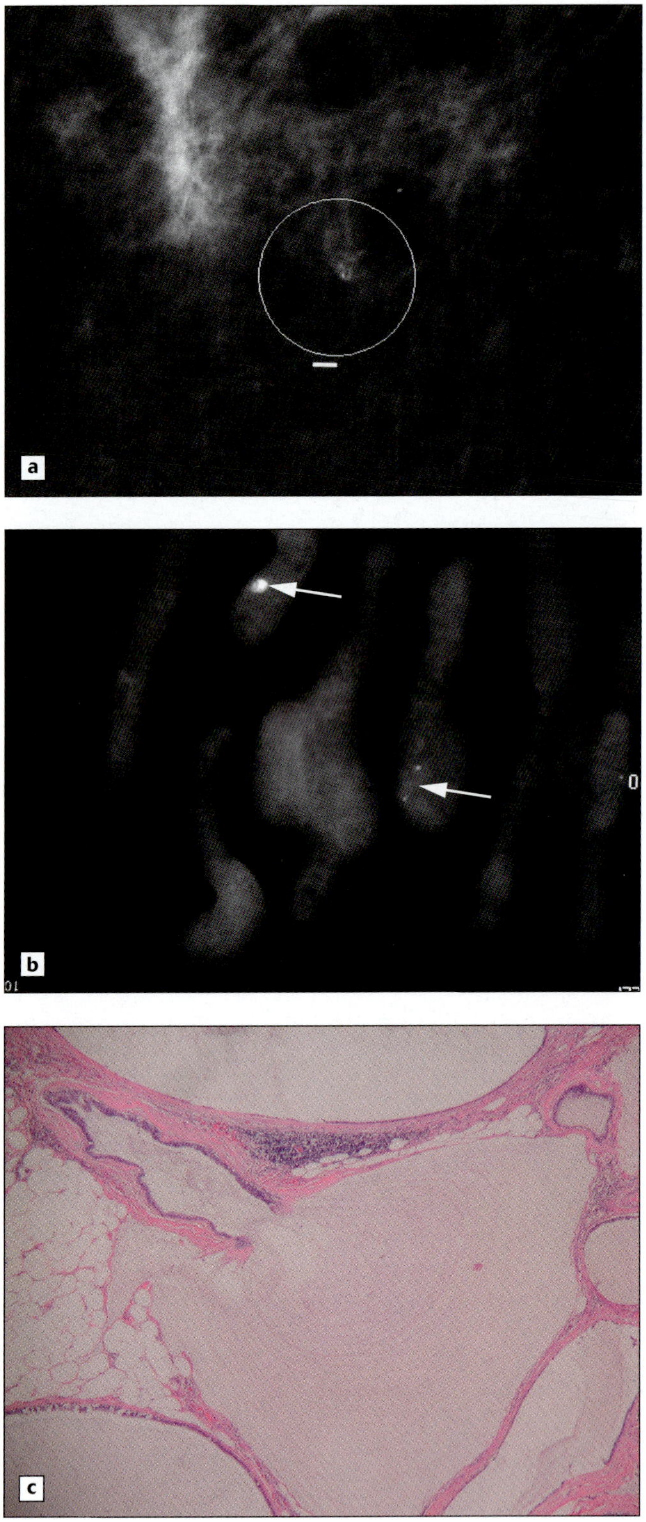

FIGURE 15.13 Mucocele-like lesion. **(a)** Routine mammography in a 57-year-old woman shows a well-circumscribed lobulated mass with associated coarse calcifications. **(b)** Specimen radiograph showing several high density clustered calcifications (arrows). **(c)** Core biopsy reveals the typical appearance of mucocele-like lesion characterized by a ruptured cyst or duct with a flat benign appearing lining and mucin that dissects into the fibrous stroma.

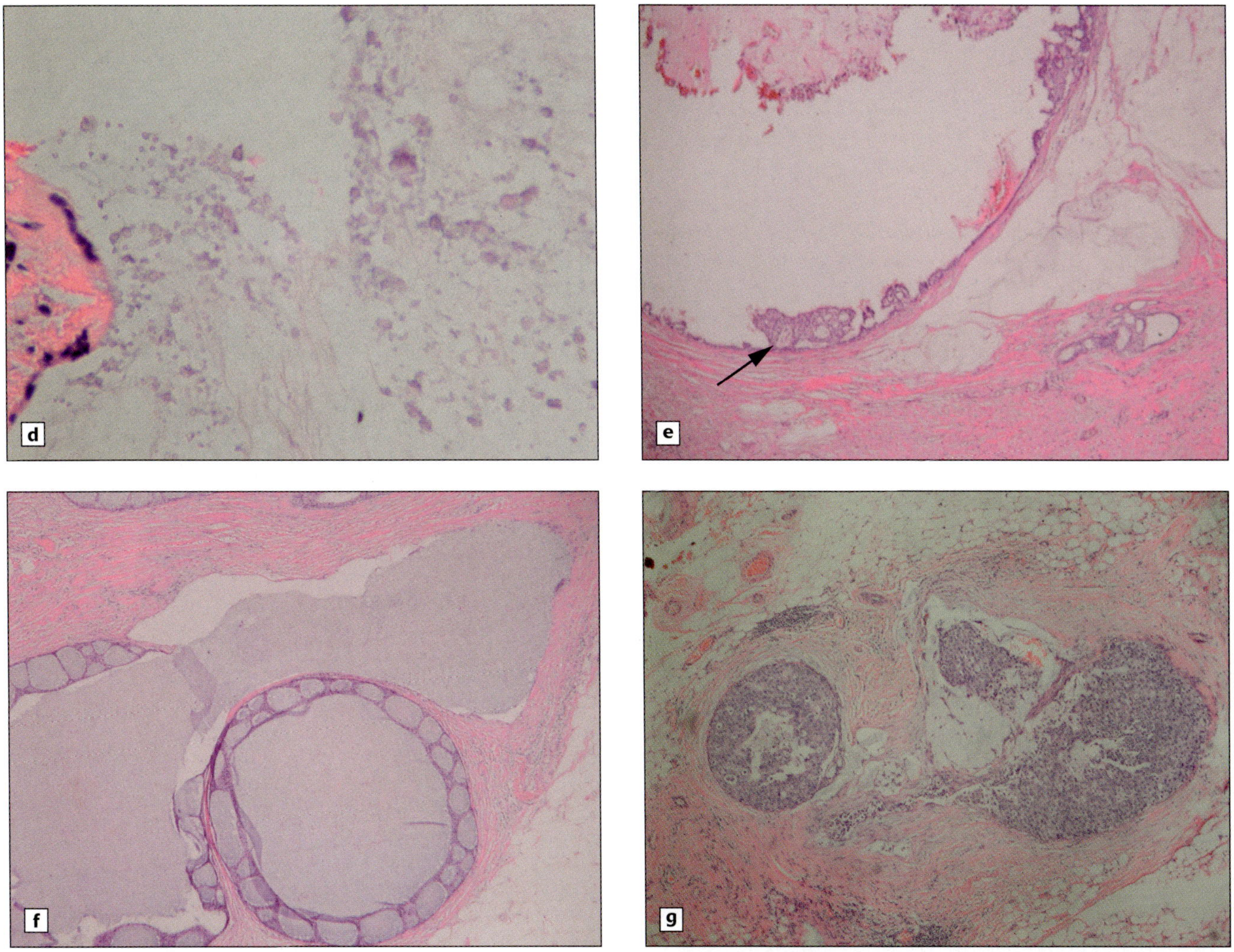

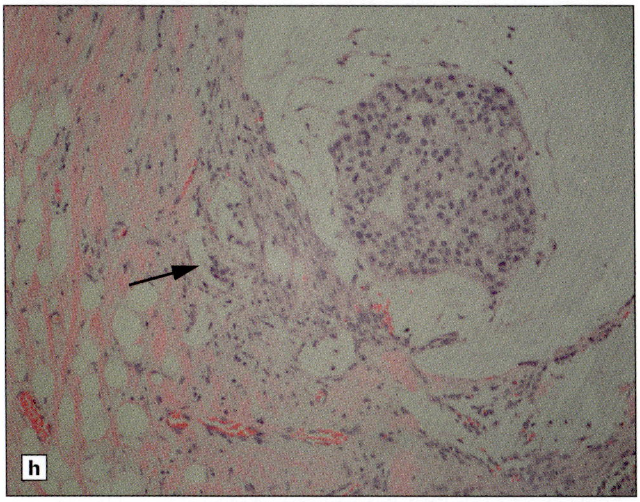

FIGURE 15.13—cont'd (d) Other areas show calcifications associated within the mucin. **(e)** Mucoceles warrant surgical excision because of their frequent association with atypical duct hyperplasia (arrow) and/or low grade cribriform intraductal carcinoma **(f).** Occasional cases will present great difficulty in differentiating mucocele from colloid carcinoma; **(g)** this field clearly demonstrates mucin-producing intraductal carcinoma in two duct spaces which have focally ruptured. The difficult question is whether the carcinoma cells in the center of the mucin represent intraductal carcinoma extruded with the mucin or true invasive (colloid) carcinoma. In such a case we would favor the former but carefully examine numerous levels and other areas **(h)** to search for clusters of tumor cells (arrow) which have lost their intraductal carcinoma growth pattern and appear to invade beyond the confines of the mucocele.

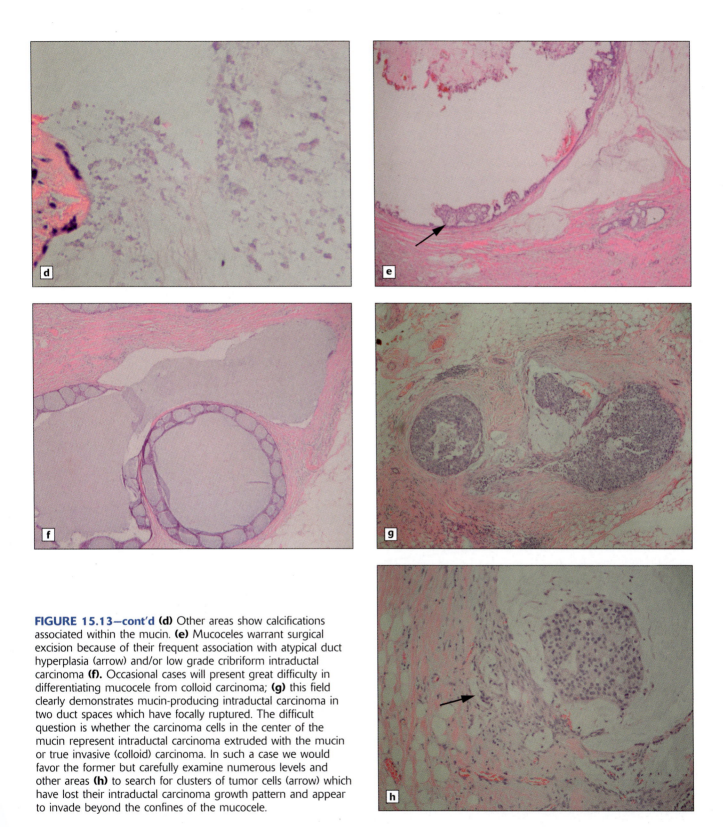

dilated mucin-producing ducts which rupture and discharge their contents into the adjacent stroma.[24] The calcifications are usually localized within the mucin. Detached epithelial cells may rarely be found floating within the mucinous substance but usually line the periphery of the cyst or duct; the cells range from being flat and benign appearing to hyperplastic, to atypical and/or frankly malignant.[25] In the largest review of mucocele-like lesions, more than half the cases were associated with either in situ or invasive malignancy.[24] It has been proposed that a continuous histologic spectrum exists, ranging from a benign mucocele-like lesion, to one with atypical duct hyperplasia, DCIS, and culminating with colloid carcinoma.[26] Support for the existence of a histologic spectrum emanates from the fact that atypical mucocele-like lesions occur a decade earlier than mucinous carcinoma. Additionally, patients with mucinous carcinoma usually have increased mucin production in surrounding normal and hyperplastic breast, suggesting a field effect of altered mucin production in the breast. Thus, earlier mammographic detection and excision may prevent progression to malignancy. While correct diagnosis within this spectrum of lesions may be difficult on excision specimens, the challenge is even greater on core biopsies. Sampling error may account for an underestimation of malignancy especially because of intralesional heterogeneity. Therefore, most authors, ourselves included, recommend excision of mucocele-like lesions even in the absence of atypia or frank malignancy.[27–29]

MYOFIBROBLASTOMA

Typically, myofibroblastoma (Fig. 15.14) is a well-circumscribed solid mass that is somewhat more frequently encountered in men,[30] sonographically heterogeneous and hyperechoic.[9] It can be a difficult diagnosis, especially on core biopsy, but particularly in rare cases in which benign glands are admixed. The usual case is composed purely of stroma with aggregations of benign spindle cells interspersed amongst dense, keloid-like accumulations of collagen. The spindle cells have a peculiar grayish cytoplasm and can occasionally appear epithelioid, greatly complicating the diagnosis. The main hindrance to making the diagnosis is the rarity of the lesion; therefore, it will not be foremost on the pathologist's mind, particularly with the limited sampling afforded by core biopsy.

NIPPLE GRANULOMATOUS ABSCESS SECONDARY TO PIERCING

The popularity of piercing the nipple for placement of rings has been associated with acute inflammation and abscesses, often granulomatous (Fig. 15.15). Cultures of

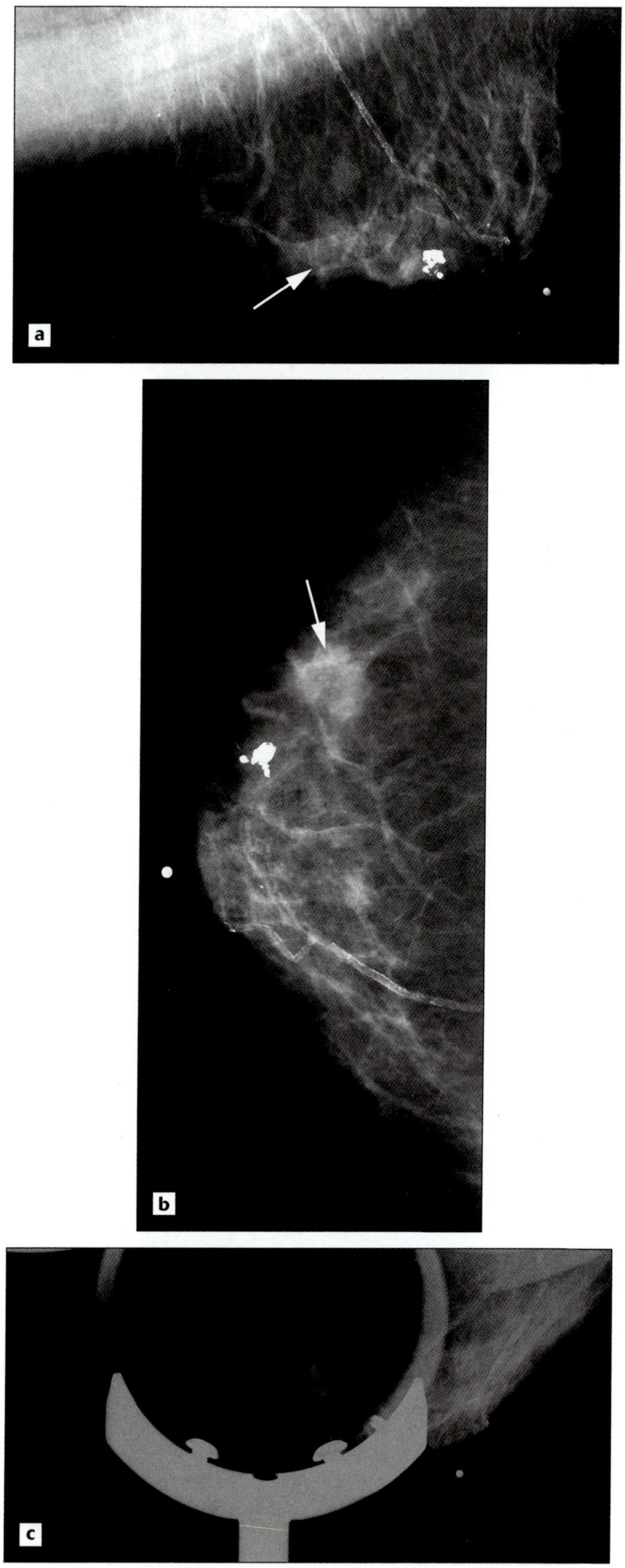

FIGURE 15.14 Myofibroblastoma. Mammography in an 84-year-old woman: Right MLO **(a)** and CC **(b)** views demonstrate an irregular mass (arrows) in the right upper outer quadrant which does not dissipate on cone compression **(c).** There are no associated calcifications.

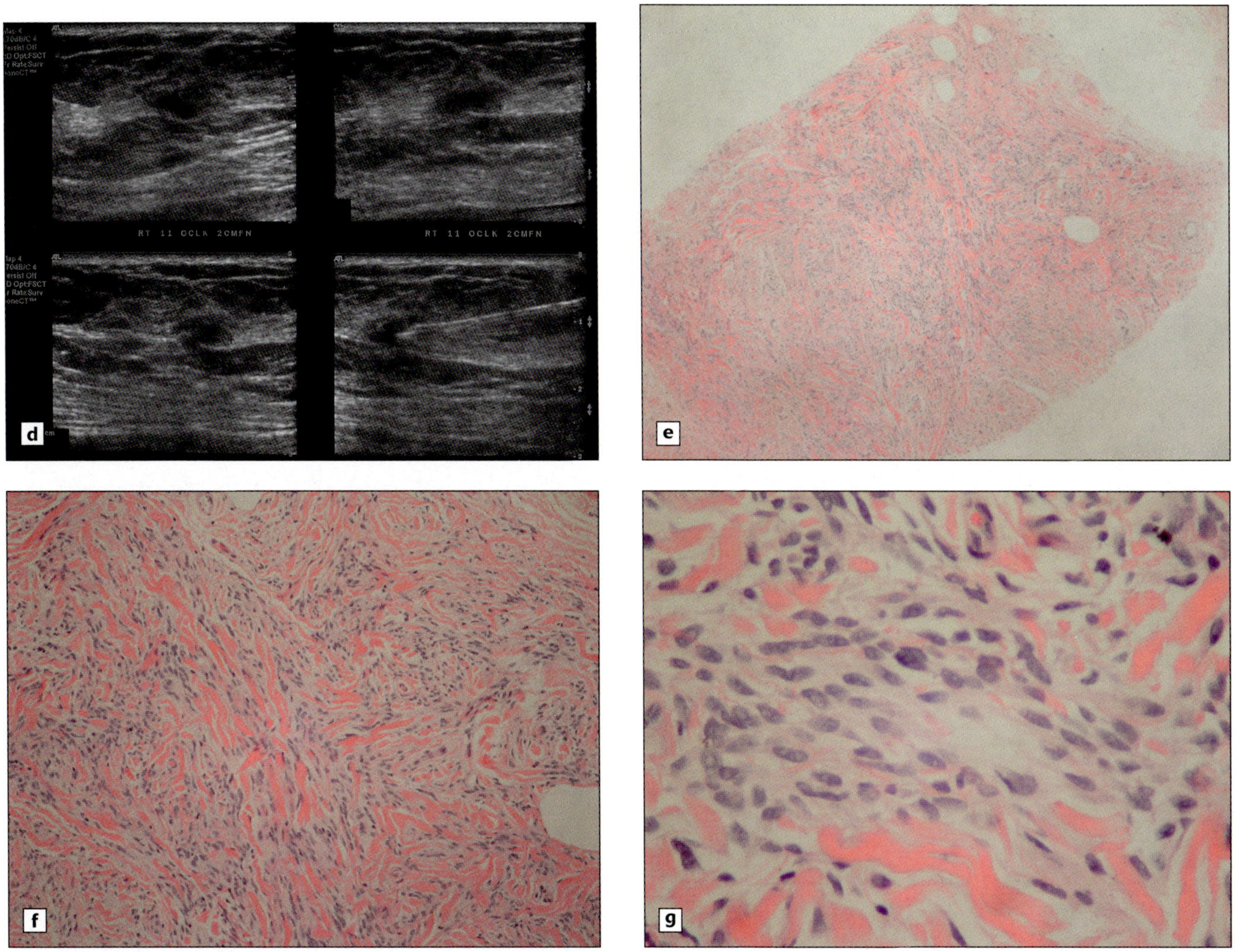

FIGURE 15.14—cont'd (d) Sonography shows a hypoechoic, lobulated but well-defined solid mass adjacent to the pectoralis muscle. There is no through transmission or posterior shadowing. **(e)** Core biopsy shows a plump spindle cell proliferation in groups and bundles adjacent to thick keloid-like collagen bundles. Note the sharply circumscribed border. **(f,g)** The spindle cells have a characteristic gray-pink cytoplasm, have bland, uniform nuclei, and lack mitotic activity.

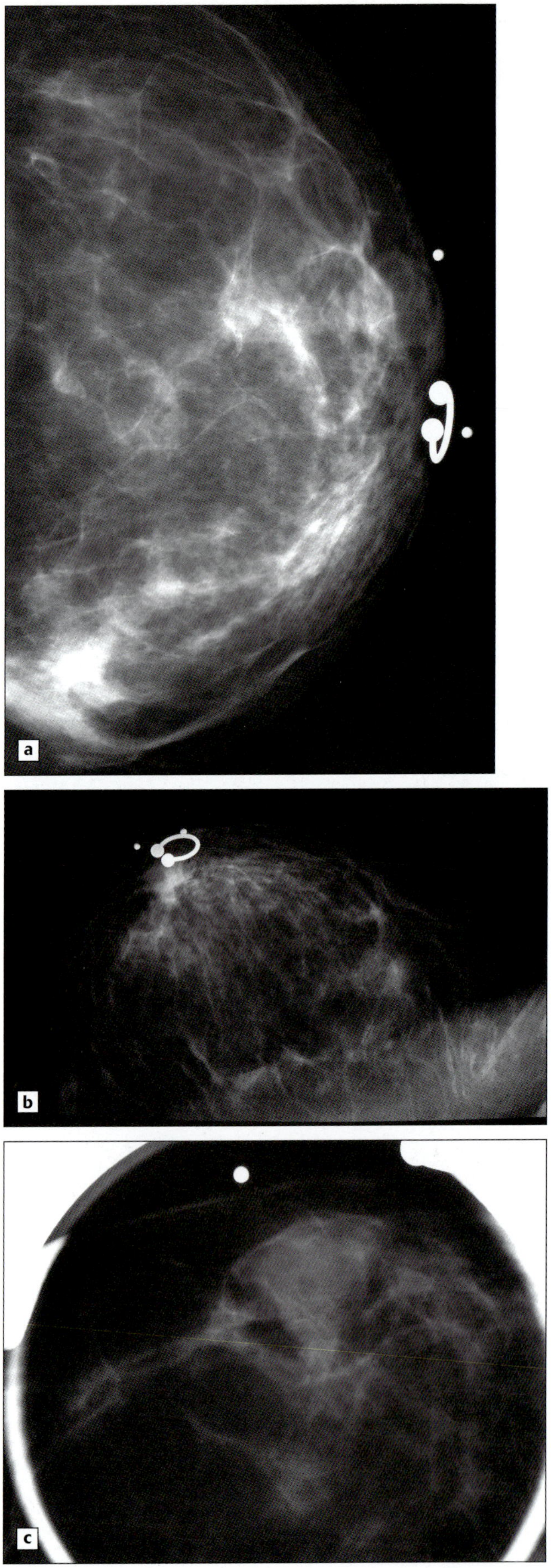

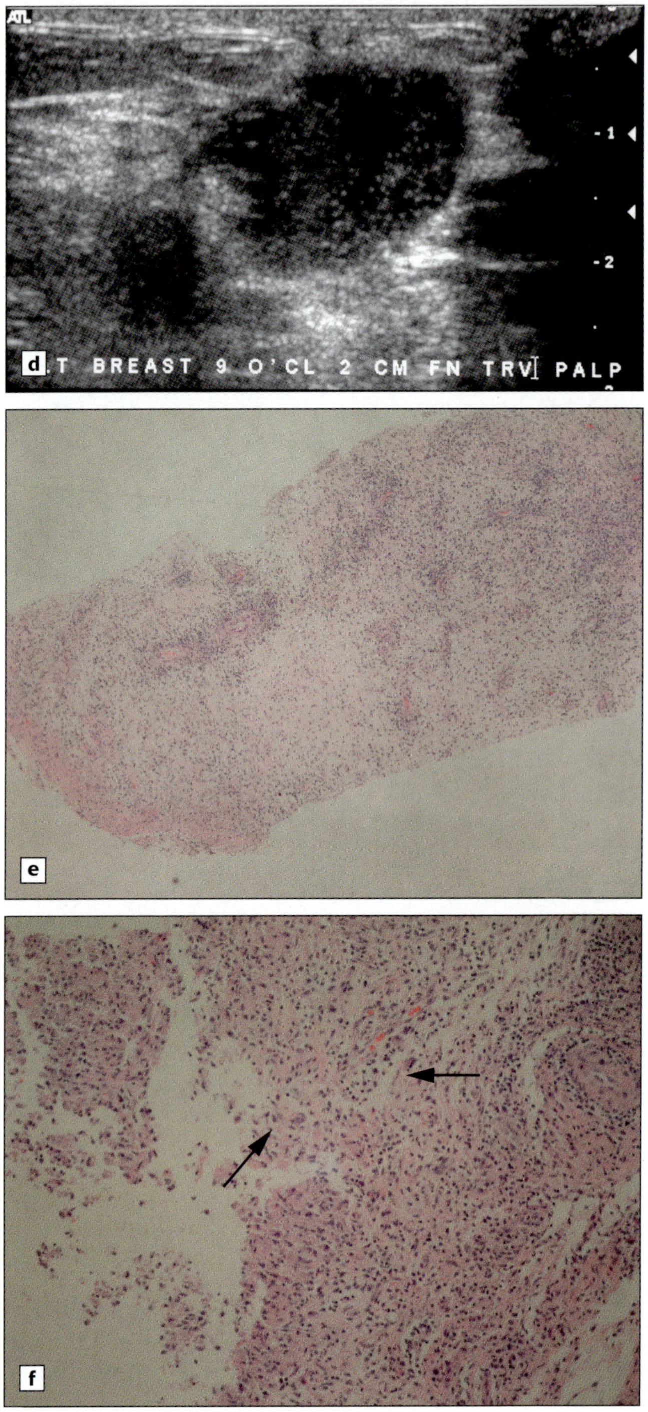

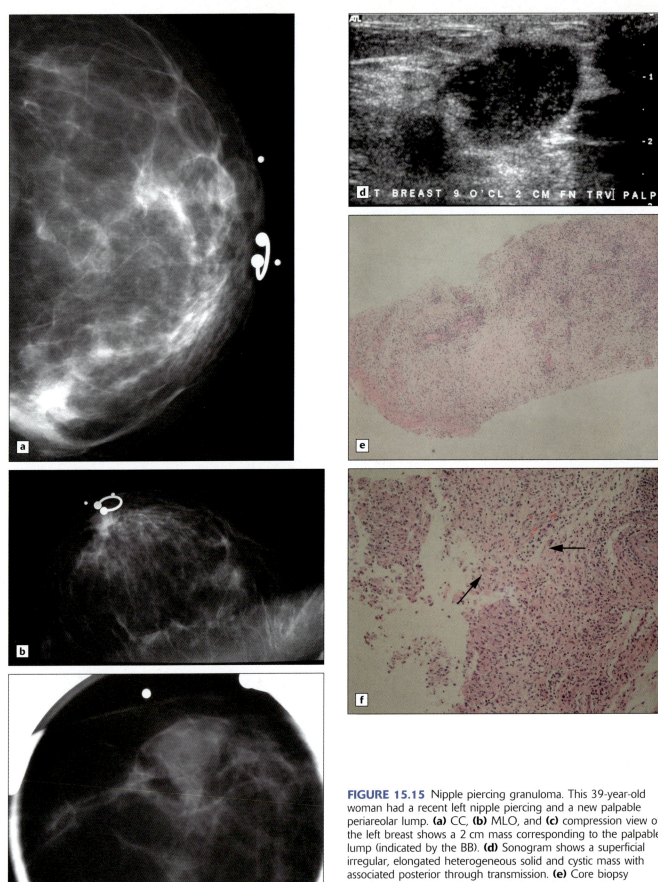

FIGURE 15.15 Nipple piercing granuloma. This 39-year-old woman had a recent left nipple piercing and a new palpable periareolar lump. **(a)** CC, **(b)** MLO, and **(c)** compression view of the left breast shows a 2 cm mass corresponding to the palpable lump (indicated by the BB). **(d)** Sonogram shows a superficial irregular, elongated heterogeneous solid and cystic mass with associated posterior through transmission. **(e)** Core biopsy is composed entirely of acute and chronic inflammation with **(f)** poorly formed granulomata (arrows). Mycobacterial culture grew *M. fortuitum*.

these lesions have grown atypical mycobacteria,[31] most frequently *Mycobacterium fortuitum*.[32] These lesions can appear sonographically as irregular, heterogeneous, and suspicious for malignancy. Treatment consists of surgery followed by antimicrobials.

OSTEOSARCOMA OF CHEST WALL

The increasing use of irradiation in the context of breast conservation as local therapy for breast carcinoma is associated with a low but real risk of sarcoma. While angiosarcoma (see above) is the most commonly reported tumor in this scenario, typically arising in the skin and secondarily involving the breast, we and others (33) have seen cases of osteosarcoma of the chest wall in a few such patients, the case illustrated herein being one we previously reported[34] (Fig. 15.16). Core biopsy of such lesions is extremely challenging since there can be extensive intratumoral heterogeneity with the correct diagnosis resting on the identification of osteoid production by malignant cells.

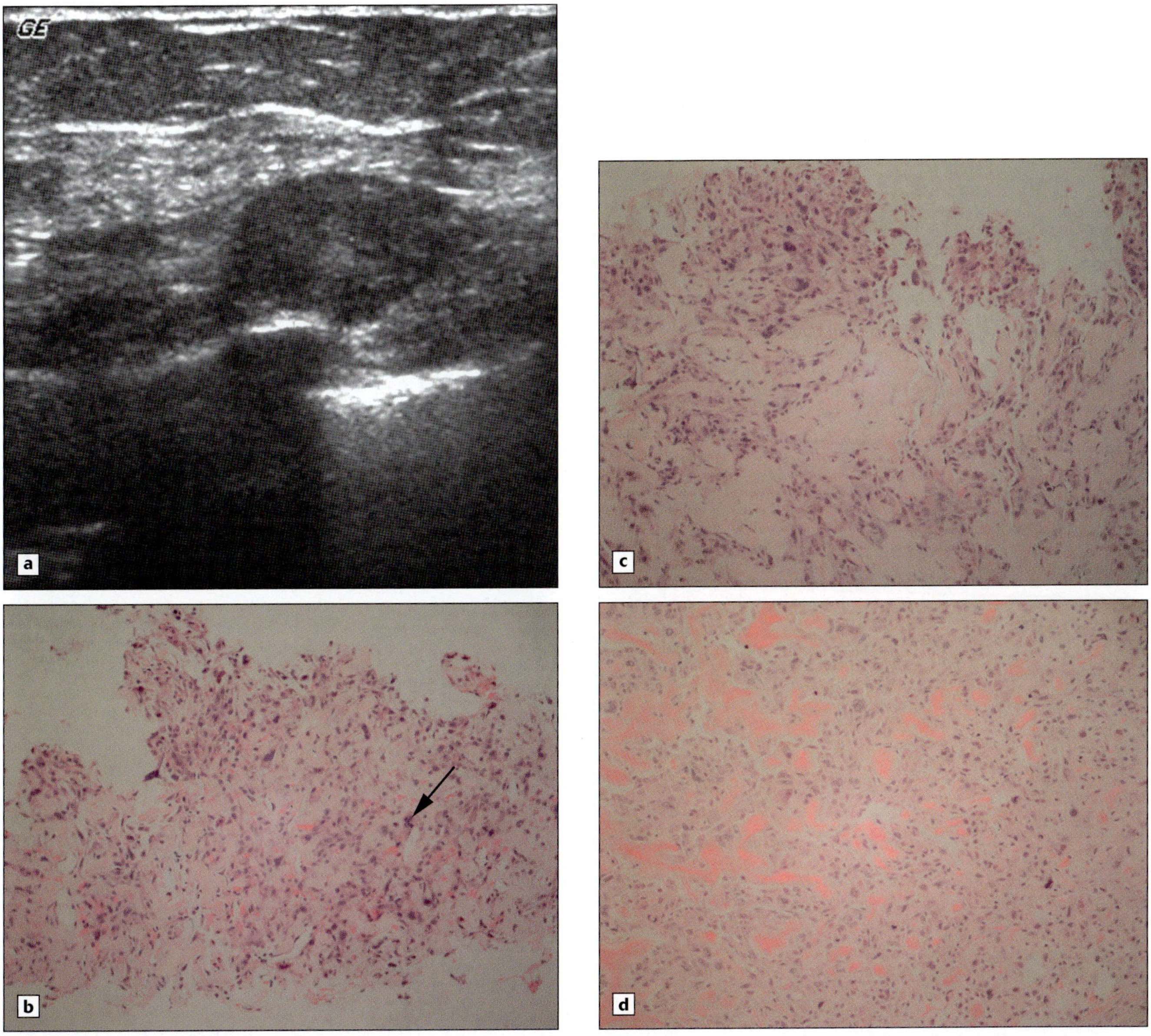

FIGURE 15.16 Osteosarcoma of chest wall. **(a)** Sonography in a 52-year-old patient who was three years post lumpectomy and radiation therapy for intraductal carcinoma shows a 1.7 cm × 1.0 cm ovoid hypoechoic solid nodule with a mildly echogenic central area and mild irregularity posteriorly. **(b)** Core biopsy reveals a population of malignant cells with an atypical mitosis (arrow) and eosinophilic stroma. The pattern of the proliferation in some areas resembled angiosarcoma but in other areas **(c)** the collagen deposition was reminiscent of osteoid. Immunohistochemical stains were negative for epithelial and vascular markers. Surgical excision **(d)** revealed osteosarcoma.

SARCOIDOSIS

When faced with a core biopsy showing well formed non-necrotizing granulomata, the pathologist should consider both sarcoidosis (Fig. 15.17) and idiopathic granulomatous mastitis (see above). While patients with such lesions in the breast will typically upon questioning relate a history of sarcoidosis, we have on occasion encountered sarcoidosis in the breast as the initial presenting lesion of the systemic disease. The radiologic characteristics are variable and can be either irregular masses or round, well-defined nodules, suggesting intramammary lymph node involvement.[35]

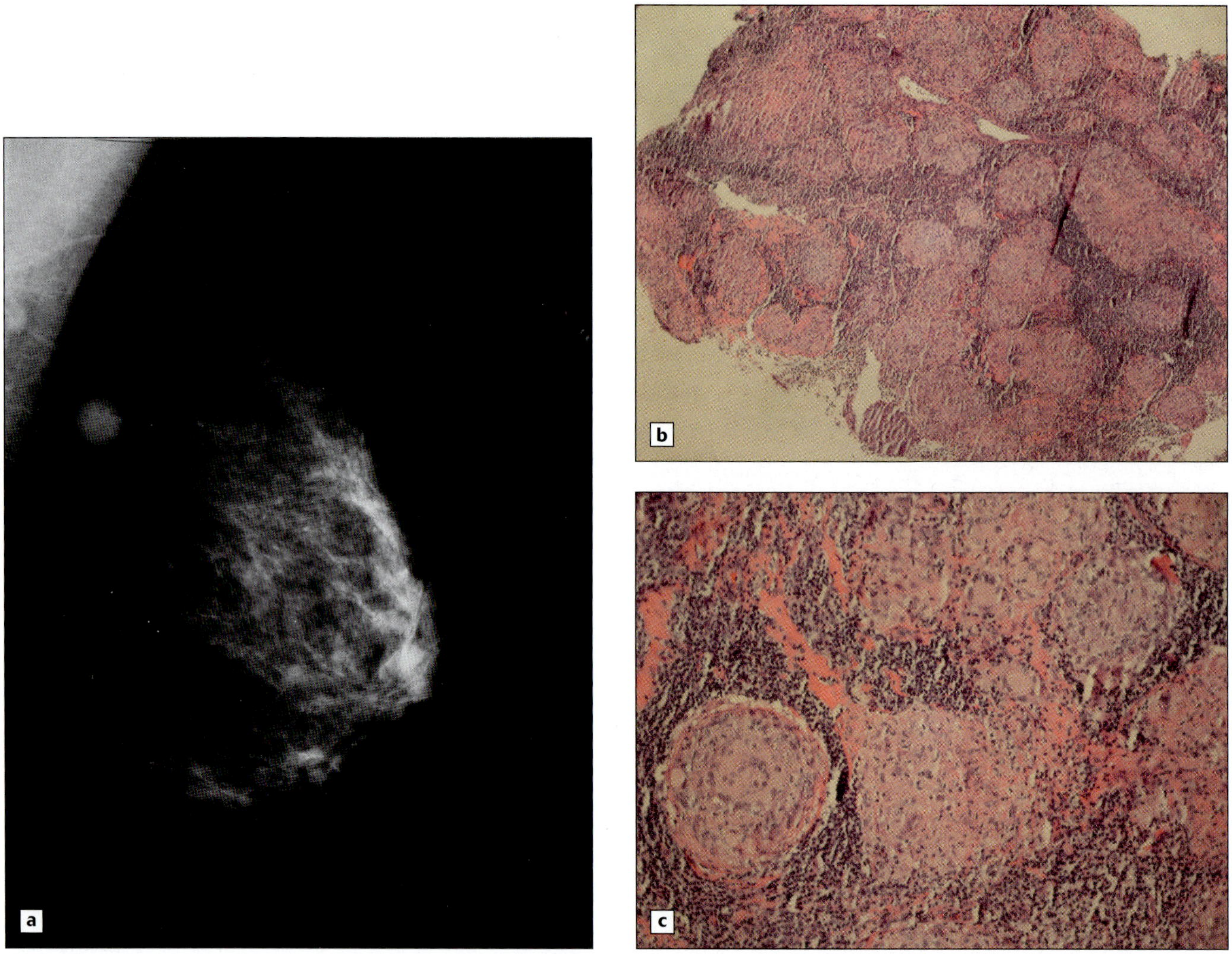

FIGURE 15.17 Sarcoidosis. **(a)** A new 1.5 cm circumscribed, round, sharply marginated mass is present in the upper outer right breast of a 47-year-old woman. **(b)** Core biopsy shows a solid proliferation of well-formed granulomata and chronic inflammation. **(c)** At higher power the granulomata contain multinucleated giant cells and are typical of sarcoidosis. It is likely that this case represents replacement of an intramammary lymph node by sarcoidosis.

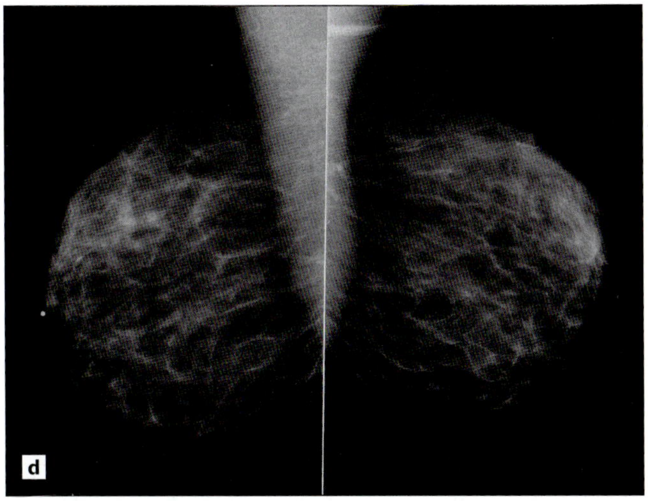

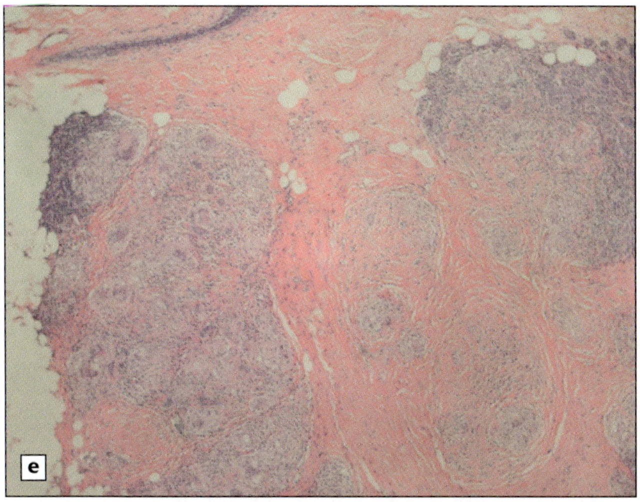

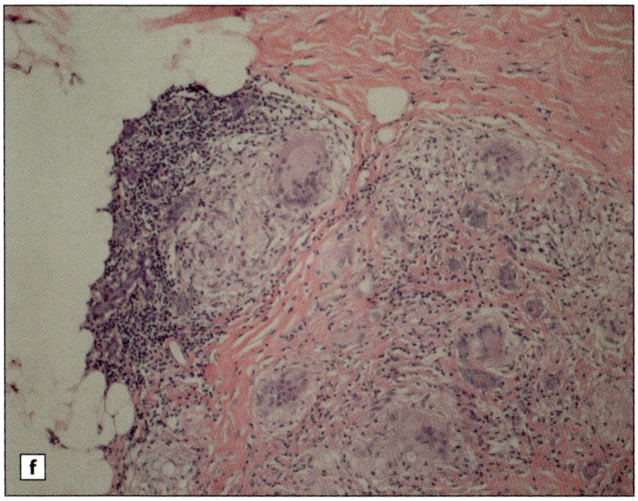

FIGURE 15.17—cont'd (d) Comparison of bilateral MLO views in a second patient shows increased heterogeneous asymmetric density in the upper part of the left breast. **(e)** Core biopsy in this case shows similarly well-formed granuloma in fibrous tissue and in surrounding normal breast parenchyma, best seen at higher power **(f)**.

SILICONE GRANULOMA

Silicone gel-containing breast implants are known to leak small amounts and can on occasion rupture, causing an intense inflammatory reaction largely composed of histiocytes (Fig. 15.18). In the past and largely in foreign countries, silicone was also injected directly into the breast for augmentation purposes. Regardless of its mode of entry into mammary parenchyma, silicone gel can be seen histologically as a colorless material that is refractile but does not polarize.[36] It is found either loose in stroma or in within deceptive histiocytes which appear to filled with fat, but actually have ingested the silicone. Echogenicity within hypoechoic masses has been a reported sonographic finding.[37,38]

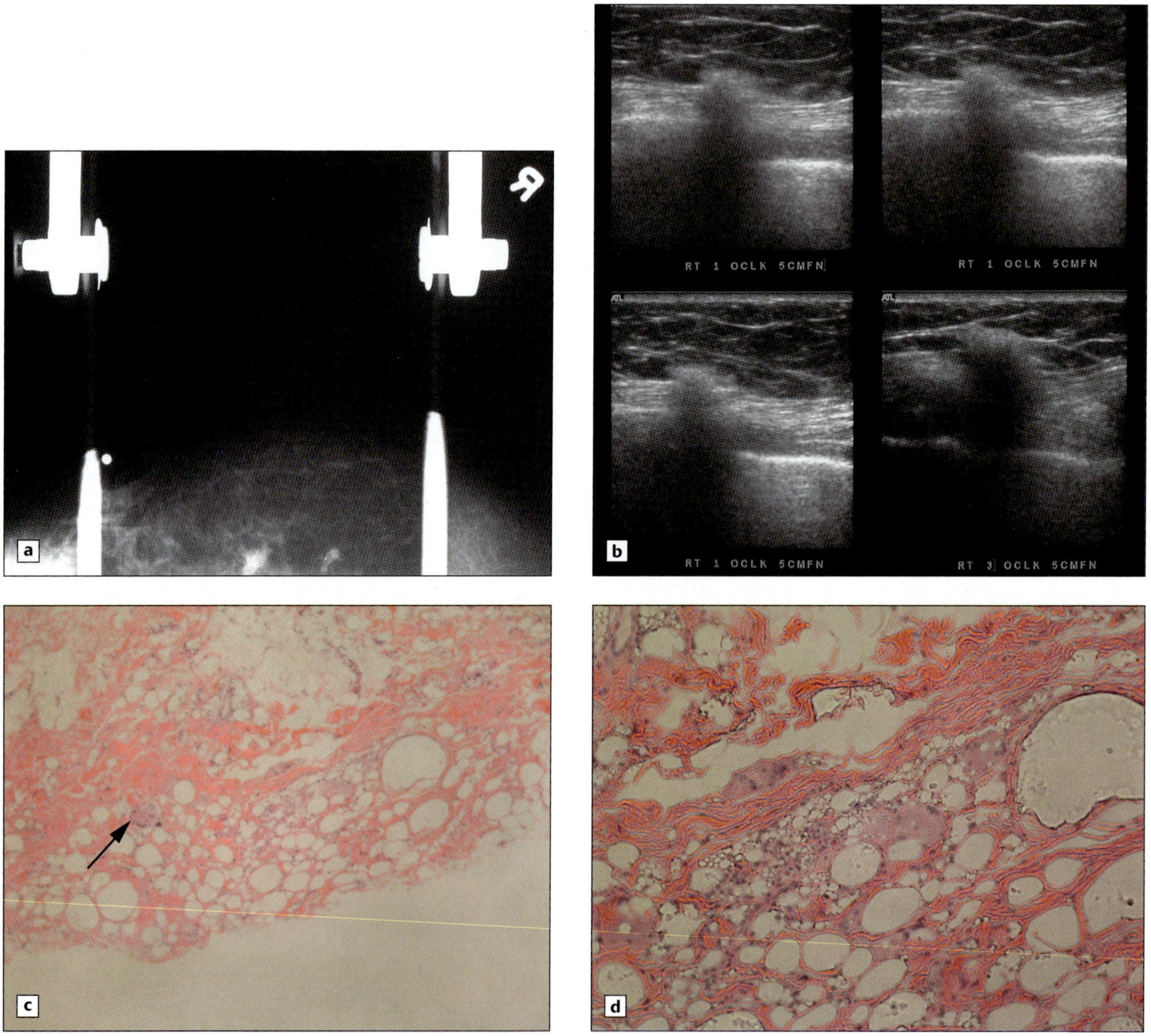

FIGURE 15.18 Silicone granuloma. This 56-year-old patient who was four years status/post removal of ruptured silicone implants presented with a) a dense, irregular mass in the right medial breast. **(b)** On sonography, adjacent to the pectoralis muscle there is a hypoechoic shadowing mass with an echogenic rim. **(c)** Core biopsy shows apparent fat necrosis (top) with foreign body giant cells (arrow) but an unusual microvesicular pattern (bottom) due to the presence of refractile **(d)** nonpolarizeable material, typical of silicone.

REFERENCES

1. Page DL. Adenoid cystic carcinoma of breast, a special histopathologic type with excellent prognosis. Breast Cancer Res Treat 93:189–190,2005.
2. McClenathan JH, De la Roza G. Adenoid cystic breast cancer. Am J Surg 183:646–649,2002.
3. Shin SJ, Rosen PP. Solid variant of mammary adenoid cystic carcinoma with basaloid features: a study of 9 cases. Am J Surg Pathol 26:413–420, 2002.
4. McLaren BK, Smith J, Schuyler PA, et al. Adenomyoepithelioma: clinical, histologic, and immunohistologic evaluation of a series of related lesions. Am J Surg Pathol 29:1294–1299,2005.
5. Zhang C, Quddus MR, Sung CJ. Atypical adenomyoepithelioma of the breast: diagnostic problems and practical approaches in core needle biopsy. Breast J 10:154–155,2004.
6. Darling ML, Bagbagbemi TO, Smith DN, et al. Mammographic and sonographic features of angiolipoma of the breast. Breast J 6:166–170, 2000.
7. Mintz AD, Mengoni P. Angiolipoma of the breast: sonographic appearance of two cases. J Ultrasound Med 17:67–69,1998.
8. Vorburger SA, Xing Y, Hunt KK, et al. Angiosarcoma of the breast. Cancer 104:2682–2688,2005.
9. Porter GJ, Evans AJ, Lee AH, et al. Unusual benign breast lesions. Clin Radiol 61:562–569,2006.
10. Goel NB, Knight TE, Pandey S, et al. Fibrous lesions of the breast: imaging-pathologic correlation. Radiographics 25:1547–1559,2005.
11. Feder JM, de Paredes ES, Hogge JP, Wilken JJ. Unusual breast lesions: Radiologic-pathologic correlation. Radiographics 19:S11–S26,1999.
12. Rosen PP, Ernsberger D. Mammary fibromatosis. A benign spindle-cell tumor with significant risk for local recurrence. Cancer 63:1363–1369,1989.
13. Mesurolle B, Ariche-Cohen M, Mignon F, et al. Unusual mammographic and ultrasonographic findings in fibromatosis of the breast. Eur Radiol 11:2241–2243,2001.
14. Sawhney S, Petkovska L, Ramadan S, et al. Sonographic appearances of galactoceles. J Clin Ultrasound 30:18–22,2002.
15. Adeniran A, Al-Ahmadie H, Mahoney MC, Robinson-Smith TM. Granular cell tumor of the breast: a series of 17 cases and review of the literature. Breast J 6:528–531,2004.
16. Damiani S, Koerner FC, Dickersin GR, Eusebi V. Granular cell tumor of the breast. Virchows Arch A Pathol Anat Histopathol 420:219–226,1992.
17. Chetty R, Kalan MR. Malignant granular cell tumor of the breast. J Surg Oncol 49:135–137,1992.
18. Tse GM, Poon CS, Ramachandram K, et al. Granulomatous mastitis: a clinicopathological review of 26 cases. Pathology 36:254–257,2004.
19. Verfaillie G, Breucq C, Sacre R, et al. Granulomatous lobular mastitis: a rare chronic inflammatory disease of the breast which can mimic breast carcinoma. Acta Chir Belg 106:222–224,2006.
20. Memis A, Bilgen I, Ustun EE, et al. Granulomatous mastitis: imaging findings with histopathologic correlation. Clin Radiol 57:1001–1006,2002.
21. Georgiannos SN, ChinAleong J, Goode AW, Sheaff M. Secondary neoplasms of the breast: A survey of the 20th century. Cancer 92:2259–2266,2001.
22. Chinyama CN, Davies JD. Mammary mucinous lesions: congeners, prevalence and important pathologic associations. Histopathology 29:533–539,1996.
23. Farshid G, Pieterse S, King JM, Robinson J. Mucocele-like lesions of the breast: a benign cause for indeterminate or suspicious mammographic microcalcifications. Breast J 11:15–22,2005.
24. Hamele-Bena D, Cranor ML, Rosen PP. Mammary mucocele-like lesions. Benign and malignant. Am J Surg Pathol 20:1081–1085,1996.
25. Fisher CJ, Millis RR. A mucocoele-like tumour of the breast associated with both atypical ductal hyperplasia and mucoid carcinoma. Histopathology 21:69–71,1992.
26. Weaver MG, Abdul-Karim FW, al-Kaisi N. Mucinous lesions of the breast: A pathological continuum. Pathol Res Pract 189:873–876,1993.
27. Jacobs TW, Connolly JL, Schnitt SJ. Nonmalignant lesions in breast core needle biopsies. To excise or not to excise? Am J Surg Pathol 26:1095–1110, 2002.
28. Carder PJ, Murphy CE, Liston JC. Surgical excision is warranted following a core biopsy diagnosis of mucocoele-like lesion of the breast. Histopathology 45:148–154,2004.
29. Ramsaroop R, Greenberg D, Tracey N, Benson-Cooper D. Mucocele-like lesions of the breast: An audit of 2 years at BreastScreen Auckland (New Zealand). Breast J 11:321–325,2005.
30. Dockery WD, Singh HR, Wilentz RE. Myofibroblastoma of the male breast: Imaging appearance and ultrasound-guided core biopsy diagnosis. Breast J 7:192–194,2001.
31. Trupiano JK, Sebek BA, Goldfarb J, et al. Mastitis due to *Mycobacterium abscessus* after body piercing. Clin Infect Dis 33:131–134,2001.
32. Lewis CG, Wells MK, Jennings WC. *Mycobacterium fortuitum* breast infection following nipple-piercing, mimicking carcinoma. Breast J 10:363–365,2004.
33. Rudman F, Stanec S, Stanec M, et al. Rare complication of breast cancer irradiation: postirradiation osteosarcoma. Ann Plast Surg 48:318–322,2002.
34. Orta L, Suprun U, Goldfarb A, et al. Radiation-associated extraskeletal osteosarcoma of the chest wall. Arch Pathol Lab Med 130:198–200,2006.
35. Sabate JM, Clotet M, Gomez A, et al. Radiologic evaluation of uncommon inflammatory and reactive breast disorders. Radiographics 25:411–424,2005.
36. Travis WD, Balogh K, Abraham JL. Silicone granulomas: report of three cases and report of the literature. Hum Pathol 16:19–27,1985.
37. Rosculet KA, Ikeda DM, Forrest ME, et al. Ruptured gel-filled silicone breast implants: sonographic findings in 19 cases. AJR 159:711–716,1992.
38. Caskey CI, Berg WA, Hamper UM, et al. Imaging spectrum of extracapsular silicone: correlation of US, MR imaging, mammographic, and histopathologic findings. Radiographics 19:S39–S51,1999.

CHAPTER

16

Complications and follow-up – after the core biopsy

Mammographic–pathologic correlation does not end after the core biopsy has been completed and a diagnosis rendered. Awareness of the original core biopsy-based diagnosis is crucial for proper pathologic handling of an excision specimen. In this vein, it is essential that core biopsies originally interpreted by an outside laboratory be reviewed prior to surgical (or other) intervention in one's own institution. Regardless of the reason for the excision, it is absolutely crucial that the pathologist identify the core biopsy site in a surgically excised specimen, i.e., lumpectomy. As is the case with core biopsies performed to evaluate calcifications, the specimen radiograph of a wire localized excision of a core biopsy site must accompany the specimen to pathology. While the clip or other marker may be evident on the specimen radiograph, it is not essential that the pathologist grossly identify it. Rather, the pathologist must identify the biopsy site histologically to confirm that the correct area has been removed, regardless of the actual diagnosis. In fact, albeit less critical, the same must be said in the context of mastectomy specimens, ensuring that a tumor (or tumors) is properly and completely evaluated pathologically. The actual histologic appearance of the biopsy site varies somewhat, depending on the nature of the marker, the material embedding the marker,[1,2] and the time interval between core and excision (Fig 16.1). The following are three examples of possible scenarios in wire-localized excision of core biopsy sites.

SUCCESSFUL WIRE LOCALIZATION OF CLIP AND BIOPSY SITE

The two examples shown in Figure 16.2 demonstrate the ideal situation in image-directed excision of core biopsy sites. The post-core biopsy clips are in obvious radiodensities adjacent to residual calcifications. The specimen radiographs also show that the localization wires have been placed accurately, immediately alongside the clips. The lesions and clips appear to be central to the lumpectomies, at least in the two-dimensional views provided by the specimen radiographs. In this scenario, the likelihood of achieving negative margins on the first surgical procedure is maximized.

UNSUCCESSFUL WIRE LOCALIZATION OF CLIP AND BIOPSY SITE

Occasionally a wire will move or become displaced in the time between placement by the radiologist and excision by the surgeon. The injection of blue dye in addition to wire placement can be helpful to the surgeon in locating the area of nonpalpable abnormality. Rarely, however, despite the best efforts on everyone's part, a specimen may be removed which shows neither the target lesion nor the biopsy site. Such cases provide evidence that surgeons should designate enough margins in an excisional breast biopsy to allow orientation in six planes by the pathologist. Such situations demand the pathologist examine all the tissue carefully for evidence of prior manipulation, largely fat necrosis, particularly at margins (Fig 16.3). Knowing the specific margin involved allows the surgeon to direct his search for the lesion by first excising that particular margin.

CLIP MIGRATION

Occasionally the clip or other marking device will migrate from its original location to an uninvolved area of the breast (Fig 16.4). Distances up to 6.5 cm have been reported.[3,4] Such cases need careful radiologic attention and surgical planning, lest the clip be removed but the cancer left in the patient, for example. Again the pathologist's role here is in histologically identifying the biopsy site, not the site of the clip. If the original core biopsy was accurate, and the surgeon successfully removes that specific lesion, the pathologist will see granulation tissue, foreign body reaction, and organizing hematoma in or immediately adjacent to the lesion, regardless of where the clip has gone.

EPITHELIAL CELL DISPLACEMENT

An occasional reported effect of needling procedures in the breast has been the iatrogenic movement of epithelial cells, both benign and malignant, out of their normal milieu, namely the duct-lobular system, and into the

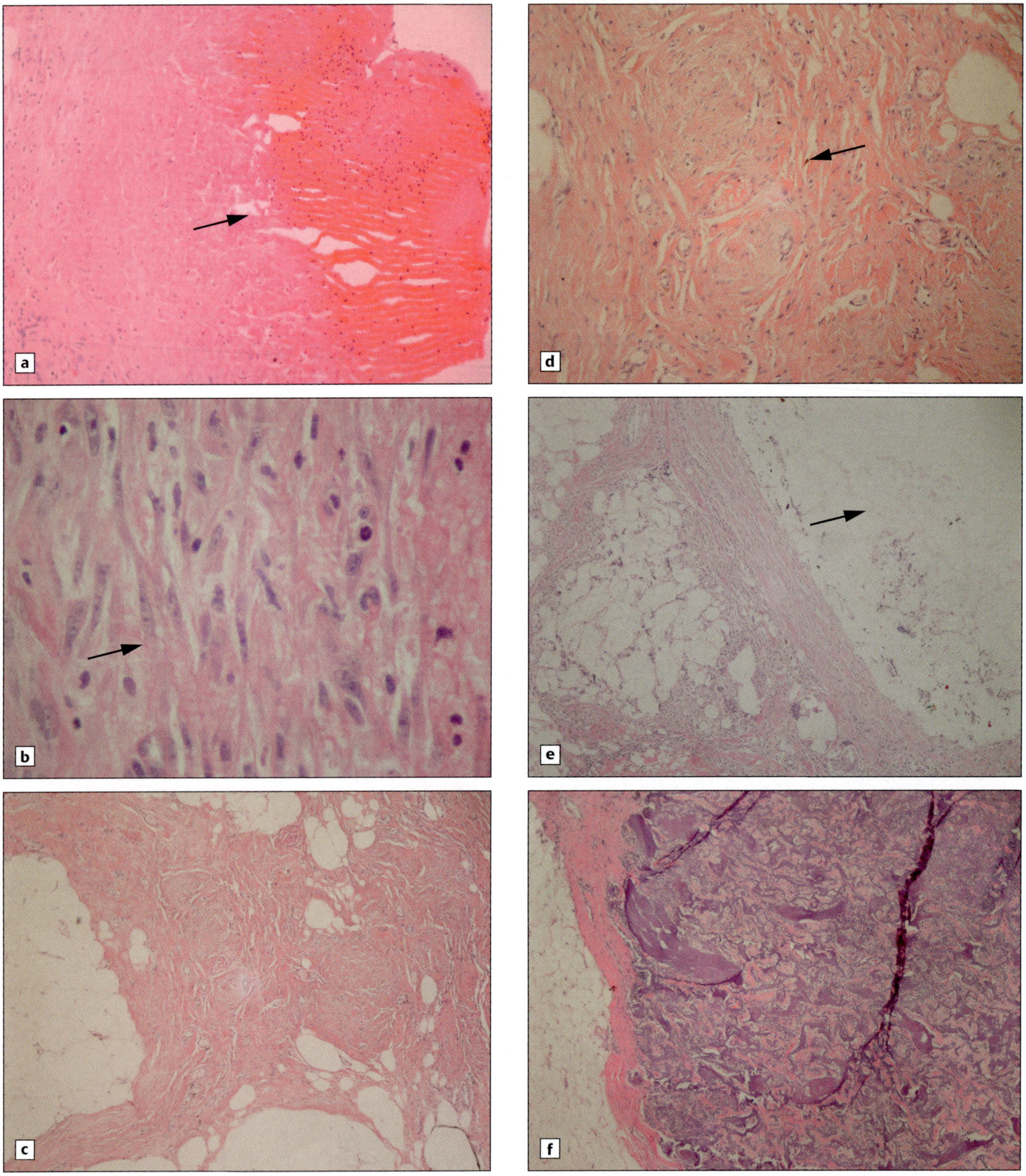

FIGURE 16.1 Histology of biopsy sites. The histologic appearance of the core biopsy site varies somewhat depending on the type of material in which the clip or marker is embedded, if any, and the time period between biopsy and excision (granulation tissue earlier, followed by scarring). **(a)** A relatively recent (about seven days) core biopsy is represented here by an organizing hematoma (arrow). Reactions such as this are more common after the larger amounts of tissue removed by mammotome biopsies; large hematomas such as this are infrequent but do occur. **(b)** A different biopsy site of approximately the same age shows granulation tissue consisting of plump fibroblasts (arrow). **(c)** After the passage of time, i.e, several weeks, nodular deposits of collagen (scarring) develop at the biopsy site; note the strong histologic resemblance to fibromatosis (see Chap. 15). Such areas can occasionally be very difficult to differentiate from fibrous stroma, particularly if there is no accompanying fat necrosis or foreign body type giant cells. **(d)** One histologic hint to the true diagnosis is the presence of hemosiderin laden macrophages (arrow), indicating prior hemorrhage. The marker materials histologically range from **(e)** almost non-staining and mucinous (arrow) in appearance with foreign body reaction to **(f)**

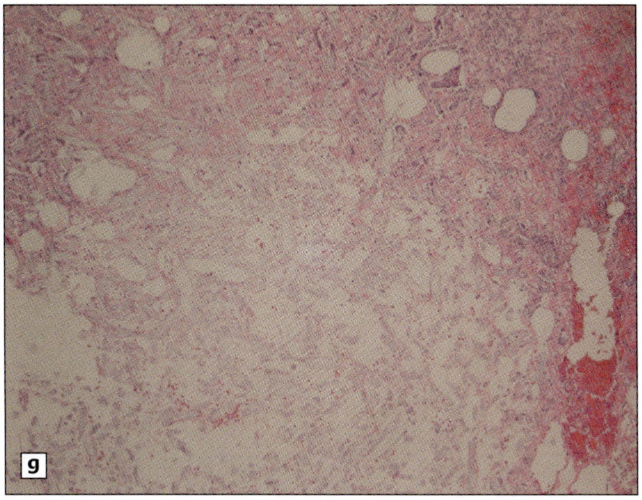

FIGURE 16.1—cont'd a purple and pink staining mass to **(g)** gray staining strands of suture-like fibers surrounded by granulation tissue and foreign body reaction.

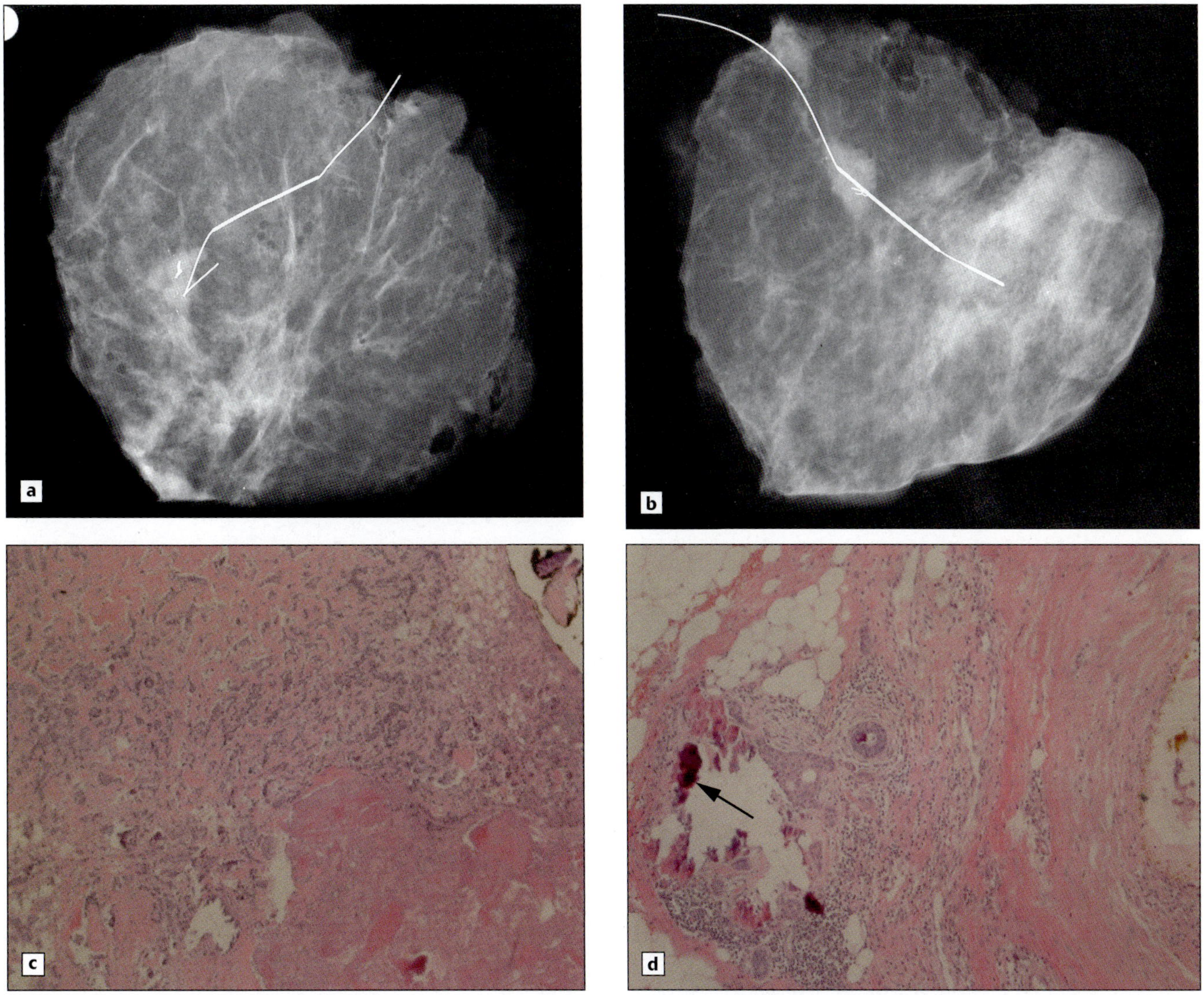

FIGURE 16.2 Biopsy site excision. **(a,b)** Two specimen radiographs serve as examples of successful wire localizations of clips. Both show the clips associated with irregular densities with calcifications. **(c)** The first case example shows invasive duct carcinoma (top) adjacent to the foreign material. **(d)** In the second example the biopsy site (right side) shows residual intraductal carcinoma with necrosis and calcifications (arrow). The density of the biopsy site was partially due to the presence of an intraductal papilloma. Negative margins were achieved despite the presence of intraductal carcinoma away from the biopsy site (evidenced by the additional calcifications on the specimen radiograph). Two microscopic areas of invasion (0.3 and 0.1 cm) were also found away from the biopsy site.

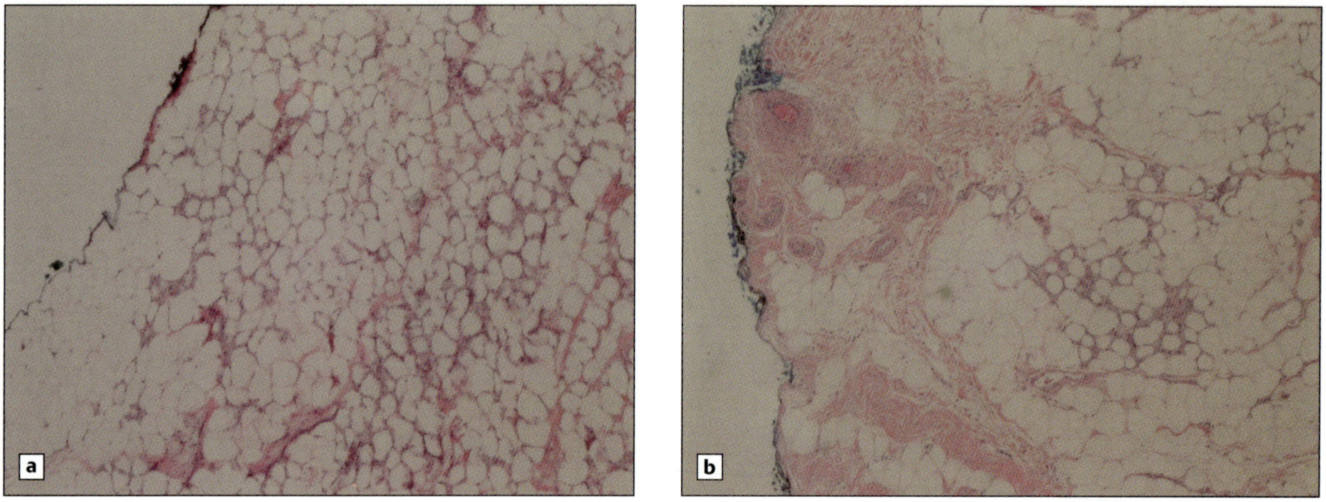

FIGURE 16.3 Unsuccessful localization of core biopsy site. In this example, the specimen radiographs did not reveal a clip. Orientation of the specimen by the surgeon allowed for multiple colors of ink to be placed on the tissue's surface. Histologically fat necrosis **(a)** was evident at an area of green ink and **(b)** adjacent to a blue ink, which had been designated to represent inferior and posterior respectively. Reexcision of the infero-posterior margins revealed the histologic biopsy site.

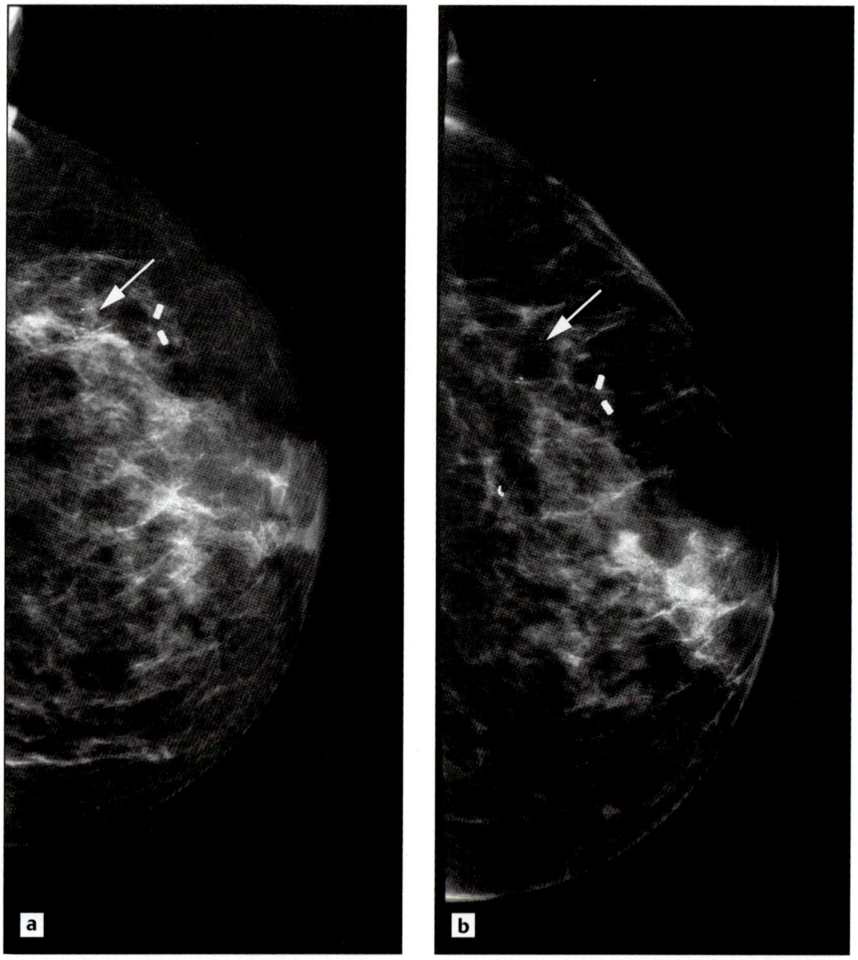

FIGURE 16.4 Clip migration. An 80-year-old woman underwent stereotactic core biopsy six months prior to this study, yielding calcifications in benign stroma. **(a,b)** In the ensuing interval there was an increase in moderately pleomorphic calcifications (arrow) spanning 4 cm. Two metallic clips mark the site of the prior biopsy. Stereotactic biopsy of the new calcifications was performed with clip deployment, eventually yielding a diagnosis of intraductal carcinoma; however, on this post-biopsy CC view the new clip has migrated 2 cm medial to the biopsy cavity (arrow). In such cases surgery should be performed as soon as possible so that the biopsy cavity can be localized easily and successfully surgically excised; the clip becomes irrelevant.

stroma of the breast or, less frequently, into lymphatic channels.[5] In our experience this phenomenon, known as epithelial displacement (Fig 16.5a), occurs almost exclusively in papillary lesions: intraductal papillomas, papillary carcinomas, or intraductal carcinomas involving intraductal papillomas.[6] In addition, we have rarely observed the phenomenon in mucinous tumors, invasive carcinomas with extensive necrosis and cystification, and invasive carcinomas containing osteoclast-like giant cells. In our view the common factor amongst these is the inherent friability of the cells or supporting structures. In papillary lesions the epithelial cells line branching fibrovascular structures which are extremely delicate and prone to fragmentation when disturbed, not unlike polyps in the colon. When such lesions are biopsied, the core biopsies themselves are fragmented (see Chap. 5). Other epithelial fragments are left behind at the core biopsy site and can be identified in the area's granulation tissue. The lymphatic drainage physiologically inherent to the healing process can even result in the presence of these fragments in lymphatic channels and in the sentinel lymph node(s),[7] the first lymph nodes to drain the area (Fig 16.5b).

LOCAL RECURRENCE VS NEW PRIMARY

An important aspect of breast conservation as therapy for breast carcinoma is follow-up imaging. Despite initial concerns by some, core biopsy is not associated with a higher than expected local recurrence rate. While strictly speaking local recurrence is limited to intraductal and/or invasive carcinoma arising at the site of previous biopsy (Fig. 16.6), the potential for a new primary carcinoma of the treated breast is also a possibility (Fig. 16.7). The latter should consist of a lesion clearly separate from the original lumpectomy site. If the patient had already been irradiated, the difference between the two is somewhat academic, since the next step in treatment, likely mastectomy, will be identical for both. Core biopsy may or may not distinguish between the two, depending on the

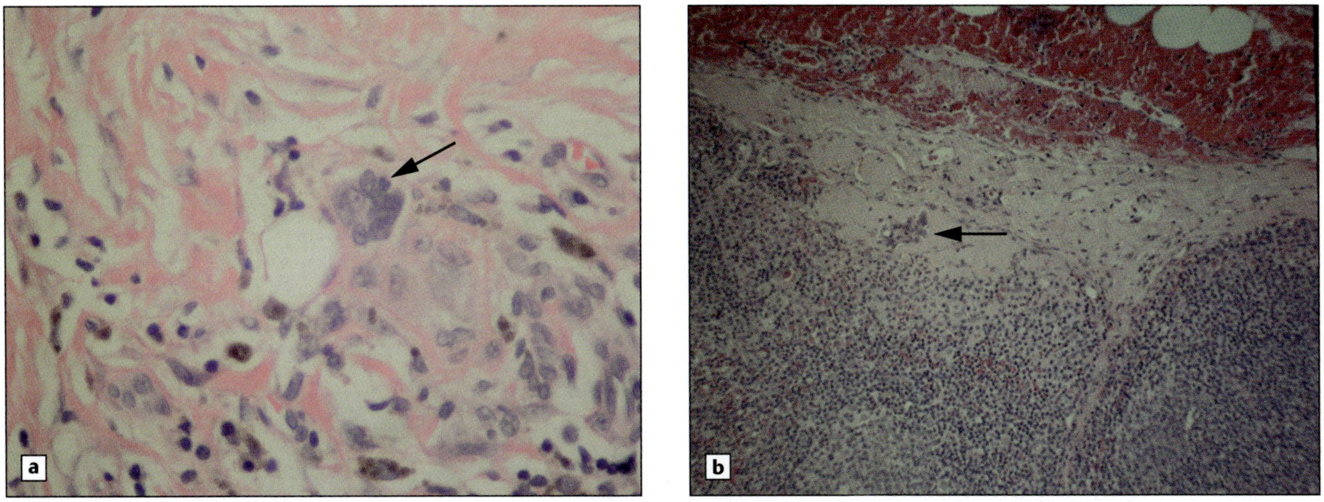

FIGURE 16.5 Epithelial cell displacement. **(a)** A focus of benign epithelial cells (arrow) present within granulation tissue of a core biopsy site. This should not be overinterpreted as invasive carcinoma. **(b)** A cluster of benign papillary cells (arrow) is present in the peripheral sinus of a sentinel lymph node in this patient who had high grade intraductal carcinoma focally involving an intraductal papilloma. The cells were cytologically and immunophenotypically completely different from those of the patient's carcinoma but identical to those of the papilloma.

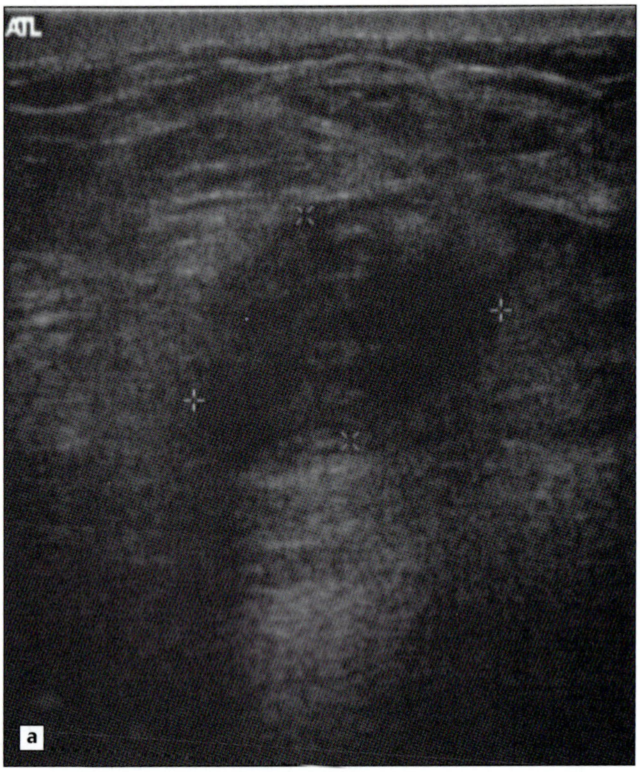

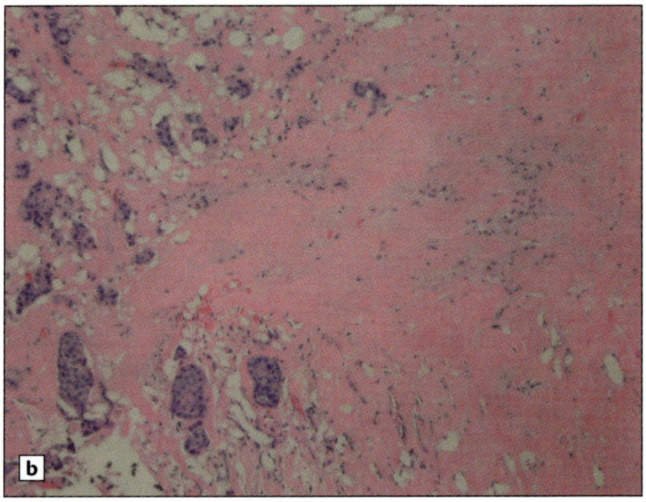

FIGURE 16.6 Local recurrence. This 81-year-old patient was being followed, having had lumpectomy, axillary dissection, and radiation for invasive duct carcinoma in 1997. **(a)** Sonography of the lumpectomy site in 2002 shows mixed echogenicity and is well defined with slightly indistinct borders at the surgical bed but no posterior shadowing (scars usually show posterior shadowing). **(b)** Core biopsy revealed infiltrating poorly differentiated duct carcinoma (left side) amidst scar and fat necrosis (center and right).

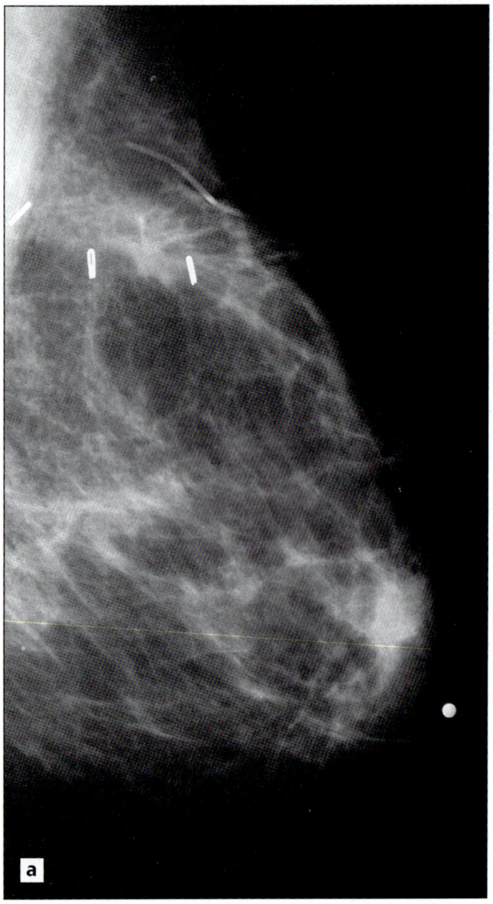

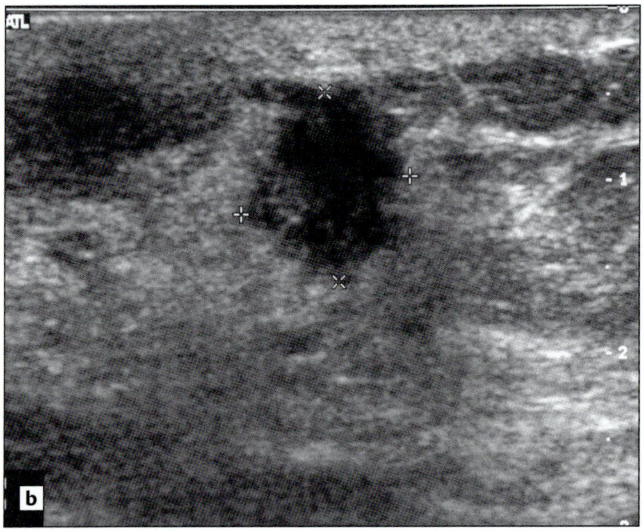

FIGURE 16.7 New ipsilateral primary carcinoma. This 49-year-old woman who was four years status post ipsilateral lumpectomy, axillary dissection, and radiation for invasive duct carcinoma palpated a periareolar mass. **(a)** Mammography shows the surgical clips, denoting the prior lumpectomy bed; however, a distinct lesion is not obvious at the area of palpable mass (note the BB). **(b)** Sonography directed to the area of the palpable mass reveals a heterogeneous, ill-defined, hypoechoic mass which was 1 cm from the nipple and was core biopsied

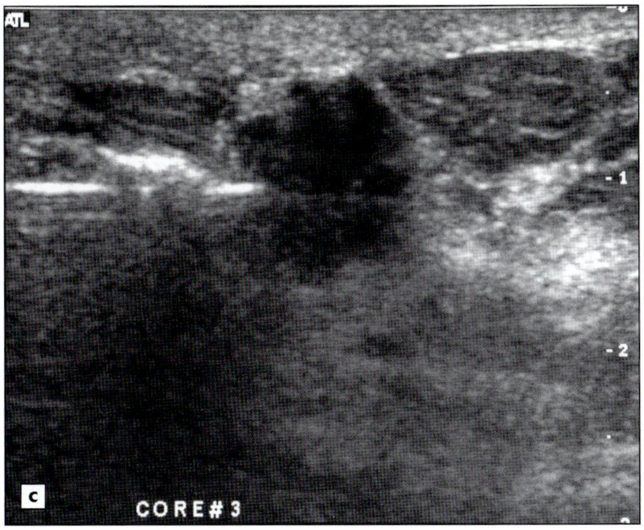

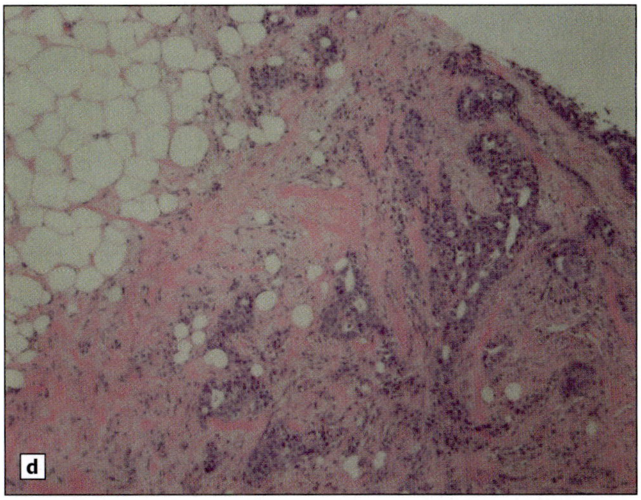

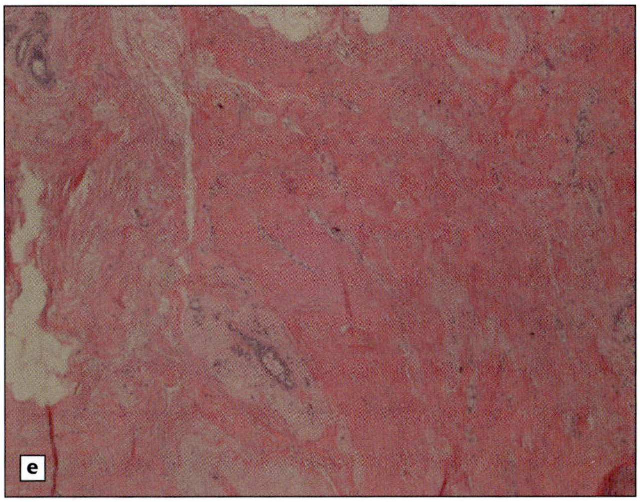

FIGURE 16.7—cont'd **(c)** revealing infiltrating poorly differentiated duct carcinoma **(d)**. Mastectomy was performed and confirmed that the tumor was separate and distinct from the prior lumpectomy site which was composed of dense scar and fat necrosis **(e)**. Both the histology and immunohistochemical phenotype of the tumor were different from those of the patient's prior tumor, consistent with a new primary carcinoma, rather than true local recurrence.

presence of a foreign body reaction and scarring in the case of local recurrence.

REFERENCES

1. Guarda LA, Tran TA. The pathology of breast biopsy site marking devices. 29:814–819,2005.
2. Crisi GM, Pantanowitz L, Otis CN. Mammotome footprints: Histologic artifacts in the era of stereotactic vacuum mammotome biopsy. In t J Surg Pathol 14:221–222,2006.
3. Birdwell RL, Jackman RJ. Clip or marker migration 5–10 weeks after stereotactic 11-gauge vacuum-assisted breast biopsy: Report of two cases. Radiology 229:541–544,2003.
4. Esserman LE, Cura MA, DaCosta D. Recognizing pitfalls in early and late migration of clip markers after image-guided directional vacuum-assisted biopsy. Radiographics 24:147–156,2004.
5. Youngson BJ, Cranor M, Rosen PP. Epithelial displacement in surgical breast specimens following needling procedures. Am J Pathol 18:896–903,1994.
6. Nagi C, Bleiweiss IJ, Jaffer S. Epithelial displacement in breast lesions: A papillary phenomenon. Arch Pathol Lab Med 129:1465–1469,2005
7. Bleiweiss IJ, Nagi CS, Jaffer S. Axillary sentinel lymph nodes can be falsely positive due to iatrogenic displacement and transport of benign epithelial cells in patients with breast carcinoma. J Clin Oncol 24:2013–2018,2006.

CHAPTER 17

Postscript

The advent of core biopsy technology has clearly changed the practice not only of breast imaging, but also of pathology and surgery. Thirty years ago even the most forward-thinking physician might not have predicted the technological advances in imaging and targeting that would allow this. While the next advance (MRI) is already upon us, others (tomosynthesis, etc.) are in development. As is certainly the case in other fields of medicine, probably the only thing that is predictable about the future is that it is unpredictable. The underlying goal of this book was to demonstrate how constant collaboration between the radiologist and pathologist can increase diagnostic accuracy and improve patient care in breast imaging, diagnosis, and treatment. Whatever future technology may hold in store for us, communication will doubtless remain our greatest single tool.

Index

N

O

P

R

S

T

U

W